Pocket Guide to Herbal Medicine

Karin Kraft, M.D.
Professor
Outpatient Clinic
University of Rostock
Germany

Christopher Hobbs, L.Ac., A.H.G.
Clinical Herbalist and Acupuncturist in Private Practice
Davis, California
USA

Foreword by Jonathan Treasure

Thieme
Stuttgart · New York

Library of Congress Cataloging-in-Publication Data is available from the publisher

Important note: Medicine is an ever-changing science undergoing continual development. Research and clinical experience are continually expanding our knowledge, in particular our knowledge of proper treatment and drug therapy. Insofar as this book mentions any dosage or application, readers may rest assured that the authors, editors, and publishers have made every effort to ensure that such references are in accordance with **the state of knowledge at the time of production of the book**.

Nevertheless, this does not involve, imply, or express any guarantee or responsibility on the part of the publishers in respect to any dosage instructions and forms of applications stated in the book. **Every user is requested to examine carefully** the manufacturers' leaflets accompanying each drug and to check, if necessary in consultation with a physician or specialist, whether the dosage schedules mentioned therein or the contraindications stated by the manufacturers differ from the statements made in the present book. Such examination is particularly important with drugs that are either rarely used or have been newly released on the market. Every dosage schedule or every form of application used is entirely at the user's own risk and responsibility. The authors and publishers request every user to report to the publishers any discrepancies or inaccuracies noticed.

This book is an authorized and revised translation of the German edition published and copyrighted 2000 by Georg Thieme Verlag, Stuttgart, Germany. Title of the German edition: Phytotherapie

Translator: Suzyon O'Neal Wandrey, Berlin, Germany

© 2004 Georg Thieme Verlag, Rüdigerstrasse 14, 70469 Stuttgart, Germany
http://www.thieme.de
Thieme New York, 333 Seventh Avenue, New York, NY 10001 USA
http://www.thieme.com

Cover design: Martina Berge, Erbach
Typesetting by Satzpunkt Ewert GmbH, Bayreuth
Printed in Germany by Druckhaus Götz, Ludwigsburg

ISBN 3-13-126991-X (GTV)
ISBN 1-58890-063-0 (TNY)   1 2 3 4 5

Traditionally, Western medical knowledge from Graeco-Roman times onward has been transmitted by means of authoritative printed texts. Today, both patient and physician may be more likely to use the Internet as a first reference source. The sheer amount of medical information available on the World Wide Web and the speed of its renewal and retrieval may outpace the Caxtonian mechanics of printed textbook production, but has done little to erode the authority of the printed word. Conversely, in fact, major medical reference texts are these days being "ported" into the memory of hand-held electronic devices or on-line databases. This development, welcomed by gadgetry enthusiasts, eliminates the hefty size and weight of the printed tome, but decreases the legibility and convenience of the printed page as well as undermining the narrative qualities of the traditional medical textbook.

However, another, and only slightly less illustrious tradition has long co-existed with that of the major medical opus. This is the "vade mecum," literally "go with me," intended as a portable tome to be kept on hand for immediate reference. To be successful, this format requires authors to possess a high degree of intimacy and fluency with their subject matter, to be able to communicate its essentials with precision and confidence, compacting prose and condensing content without sacrificing narrative. The size of the resultant printed volume must be compact enough to make it easily portable, which nowadays translates as "pocket guide."

The present pocket guide is a medical vade mecum devoted specifically to the field of phytotherapy (herbal medicine), authored by the German physician and phytotherapist Karin Kraft. Prof. Kraft is a member of the Commission E (the official expert committee which originally considered the safety and efficacy of phytomedicines in Germany), and is currently a member of the supervising editorial board of ESCOP (European Scientific Cooperative on Phytotherapy). ESCOP produces the scientific monographs that provide the official core data for herbal medicines in the EU.

In Germany, phytotherapy enjoys a higher degree of integration into general medical practice than in any other European country, with physicians regularly writing millions of prescriptions for approved phytomedicines on a daily basis. In the original German edition of this pocket guide, Prof. Kraft provides the busy general practitioner with a compact and practical reference guide that includes a materia medica of herbs, a prescriber for many conditions, and extensive data on dosage, forms of administration, safety data and technical standards for German commercial herbal products. (Special mention should made of Prof. Kraft's inclusion of an often neglected area, that of topical applications of herbal medications such as poultices and compresses, more popular in Europe than in the USA).

In North America, herbal medicine is a more marginal discipline, ultimately the legacy of a period of political opposition between medical factions at the turn of the 19th century which resulted in the effective outlawing of botanical medical practice following the Flexner Report of 1910. Although the majority of "official" medicines in the United States Pharmacopoeia were originally botanicals or botanically derived, there remains a sharp discontinuity between standard practice medicine today and its botanical past. The once widespread schools of physiomedical and eclectic botanical medicine were preserved partly through their migration to the United Kingdom, where an unbroken tradition today enables qualified British medical herbalists to diagnose and treat conditions with phyto-medicines, alongside their conventional medical colleagues. The British model is distinct again from the German experience and emphasizes the importance of understanding different cultural and national expressions of traditional herbal medicine, education, and practice.

Sensitive to such cultural variations, Thieme wisely enlisted the aid of Christopher Hobbs, a fourth-generation American herbalist, to help render the translation of Prof. Kraft's German text into the US cultural context. Hobbs, one of the most highly regarded herbal practitioners in the US, addressed this challenging task by reviewing every line of the text. Hobbs has replaced some herbs in the materia medica, suggested more appropriate local equivalents for herbal products, and annotated bi-cultural comments where relevant. He has also rewritten doses into the typically higher US forms. Meanwhile, Hobbs has deftly preserved the nuances of the German text; Prof. Kraft actively participated in, and agreed to, all the changes. The result of this bi-cultural collaboration is an almost seamless representation of the German original harmonized to the North American audience.

As more physicians in this country recognize the need to investigate the CAM (complementary and alternative medicine) modalities that are being espoused by many of their patients, a premium is inevitably placed upon reliable sources of data and clinical information about CAM. Botanical medicines in particular have sadly been the subject of excessive amounts of published secondary and tertiary "information" devoid of clinical context, and largely irrelevant to the primary care provider. By contrast, Karin Kraft and Christopher Hobbs present us with a succinct and authoritative survey of herbal medicine that is accessible to the physician and can readily be applied to everyday clinical practice. The "pocket guide" represents a unique cross-cultural and trans-disciplinary blend of reliable, accurate, and accessible information about phytotherapy; it is a mini-masterpiece of integrative medicine.

March 2004

Jonathan Treasure
Medical Herbalist
Ashland, Oregon, USA

The use of medicinal plants to treat everyday complaints and illnesses is becoming ever more popular. This pocket guide is aimed not only at doctors and members of the various healing professions interested in phytotherapy, but also in particular at interested lay people, for whom this book is intended as a practical guide in the often confusing self-treatment market. This pocket guide is based on experiences and prescriptions that have been used in Germany for many years or even decades. If necessary, they have been supplemented by US-American remedies and suggestions for use. Where possible, available scientific literature has also been taken into account. The book includes the medicinal plants most widely used in Germany, almost all of which are also used in the US, as well as their use in the treatment of major syndromes. A general section in which production processes, quality characteristics, and legal backgrounds are explained is followed by portraits of the most important medicinal plants with references to more recent scientific literature. Illnesses and possibilities of treating them with medicinal plant preparations as well as a critical evaluation of the significance of this therapy make up the next section. A specialty of this checklist is the section "Care Involving Medicinal Plants." Here special value was attached to practicability. A tabular section divided up into medicinal plants with brief summaries of remedies and references follows. Contact addresses and lists of manufacturers as well as a comprehensive table of contents round off the guide.

Ms Angelika-M. Findgott from Thieme International has done a first-class job of coordinating the work of both authors and editing the manuscripts. We, the authors, know that we echo her sentiments in wishing that this pocket guide will be a practical aid to all those who are interested in using medicinal plants and will contribute to the alleviation and curing of illnesses and complaints.

Rostock in Spring 2004   Karin Kraft

Contents

Appendix: Glossaries, Dosages, Addresses, References, and Index

1.1 Characteristics and Status of Herbal Medicines

Preliminary Remarks

➤ Herbal medicine is a scientifically recognized complementary and alternative treatment method with proven efficacy.
➤ In North America, herbal remedies are considered dietary supplements by law and are considered safe unless proven otherwise. Manufacturing standards are not as stringent as required for pharmaceutical drugs. While only a few "structure and function" claims (such as "benefits digestion") can be made by manufacturers, many work around that limitation by making extensive use of "third-party" advertising in magazines and through company representatives.
➤ In Germany, herbal remedies are defined as medicinal products by German Drug Law.
➤ German legislators regard herbs and herbal remedies as medicinal products with specific pharmaceutical characteristics. Together with homeopathic and anthroposophic medicines, herbal medicines are classified as drugs of a special system of therapeutics.
➤ According to German law, every physician must be knowledgeable about herbal medicine. North American physicians are not required to have this training, and few classes are offered in herbs or natural medicine in medical school.
➤ The public interest in alternative therapies for general health maintenance and supportive treatment of chronic diseases has increased tremendously.

Distinctions Between the Different Types of Therapeutic Preparations

➤ **Herbal products:** One of the main distinguishing features of herbal preparations is their complex chemical composition.
➤ **Chemical or synthetic drugs:** Chemically defined drugs in general contain precisely definable quantities of usually one particular active ingredient and also accompanying substances.
➤ **Homeopathic remedies:** Homeopathic products are prepared according to special formulation techniques and are prescribed according to the principles introduced by Samuel Hahnemann in the early nineteenth century. His "Law of Similars" states that the remedy prescribed, in a more or less highly diluted form, to cure a given condition or disease should be a substance that induces similar symptoms in healthy individuals when given in much higher amounts.
➤ **Anthroposophic remedies:** Anthroposophic remedies are prepared according to the ideas and teachings of Rudolf Steiner.

Definitions

➤ **Herbal medicine:** A time-honored system of healing practiced in every culture in the world. Science has modernized the system using analytical and pharmaceutical testing. The science-based practice of herbal medicine is now called *phytomedicine* or *phytotherapy*, which is a system of therapeutics in which diseases and disorders are treated with medicinal plants and preparations made from them using scientific principles.
➤ **Medicinal herbs:** Medicinal products whose active ingredients consist exclusively of medicinal plants and preparations made from them. Using modern chemical and pharmaceutical methods, a number of popular herbal remedies are nowadays "standardized" to provide consistent levels of proven identified active compounds.

1.1 Characteristics and Status of Herbal Medicines

> **Phytochemistry:** The study of plant chemistry, including the identification, isolation, analysis, and characterization of plant constituents, and determination of the chemical structures of plant constituents.

> **Pharmaceutical biology:** The field of research concerned with the extraction and development of biogenic drugs from plants and other living organisms as well as the processing and application of these drugs.

> **Phytopharmacology:** The study of the uptake, distribution, and effect of herbal preparations and of their elimination from the body.

> **Active principles:** Substances or substance groups definable by chemical analysis that essentially contribute to the therapeutic action of a medicinal herbal preparation.

> **Active ingredients of medicinal herbal preparations:** Plant ingredients in their natural states and preparations made from them.

> **Minor constituents:** Substances that have an indirect or slight effect on the therapeutic action of an herbal drug.

> **Single-herb herbal preparation:** Herbal medicinal preparation from one medicinal plant.

> **Target constituents:** Herbal drug preparation constituents definable by chemical analysis that are used as parameters of in-process quality control and may contribute to a characteristic pharmaceutical property.

> **Species, genus, family:** Taxonomic terms classifying a plant. A genus may include one or more species, and a family may include one or more genera.

Research on Herbal Remedies: State of the Art

> Remarkable advances in phytotherapeutic research have been made within the past 15 years.

> The worldwide interest in herbal drug research is steadily increasing.
>   - Collaboration between universities, the dietary supplement and herbal industry, and the pharmaceutical industry is essential to promote the success of this research. In North America, government funding of human studies on the efficacy and safety of herbal preparations is just beginning.
>   - Comparable to research on chemically defined drugs, research on herbal preparations is also carried out using molecular biological, pharmacological, and clinical techniques of investigation.
>   - The findings of herbal research are published in recognized medical journals such as *JAMA*, the *British Medical Journal*, and *Arzneimittelforschung*.
>   - Researchers are developing high-quality standardized extracts with proven efficacy.
>   - Both basic research and clinical studies have repeatedly shown that whole-drug complexes are superior with respect to range of action and tolerability to isolated chemical constituents.

German Drug Law Provisions

> **Phytopharmaceutical standards:** In Germany, manufacturers of herbal preparations are held to much higher standards than their counterparts in North America. According to the German Drug Law (*Arzneimittelgesetz*), herbal "drugs" (preparations) must meet the same standards as chemically defined drugs with respect to pharmaceutical quality, efficacy, and safety, whereas in the United States they are considered dietary supplements.

➤ **Marketing authorizations for herbal medical drugs:** In Germany, applications for marketing authorization must be submitted to the Federal Institute for Drugs and Medicinal Products, accompanied by the following documents:

1. Results of physicochemical, biological and microbiological tests and a description of the testing methods (analytical testing, assessment of pharmaceutical quality)
2. Results of pharmacological and toxicological tests (assessment of drug efficacy and safety)
3. Results of clinical studies (efficacy and safety)

– If the beneficial and adverse effects, and the side effects of a preparation are already known, empirical evidence acquired by scientific methods can be submitted instead of items 2 and 3.

– Until 1994, the Commission E, a diverse group of scientists, physicians, pharmacists, physiatrists, biostatisticians, and representatives of the pharmaceutical industry was charged with the task of preparing monographs on the various medicinal plants. In this capacity, the Commission issued summaries and assessments of the published data on the pharmacology, toxicology, and clinical efficacy of 360 herbal medical preparations. These monographs are available in English, published by the American Botanical Council (see list of references, p. 479).

– This valuable and influential effort should not be overrated however. The monographs are not referenced with the primary literature, and so cannot be peer-reviewed or critically evaluated, especially since, recognizing the explosion of recent scientific work, they have not been revised in nearly 10 years.

– The German Cooperative on Phytopharmaceuticals (Kooperation Phytopharmaka) took over responsibility for revising the existing monographs in Germany in 1994. The revised monographs included a comprehensive review of the recent literature. Some of them are available in English.

– In 1994 also the ESCOP (European Scientific Cooperative on Phytotherapy) was constituted in order to actualize the monographs on an European base (see list of references, p. 479)

– This valuable and influential effort should not be overrated however. The monographs are not referenced with the primary literature, and so cannot be peer-reviewed or critically evaluated, especially since, recognizing the explosion of recent scientific work, they have not been revised in nearly 10 years.

– According to the simplified reauthorization procedure for traditional medicines, traditional medicines must be labeled as follows: Traditionally used (a) as a roborant (strengthening agent) in ...; (b) for improvement of general feeling in ...; (c) to enhance organ function ...; (d) to prevent XYZ ...; or (e) as a mildly effective medical drug in case of .... Specific diseases must not be mentioned as indications for the traditional preparation.

1.2 From the Plant to the Remedy

Origins of Medicinal Plants for the Manufacture of Herbal Products

➤ **Wild harvested herbs**
- Half of all medicinal plants on the market and two-thirds of all plant species are harvested from the wild.
- For economic reasons, wild harvested herbs are preferably used in the cases of certain slow-growing plants and of plants of which there is a naturally abundant supply.

➤ **Cultivated herbs**
- Cultivated herbs are used when the natural supply is not sufficient to meet demand or if a herb required for medicinal purposes is a protected plant species, such as purple coneflower, *Echinacea purpurea,* and goldenseal, *Hydrastis canadensis.*
- *Advantages of controlled farming*
  • Uniform seed material, optimal growing conditions and harvesting times
  • Reduced risk of mistaken identity or adulteration
  • Reduction of impurities, microbial contamination, and residues from pesticides and heavy metals (especially in plants imported from developing countries)
- *Organic farming:* Ensures the maintenance of natural growing conditions and is environmentally friendly.

➤ **Cultivation of special crops**
- Mainly used to enrich and optimize the primary constituents of medicinal plants. A way of standardizing active constituent levels.
- Reduces the number and quantity of undesirable substances in the plants.
- Enhances the resistance of the plants to atmospheric influences, diseases, and pests.

Quality Assurance

➤ **Homogeneous starting materials**
- Homogeneity is achieved by optimization and wide-scale standardization of growing conditions (e. g., in cultures), and asexual propagation
- *Note:* The concentrations of constituents in a given plant (e. g., ginseng or arnica) tend to vary according to location of origin, season of harvesting, and age.

➤ **Standardized preparation process**
- Manufacturers use exact specifications for analyzing parent substances—meaning the herbs and their parts used—and herbal extracts made from them, using solvents such as ethanol. Specifications for assaying the content of target or primary constituents are just as exact and are designed to ensure that the chemical composition of the herbal extracts remains consistent from batch to batch.
- Standardization ensures that the quality of medicinal plants and extracts made from them are reproducible and consistent.
- Minimum concentrations of active principles in raw (unprocessed) herbs are specified in sources such as the German and European Pharmacopeias and, lately, the US Pharmacopeia.

◉ *Note:* Insofar as the manufacturers of phytomedicines use different methods of processing, the final products may vary greatly with respect to the type and/or concentration of their ingredients. This is especially true of liquid tinctures of all kinds, including glycerites, and herb products that contain powdered herbs.

➤ **Chemical standardization:** Many manufacturers today sell products that contain standardized extract powders in capsule and tablet form, and the levels of identified active constituents vary much less in these products.

➤ **Quality** is ensured through good harvesting, drying, processing, and storage practices of both herbs and preparations (see also section on storage):
   – Good harvesting practice takes into account the growth phase (time of year) and best time of day to harvest a given plant.
   – The drying process should be performed at a suitable temperature, without overheating, and under appropriate lighting conditions.
   – The plant material should be cut, cleaned, and stored without direct light exposure at an appropriate temperature in accordance with the rules of good professional practice. Herbal preparations such as liquids, capsules, or tablets should be stored away from heat and direct sunlight, preferably in glass containers that exclude oxygen.

➤ **In-process controls:** The manufacturer should monitor each step of the process of converting raw materials into finished medicinal products by applying the appropriate analytical tests.

➤ **Drug safety for herbal medicinal preparations**
   – In Germany, herbal medicinal preparations are subject to essentially the same standards for toxicity, teratogenicity, and mutagenicity/carcinogenicity as chemically defined drugs. End user suppliers and storage specifications are described below.
   – The processed plant material must be tested for a wide variety of different pesticides. In North America, manufacturers of herbal products must follow good manufacturing practices based on regulations for food products regarding cleanliness and safety. The Food and Drug Administration (FDA) does not currently require manufacturers to test herbal medicines that are generally recognized as safe (GRAS) and have been used in food products before 1 January 1958 for toxicity in the same way as pharmaceutical drugs, since manufacturers are allowed to make only minimal "structure–function" claims for herbal preparations.
   ◉ *Note:* Plants collected in the wild, as well as plants raised in conventional (nonorganic) farms, may have high concentrations of pesticides and/or heavy metals.

➤ **End user suppliers:** Pharmacies, supermarkets, health food stores, web-based suppliers, or by direct order from certain suppliers.

➤ **Storage**
   – Store in a cool (not cold), dark place, out of the reach of children.
   – Discard after the expiration date.
   – Factors that can reduce the shelf life of herbal medicines:
      • Exposure to air (keep in airtight bottles)
      • Humidity
      • Heat
      • Light (leading to oxidation-related decomposition)

- Fungal or bacterial contamination (leading to formation of poisonous metabolites)
- Evaporation

◎ *Note:* Plants infested with pests or mold must be destroyed.

- In order to identify plants that are spoiled or infested, the plant material should be inspected for mold, altered or unpleasant odor, insects, and traces of insects (cobwebs, etc.).
- The pharmacist should be able to furnish information on the shelf life of herbal medicines (e.g., teas and other herbal remedies prepared in the pharmacy).
- Herbal preparations should be stored in containers that are airtight, waterproof, lightproof, and fragrance-free.
- Storage temperature: 10 – 20 °C (50 – 68 °F).

Comparison of Efficacy

➤ It is virtually impossible to compare the efficacy of herbal remedies prepared by different manufacturers, even when they are derived from the same plant species, because different companies use different drying, processing, and manufacturing processes, and because plants from different populations vary in constituent levels.

➤ The therapeutic efficacy of herbal remedies with comparable concentrations of primary constituents but produced by different manufacturers may vary because of the differences in the content of minor constituents.

➤ In the future, individual pharmaceutical companies will be required to test the efficacy and tolerability of plant extracts prepared by different manufacturing processes.

Primary and Secondary Metabolism

➤ A distinction is generally made between primary and secondary plant metabolism. The products of primary metabolism maintain the plant's vital functions, whereas the products of secondary metabolism, as far as is currently known, are not essential for the plant's immediate survival.

➤ **Products of primary metabolism:** Carbohydrates, fats and proteins are basic nutrients for humans and animals, but are rarely relevant as pharmacologically active substances. Nonetheless, they may have a positive or negative effect on the efficacy of the active principles in drugs.

➤ **Products of secondary metabolism:** Many secondary plant substances protect plants from feeding damage, act as storage or waste products, or ward off pests and diseases. Some are pharmacologically active.

Examples of Products of Primary Metabolism

➤ **Pectins**
  – *Substance group:* Carbohydrates.
  – *Example:* Apple pectin.
  – *Structural properties:* High-molecular weight compounds comprising sugarlike molecules.
  – *Plant sources:* Found in many kinds of fruit, especially when unripe.
  – *Pharmacological properties:* Pectins cannot be digested by endogenous intestinal juices and have a high water-binding capacity.
  – *Indications:* Diarrhea.
    • Pectins lower the pH of the bowel because they encourage growth of beneficial bacteria. This produces less favorable living conditions for the pathological bacteria that cause diarrhea (see p. 190, "Diarrhea").

➤ **Essential omega-3 and omega-6 fatty acids**
  – *Substance group:* Fats.
  – *Examples:* Alpha-linolenic acid and gamma-linolenic acid.
  – *Plant sources:* Flaxseed, rape seed, evening primrose seed, etc.
  – *Structural properties:* Fatty acids.
  – *Pharmacological properties:* Used in the synthesis of tissue hormones of the eicosanoid, prostaglandin, and thromboxane groups.
  – *Indications:* Symptoms and ailments involving inflammation.

Products of Secondary Metabolism

➤ **Alkaloids**
  – *Examples:* Atropine, caffeine, morphine, colchicine, nicotine, berberine.
  – *Plant sources:* Mainly in nightshades such as belladonna, bittersweet, and thornapple, but also in papaveraceous plants (opium poppy, greater celandine), the borage family (coltsfoot, comfrey), and the spea family (*Crotalaria*).
  – *Structural properties:* Alkaloids contain nitrogen have complex structures, and undergo alkaline reactions.
  – *Pharmacological properties:* Most alkaloids have a potent effect on the central nervous system, e. g., sympathomimetic or parasympatholytic effect.
  – *Indications*
    • Isolated alkaloids used in pure form (e. g., atropine) are highly potent drugs that are available by prescription only.

1.3 Constituents and Active Principles

- Chelidonine (celandine), berberine, caffeine, and theophylline are less potent alkaloids.
- Pyrrolizidine alkaloids (present in members of the borage and aster family): Their significant toxicological features are hepatotoxicity and mutagenicity.

➤ **Essential oils**
- *Examples of individual essential oil components:* Menthol, thymol, α-pinene, eugenol, chamazulene. Essential or volatile oils are highly complex mixtures of monoterpenes (containing 10 carbon atoms) and other types of compounds.
- *Plant sources:* Found in a variety of plants, such as conifers, and members of the mint and parsley families.
- *Structural properties:* Monoterpenes (e. g., menthol, thymol), sesquiterpenes (e. g., constituents of chamomile such as bisabolol), sesquiterpene lactones (parthenolide in feverfew), iridoid substances (gentopicrin in gentian root), and phenylpropane (e. g., chemicals in ginger root, eugenol).
- *Pharmacological properties:* Essential oils are aromatic, highly volatile, fat-soluble substances that stimulate chemoreceptors. They are readily absorbed in the gastrointestinal tract and by the skin (e. g., when used in bath salts and liniments).

➤ **Bitter substances**
- *Examples:* Gentianin, gentiopicrin, cynaropicrin.
- *Plant sources:* Members of the Aster (artichoke, dandelion) and Gentian (gentian, centaury) families.
- *Structural properties:* Mainly derivatives of terpenes and seco-iridoides.
- *Pharmacological properties:* Bitter substances stimulate the reflex production of gastrointestinal secretions (especially saliva and gastric juices) via lingual taste buds.
- *Indications:* For treatment of dyspeptic complaints; to stimulate appetite and improve digestion and assimilation of nutrients.

➤ **Carotinoids**
- *Examples:* β-carotene, lycopene, lutein.
- *Plant sources:* Colored fruit, leafy vegetables.
- *Structural properties:* Tetraterpene derivatives.
- *Pharmacological properties:* Antioxidants and immunomodulators; vitamin A precursors (β-carotene).
- *Indications:* Inflammation, immunodeficiency, photodermatosis.

➤ **Flavonoids**
- *Examples:* Rutin, silymarin, kaempferol, quercetin.
- *Plant sources:* Found in a wide variety of plants.
- *Structural properties:* Flavonoids have a molecular skeleton consisting of acetic acid units and a phenylpropane group. Their pharmacological properties are determined by those of their substituents.
- *Pharmacological properties:* Flavonoids have a nonspecific protective effect on the capillaries, act as radical scavengers, and stabilize the cell membrane. They additionally have anticonvulsant and diuretic effects and increase the tolerance of cells to oxygen deficiency.
- *Indications:* For treatment of varicose veins, inflammations, edema, dyspeptic complaints and liver disorders; to stimulate bile secretion.

➤ **Tannins**
- *Examples:* Proanthocyanides; phenolcarboxylic acids such as chlorogenic acid, cynarin, and ursolic acid.
- *Plant sources*
  - Relatively high concentrations can be found in many parts of woody plants (e.g., oak bark) and in rose plants, blackberries, silverweed (goosewort), stag-horn, blackthorn, and tormentil.
  - Lower concentrations are present in many plant-based foods and beverages (black and green tea, bilberries [blueberries]).
- *Structural properties*
  - Phenolcarboxylic acids are derived from caffeic acid, salicylic acid, and bile acid.
  - Condensed proanthocyanides consist of catechinic acids.
- *Pharmacological properties*: Tannins irreversibly link protein chains and have astringent action on the skin and mucous membranes. Hence, they have anti-inflammatory, styptic, counterirritant, and weakly antibacterial effects and prevent the excess secretion of mucus.
- *Indications:* External uses: for irritations of the skin and mucous membranes. Internal uses: for acute unspecific diarrhea.

➤ **Glycosides**
- *Examples:* Cardiac glycosides, anthranoids, flavonol glycosides.
- *Plant sources:* Found in many members of the plant kingdom.
- *Structural properties:* Contain one or multiple sugar molecules as well as a nonsugar component that determines their pharmacological activity.
- *Pharmacological properties*
  - Positively inotropic (cardiac glycosides); laxative (anthranoids); improve circulation (flavonol glycosides in ginkgo leaves).
  - Higher doses can induce severe side effects and, in some cases, poisoning (cardiac glycosides, anthranoids).
- *Indications:* Cardiac failure, constipation; to improve the circulation.

➤ **Phytosterins** (phytosterols)
- *Examples:* β-Sitosterol.
- *Plant sources:* Pumpkin seed, nettle root, saw palmetto fruit.
- *Structural properties:* Very similar to those of cholesterol.
- *Pharmacological properties:* Phytosterols occupy cholesterol receptors and thus lower cholesterol levels. They also stabilize cell walls and inhibit the synthesis of mediators of inflammation.
- *Indications:* To counteract elevated concentrations of lipids (antilipemic); for treatment of benign prostatic hyperplasia.

➤ **Saponins**
- *Examples:* α-Hederine (ivy), diosgenin (wild yam), glycyrrhizic acid (licorice).
- *Plant sources:* Widely distributed in plants such as ivy (leaf), licorice (rootstock), and horse chestnut.
- *Structural properties*
  - Consist of a water-soluble sugar chain and a fat-soluble component (aglycone or genin).
  - Triterpene, steroid, and steroidal alkaline saponins are distinguished by their aglycone component.

1

1.3 Constituents and Active Principles

- *Pharmacological properties:* Saponins induce local tissue irritation and reflex expectoration, inhibit the growth of microorganisms, especially fungi, and have partial anti-inflammatory and antiedematous effects.
- *Indications:* To emulsify watery and oily solutions and to promote the dissolution of substances that are not easily absorbed.

◉ *Note:* Most saponins retain their hemolytic properties, even when highly diluted. Hence, they should not be used to treat injuries or inflammations of the digestive organs.

➤ **Mucilage**
- *Examples:* Arabinolactans, glucans, lichenin.
- *Plant sources:* Marshmallow root, Iceland moss, ribwort, linden flower.
- *Structural properties:* Polysaccharides.
- *Pharmacological properties:* Mucilaginous substances swell when added to water, forming viscous solutions or gels. Water-soluble mucilages are demulcent and reduce inflammation. Insoluble mucilages swell in the gastrointestinal tract and regulate the bowels.
- *Indications:* To soothe irritated mucous membranes of the mouth, throat, and gastrointestinal tract; to alleviate dry cough and to regulate the bowels.

➤ **Mustard oils**
- *Examples:* Sinalbin, glucobrassicin.
- *Plant sources:* Black radish, mustard, great nasturtium.
- *Structural properties:* Steam-volatile, pungent compounds formed by organosulfuric acids.
- *Pharmacological properties:* Mustard oils have antibacterial effects and induce hyperemia of the skin.
- *Indications:* Used externally to increase the blood flow.

General Formulations

➤ **Objectives of processing**
  – To increase the concentrations of active principles.
  – To eliminate undesirable constituents.
  – The pharmacologically active principles of different species of a medicinal plant genus can differ. The goal is to obtain high-quality extracts from a *defined* plant species with the highest possible concentrations of the active principles.

➤ **Starting materials**
  – In some cases the whole plant, but usually only the plant component with the highest concentration of active principles (i. e., flowers or roots).
  – The composition of extracts made from the same plant may vary according to which part of the plant was used for its preparation (e. g., nettle leaf extract vs. nettle root extract).

➤ **Traditional dosage forms** (result of processing of the herb)
  – Tea (*species*)
  – Decoction (*decoctum*)
  – Infusion (*infusum*)
  – Maceration (*maceratio*)
  – Juice (*succus*)
  – Syrup (*sirupus*)
  – Tincture (*tinctura*)
  – Extract (*extractum*)

➤ **Modern pharmaceutical preparations** (made with pharmaceutical excipients)
  – Capsules
  – Tablets
  – Film-coated tablets
  – Sugar-coated tablets
  – Ointments
  – Creams

Preparations from Fresh Plant Material

➤ **Plant juice**
  – *Definition:* The liquid obtained by pressing and crushing freshly harvested plant material (plant parts).
  – *Preparation:* Prepared from freshly harvested plant parts. Expressed juice primarily contains water-soluble plant constituents.
  – *Storage:* Once opened, the bottle should be closed and stored in a refrigerator and the rest discarded after one week. The contents should be discarded after the expiration date specified on the label.
  – *Medicinal action:* Usually relatively weak, except in rare cases (expressed Echinacea juice, for example).

➤ **Distillates**
  – *Definition:* Formulations obtained by extracting active principles from fresh or dried plant material by steam distillation.
  – *Preparation:* Obtained by separating the steam-volatile constituents of fresh or dried medicinal plants by vaporization.
  – *Storage:* See p. 5.
  – *Medicinal action:* Determined by the water-volatile constituents (e. g., mustard oils, essential oils) contained in the distillate.

1.4 Herbal Formulations

- ➤ **Oily extracts**
  - *Definition:* The preparation obtained by dissolving the fat-soluble constituents of a medicinal plant in, for example, olive oil, almond oil, or peanut oil.
  - *Preparation:* Prepared by immersing the freshly cut or dried plant parts in a vegetable oil and allowing them to stand, usually at room temperature, until the fat-soluble constituents have been extracted.
  - *Storage:* These preparations are relatively unstable and should therefore be prepared in small quantities (see p. 5 for storage instructions).

Extracts

- ➤ **Definition**
  - Extracts are prepared by dissolving medicinal plants in a solvent to separate their active principles from extraneous substances.
  - The type of formulation (aqueous, alcoholic) depends on the type of solvent used (water, alcohol).
  - Extracts are characterized as either dry or liquid depending on the concentration of residual solvent in the final product.
  - 🔾 *Note:* The composition of and uses for preparations from the same plant may differ between the various preparation techniques. Hence, any extract produced by a special preparation technique is a unique active substance.
- ➤ **Process of manufacturing plant extracts:** See Fig. **1**.
- ➤ **Aqueous extract**
  - *Definition:* An extract prepared using water as the extracting agent. These extracts mainly contain water-soluble constituents and few lipid-soluble components.
  - *Disadvantages:* The individual constituents are relatively unstable, and microorganisms can multiply rapidly.
- ➤ **Alcohol extract**
  - *Definition:* An extract prepared using ethanol and water mixed at various ratios and concentrations, called the *menstruum*.
  - *Preparation*
    - In Germany the standard procedure calls for the plant material to be cut into pieces and then steeped in the menstruum (macerated) for several hours; in the North American standard the fresh or dried and powdered plant material is macerated in the menstruum for a week to 10 days and the liquid is then pressed out with a hydraulic press (if available).
    - The drug is repeatedly steeped in the menstruum, strained and concentrated (percolation) until completely extracted.
  - *Advantages*
    - Ethanol (grain alcohol) is an excellent extracting agent. At higher volume concentrations, it can also extract lipophilic drug constituents, such as essential oils.
    - Alcohol preserves the extracts for a longer times (up to 2 to 3 years).
    - Alcohol assists rapid absorption of the active ingredients.
- ➤ **Tincture**
  - *Definition:* A solution prepared by macerating or percolating a medicinal herb in various concentrations of ethanol.
    - According to the German Pharmacopeia (DAB 1996), dry extracts made by using suitable concentrations of ethanol are also defined as tinctures.

Transforming Freshly Harvested Plants into Extracts

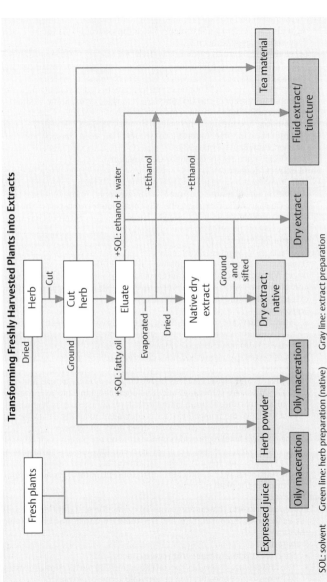

Fig. 1 The process of manufacturing plant extracts.

SOL: solvent   Green line: herb preparation (native)   Gray line: extract preparation

1.4 Herbal Formulations

- *Preparation:* Tinctures are prepared using 1 part drug and 5 parts extractant or, with high-potency constituents like atropine from belladonna, 1 part drug and 10 parts extractant.
- *Labeling:* Dried herb to extract ratio (HER) = 1 : 5 or 1 : 10 means that the preparation was prepared using 1 part plant material and 5 or 10 parts of the menstruum.
- *Storage* (see p. 5): Should not be stored for more than one year owing to the potential instability of certain compounds in the extract. Some studies by Bauer, a leading authority on echinacea, and co-workers show the stability of echinacea tincture under normal conditions to be 2 to 3 years with about 30 % reduction in some important constituents per year. (Personal communication, Rudi Bauer, PhD, 1987.)
- ◉ *Note:* Many tinctures should not be used undiluted.

► **Fluid extract** (fluid extract)
- *Definition:* An alcoholic preparation of a medicinal herb containing higher concentrations of plant constituents than are found in conventional tinctures. One part of fluid extract generally corresponds to one part of the parent herb calculated on a dry-weight basis. This concentration has to be achieved by evaporating off some of the alcohol.
- *Preparation:* As for tinctures.

► **Dry extracts** (powdered extracts)
- *Definition:* Solid preparations obtained by condensing and drying fluid extracts. A powdered extract contains generally 95 % solids and 5 % water residue (moisture). A native extract or native dry extract contains only plant extract material and is free of additives.
- *Preparation*
  • Fluid extracts are separated from solvents by carefully heating the extract and allowing the solvent to evaporate, often in a vacuum chamber by freeze-drying or spray-drying.
  • The selected drying method has a decisive effect on product quality; for example, excessive heat degrades some active constituents.
  • Adjuvants and carriers such as highly dispersed silica, lactose, and methylcellulose are sometimes added to prevent caking and to adjust the final extract concentration. Extracts that are adjusted to 5 : 1 (meaning that 1 part of the finished extract is equivalent to all the desirable and active constituents of 5 parts of the dried herb) are typical.
  • The package labeling provides information on the parent plant or plant part, the extractant, and the dried herb/extract ratio (HER). An HER of 10 : 1 means that 10 parts of the plant material yielded 1 part extract. A low HER (such as 1 : 2) indicates a high concentration of the active compounds in the plant material.

► **Special extracts**
- *Definition:* Extracts that undergo special extraction and purification processes to separate, concentrate, and free them from toxic and undesirable substances.
- *Preparation*
  • Special extracts are made from raw extracts.
  • The raw extract undergoes special extraction and purification processes to increase the concentration of desirable active principles.

- Toxins and undesirable substances that do not contribute to the medicinal action of the preparation are removed.
- This treatment reduces the risk factors associated with the native material, and often provides a finished product that is many times more concentrated in one or more active constituents than is the parent herb, such as the highly concentrated and standardized ginkgo extract typically sold in consumer products (50 : 1). Hence, the effects of the special extract can no longer be compared with those of the raw materials.

Medicinal Teas

➤ **Definition**: Herb teas, such as orthosiphon or lobelia, with a strong medicinal action. Best used under the guidance of an experienced health care professional such as a naturopathic practitioner or herbalist. Many milder teas like ginger, peppermint, and chamomile have some medicinal qualities, but are usually considered safe to use at home with care. The use and sale of many of these herb teas fall under the food laws in North America; beverage teas, see p. 479).

- The concentrations of active principles in medicinal teas are determined by the relative proportion of the herbs to extractant (water), the degree of cutting or grinding of the herb, the recommended water temperature, and the steeping time.
- *Disadvantages:* It is difficult to determine the exact dosage; combined components may become separated. Cutting or powdering of herbs often drastically reduces their shelf life by allowing oxygen to reach and degrade active constituents.
- *Suppliers of medicinal teas:* Pharmacies, drug stores, health food stores, herb shops, and supermarkets.
- *Preparation:* Leaves, flowers, and other plant materials are cut coarsely to finely. Wood, bark, and root materials are cut finely or pulverized.
- *Storage:* Keep dry and store in metal tins or dark jars to prevent direct light exposure. The expiration date should be indicated on the label.

➤ **Types of tea preparations**
- **Loose tea:** Available as single-herb preparations and as tea mixtures. Tea mixtures do not usually contain more than seven different plant species. Traditional Chinese tea formulas often contain 6 to 15 different herbs. Those with as many as 20 to 30 herbs cannot reliably be used to achieve selective or specific effects.
- **Tea bags**
  - *Definition:* Small filter bags in which finely chopped herbal teas are enclosed.
  - *Suitability:* All herbs with constituents readily extractable with boiling water.
  - *Advantages:* The small particle size of the tea yields a high degree of extraction of the constituents. Tea bags are easy to use and ensure uniformity of dose and composition.
  - *Disadvantages:* Some of the volatile substances are lost during preparation and storage and certain constituents undergo oxidation upon exposure to the air.
  - The individual tea bags should be separately wrapped in airtight packets.

- **Instant teas**
  - *Definition:* Tea preparation that readily dissolves in water. Powdered teas contain around 8–10 % extractable plant constituents in addition to fillers, carriers, flavor enhancers, and colorants (e. g., sugar, dextrin, gelatin, acacia). To prepare tea granules, liquid drug extracts are sprayed onto a carrier and dried. Tea granules consist mainly of sugar, with plant constituents comprising only 2–3 % of the final product. Many Chinese medicinal tea blends are available in this form.
  - *Note:* Diabetics must be aware of the relatively high sugar content. Since essential oils are lost during the comminution process, they are sometimes added at a later phase of the manufacturing process.

➤ **Methods of tea preparations** (see also p. 27)
  - **Infusion:** Preparation made by pouring boiling water onto the fresh or dried herbs and allowing them to steep in order to extract their medicinal principles. Suitable for the preparation of delicate or finely chopped herbs (leaves, flowers, seeds, bark, and roots) with volatile and thermolabile constituents (e. g., essential oils).
  - **Decoction:** Prepared by boiling fresh or dried herbs in water for 10 to 60 minutes to extract their medicinal principles. Suitable for the preparation of hard or very hard plant materials (woods, barks, roots) or herbs with sparingly soluble constituents (e. g., silicic acid).
  - **Maceration (cold extract):** Prepared by allowing a tea herb to steep in cold water for several hours to extract its active principles. Suitable for the preparation of mucilage-containing herbs such as flaxseeds or psyllium seeds whose high concentrations of starches and pectins would cause them to gelatinize if prepared with boiling water. Also used to prevent the extraction of undesirable constituents that dissolve in hot water.

➤ **Prescription and reimbursement of costs**
  – In some European countries, as well as China, properly-prescribed herbal preparations are reimbursable by law.
  – In North America, herbal preparations, even when prescribed by a licensed practitioner, are not reimbursable by insurance companies or HMOs. This is slowly changing, as more research-based evidence of the cost-effectiveness of herbal remedies emerges.

➤ **Reading and writing prescriptions**
  – The Latin terminology should be used in written prescriptions so that the medicinal herb in question can be readily identified at the pharmacy, where the drug containers are labeled with the Latin terms.
  – The English and Latin terms for the most important plant parts are listed in Table **1**.

Table 1 English and Latin names and abbreviations of plant parts

English Name	Latin Name Singular (Plural)	Abbreviation
Leaf	folium (folia)	fol.
Flower	flos (flores)	flor.
Fruit	fructus (fructus)	fruct.
Herb	herba (herbae)	herb.
Root	radix (radices)	rad.
Rhizome	rhizoma (rhizomae)	rhiz.
Bark	cortex (cortices)	cort.

➤ **Writing prescriptions for teas, tinctures and other special preparations:** The prescription must tell the pharmacist how much of which drugs to use, which ratio of each drug to use, and so forth.

➤ **Prescription format:** The standard Latin abbreviations should be used in written instructions for the pharmacist. The most important terms and abbreviations used in written prescriptions are summarized in Table **2**.

Table 2 Latin terms and abbreviations used in prescription writing

Latin Abbreviation	Derivation	English Equivalent
Aa	ana partes aequales	(equal parts) of each
aqu.	aqua	water
add.	adde	add
aut simil.	aut similia	or similar
c.	cum	with
cc, conc.	concisus	cut
cont.	contusus	crushed
d.	da	give

Continued

1.5 Prescribing Herbal Medicines

Fundamentals of Phytotherapy

Table 2 Continued

Latin Abbreviation	Derivation	English Equivalent
d.s.	detur signetur	give and label as follows
Ft	fiat	make, prepare
Gtt	gutta, guttae	drops
Inf	infunde	make an infusion
m.	misce	mix
M ft spec.	misce fiat species	mix and make a tea
M ft ungt.	misce fiat unguentum	mix and make an ointment
M. D. S.	misce, da, signe	mix, give, label as
p.c.	post cibum	after meals
pulv.	pulvus, pulveratus	powder, pulverized
Rx	recipe	take
S.	signa	label, mark
spec.	species	tea
supp.	suppositorium	suppository
tal. dos.	tales doses	such doses
tct., tr.	tinctura	tincture
ungt.	unguentum	ointment

➤ The proper dose in herbal medicine is always a matter to be considered in clinical practice.

➤ Several factors should be taken into account when determining the proper dose, as follows.
  – The cultural context in which the herb is used
  – Federal or state regulations
  – The potential toxicity or strength of each herb
  – The relative concentration or strength of the product
  – The dose form, i. e., tincture, standardized extract, etc.
  – The age, strength, and needs of the individual taking the preparation
  – The duration of administration

➤ Cultures vary as to how much of an herb or herb preparation is taken at a dose, and over how long a period.
  – For instance, native Americans were used to drinking several cups of strong teas made by boiling the herbs. Consumption leading to vomiting was common as a means of cleansing the system. This would not be acceptable in most technologically developed nations today.
  – In China, a common herb prescription contains from 5 to 10 herbs, and the daily dose for each is in the range of 3–12 grams. Many herb tea prescriptions given for therapeutic use contain about 60–200 grams of dried herbs. These are to be boiled for up to an hour and 2–3 cups of the strong brew are consumed over the course of a day.

➤ In Germany and other European countries, as well as North America, standardized extracts are commonly prescribed in tablets and capsules, as well as teas and hydroethanolic tinctures. Some standardized extracts are highly concentrated. For instance, *Ginkgo biloba* leaves are extracted to produce a 50 : 1 concentrate. One part of the finished extract represents the active flavonoids and terpenes from 50 parts of the leaves.

➤ Teas and tinctures in Europe tend to be of lower concentration than in North America, and the recommended daily dose also seems to be lower. In Germany and Europe, mother tinctures made with an extract ratio of 1 : 10 are often favored. This means that 10 parts of the finished tincture represent most of the desirable and active constituents from only 1 part of the herb. This is called a "mother tincture." For instance an ounce of echinacea mother tincture made at this concentration would represent 1/10 of an ounce of dried echinacea root or leaves, or about 3 grams. If the recommended dose were 1–2 mL, 3 times/day, the patient would receive the equivalent of about 100–200 mg of dried herb, 3 times/day, or up to 600 mg/day. By comparison, a common daily dose of Chinese herbs can be up to 200 *grams* of herbs boiled and consumed as a tea. While it has been argued that hydroalcoholic tinctures are more absorbable by the body and so have a stronger impact than teas, the difference would be slight compared with the great difference in doses between the two cultures.

➤ In North America, as in Europe, standardized extracts are commonly sold and prescribed by practitioners. Chinese herb tea and tablet prescriptions are also widely used.

➤ Hydroalcoholic tinctures are usually manufactured at a concentration of anywhere from 3 : 1 to 10 : 1, and most are around 5 : 1. The recommended dose listed on bottles of these tincture products tends to be 20 to 80 drops, several times daily. More experienced western herbal practitioners tend to prescribe up to 5 mL of a hydroalcoholic tincture, 3 to 5 times/day, as an initial therapeutic dose, and about 1–2 mL, 2 to 3 times/day as a maintenance dose.

➤ Based on all these differences, how is one to best determine the dose for each individual for any given clinical encounter? This has to be determined on the basis of a knowledge of the strength of the herb, the strength of the preparation, the quality and freshness of the herbs that went into the product, and of course the size, weight, age, and needs of the patient.

➤ In Table 5 , usual German doses are given, along with the usual North American dose. We recommend that you adjust the dose within this range of doses, again based on the individual situation. Use common sense. Smaller people need a smaller dose than a very large person. Young children need a smaller dose than an adult. Very young children usually need only a few drops to obtain a therapeutic response. Weak or sensitive individuals need (or can tolerate) a smaller dose than a robust, healthy person. Do not think of the dose as static and fixed for all circumstances. Use your best judgement, taking account of the situation, and always adjust the dose rather than dispensing an herb in the same dose for every situation and person.

➤ In the plant summaries this book maintains the German dosages of the original, however, please refer to the dosage table 337 f for American doses.

➤ Usually it is best to start a person on a new herb or formula at the minimum dose to check for sensitivity and response before going on to a larger dose if no response is noted. For long-term use the dose can often be half of the therapeutic dose as a maintenance dose.

Clinical Applications of Herbal Medicine

➤ **Primary indications**
- Gastrointestinal diseases
- Colds and flu
- Liver and gallbladder diseases
- Psychovegetative diseases
- Circulatory problems and decreased mental performance
- Sleep disorders
- Diseases of the kidney and efferent urinary passages
- Prostatic diseases
- Diseases of the female genital tract
- Varicose veins
- Convalescent care
- Prevention of degenerative diseases
- Supportive (adjuvant) treatment

➤ **Indicated for adjuvant therapy only in**
- Severe diseases
- Infectious diseases
- Emergency medicine

➤ **Advantages of herbal medcines**
- Although recent reports highlight a few problems with herb–drug interactions such as St. John's wort reducing plasma levels of antirejection and antiretroviral drugs, the overall chance of most herbal preparations interfering with the safety and efficacy of synthetic drugs is small, on the basis of actual human reports. Many published comments about herb–drug interactions in the literature and popular press involve theoretical interactions only. More work needs to be performed in this new area of research.
- Herbal medicines have a wide therapeutic range (the gap between therapeutic and toxic doses is very large) and, thus, a superior risk-to-benefit ratio. A number of recent published studies involving thousands of patients show that patient reports of adverse effects are close to those reported for placebo.
- Herbal medicines provide a high level of treatment safety.
- When given a choice, patients with the conditions listed above tend to accept them more readily than synthetic drugs, thereby increasing compliance.
- Herbal medicines facilitate the transition from acute short-term to chronic long-term treatment.
- Herbal medicines can replace some of the conventional synthetic drugs used to treat patients with chronic diseases, such as chronic fatigue syndrome, and multiple morbidity syndromes. This is important because their synthetic counterparts often have considerable side effects.

➤ **Disadvantages of herbal medicines**
- Herbal medicines are often not potent enough to treat severe illnesses by themselves, except sometimes with a long-term course.
- Diseases may be drawn out unnecessarily when self-prescribed herbal drugs are taken improperly.
- The improper long-term use of certain herbal preparations, such as the pyrrolizidine alkaloid-containing herb comfrey, can lead to severe side effects.

2.1 Potentials and Limitations

Self-Care Management

➤ Owing to budget restrictions and the reduced number of drugs covered under many health insurance plans, the role of herbal self-treatment is increasing.
➤ In self-care management, the responsibility for correct herb use and dosage lies with the patient.
➤ As a result, side effects and interactions with other drugs are more likely to go unnoticed by these patients.
➤ It is therefore imperative that all herbs and herbal remedies be accurately labeled with adequate instructions and warnings. Ideally, the patient will consult a qualified health care professional such as a physician trained in herbal medicine, trained herbalist, or naturopathic physician before initiating self-treatment with any herbal remedy. The advice of a physician should also be sought when herbal preparations are used together with pharmaceutical drugs, and obviously with severe ailments.
➤ In North America, according to recent studies, most patients do not inform their physician about herbal use. This may be because most medical doctors are uninformed about some of the current research regarding the safety and efficacy of herbal preparations. This is not surprising, since they rarely receive training or continuing education in this area. Perceived disapproval from a physician may also play a role in this choice.

Role of the Physician

➤ The physician should be informed of the use of herbal remedies to avoid unnecessary or excessive treatment and unwanted interactions with synthetic drugs (physician-supervised self-care management).
➤ Since physicians should be able to advise patients about the limitations of self-care management, doctors must have a solid knowledge of herbal medicine. Patients often tend to be more responsive about informing physicians concerning herbal use when they feel the physician is knowledgeable and, as far as possible, unbiased.

◎ *Note:* Not all herbal medicinal products are safe and gentle. The improper long-term use of certain herbs can lead to serious side effects. Therefore, herbal remedies should not be used for extended periods without the supervision of a physician or other appropriately experienced health care provider.

Preliminary Remarks

➤ Owing to their low rate of side effects, the use of herbal remedies is increasing in certain patient groups, particularly in chronically ill children, pregnant and nursing mothers, and senior citizens.
➤ Certain precautions may be observed when treating allergy sufferers and intensive-care patients with herbal remedies.

Infants and Children

➤ Pharmacokinetics
  – The pharmacokinetic and pharmacodynamic responses of infants and small children to herbal remedies are different from those of adults. As a result, the therapeutic range of an herbal drug will also differ in children and adults.
  – These differences are attributable to the underdevelopment of organ structure and function in children and differences in receptor structures.
  – Drugs are retained longer in a child's body owing to the lower rates of excretion and metabolism.
➤ **Basic rules for treatment of pediatric patients**
  – The treatment of pediatric patients with herbal medicinal preparations should be carried out under the supervision of a physician and/or other appropriately experienced health care provider, if the persons who take care of the child are not experienced in herbal medicine, or the disease is more serious or longer lasting. A herbal remedy suitable for use in children should be selected and administered at the lowest dose possible.
  – Generally, the herbal preparation should be administered according to the supplier's recommendation.
  – For preparations without dose recommendation a formula for calculation of reduced dosages for children and infants based on body weight may be used: children's dose = (adult dose/110) × (1.5 × weight in kg).
➤ **Practical dosage recommendations for administration of teas (or diluted tinctures) to pediatric patients**
  – *Infants:* 5 drops or 1 to 2 droppersful of a tea, or 1 part of tincture (ca. 1 : 5) diluted with 10 parts water, several times a day.
  – *Children 1 to 5 years:* 1 to 2 teaspoons of a tea infusion 3 to 5 times a day (or a liquid made by diluting 1 part of tincture with 10 parts of water).
  – *Children 6 to 10 years:* 1/4 to 1/3 of the adult dose.
  – *Children 11 to ca. 16 years:* 1/2 of the adult dose.
  – *Children over 16 years:* Generally the adult dose, but used with greater caution.
  – It is important to start with the smallest dose for the first day and work up to a higher dose, if no adverse reactions are apparent.
➤ **Administration:** Teas, highly diluted alcoholic tinctures, and flavored liquid glycerites are preferably used with pediatric patients because they contain low doses of the active constituents.
◉ *Note:* Instant teas containing saccharose promote the formation of dental caries.
  – Alcohol-free herbal preparations, such as flavored glycerites, are preferable for pediatric medicine. Liquid herbal remedies often contain alcohol as a preservative; the ethanol content must be indicated on the label.

2.2 Special Patient Groups

⊙ *Note:* In Germany, many herbal remedies, even those that have been taken by pediatric patients for years without adverse effects, are labeled with statements such as "Owing to the lack of sufficient scientific data on the use of this preparation in children, it should not be used in children under 12 years of age". Such statements are intended to indicate a residual risk. In this case, it is important to obtain the advice of a physician in selecting the proper remedy. On the other hand, remedies labeled with the statement "Children under 12 years of age should not take this preparation" are clearly contraindicated in pediatric patients. In North America, many preparations are not labeled with recommendations for pediatric use, which is why special children's herbal products are increasingly popular. These are mild and pleasant-tasting.

➤ **Value of herbal medicine:** The rate of spontaneous healing is much higher in infants and children than in adults. This makes it more difficult to assess the effectiveness of herbal medicines in pediatric patients.

Geriatric Patients

➤ **Preliminary remarks:** Around 27 % of all individuals over the age of 65 are afflicted by one chronic disease, 20 % by two chronic illnesses, and 3 % by three or more. In some cases, the symptoms of organ dysfunction precede the clinical manifestation of a disease by several years. Many of these patients respond well to herbal remedies.

➤ **Pharmacokinetic changes of aging**
  - Impairment of blood pH regulation
  - Decreased absorption of oxygen in the blood
  - Decrease in the respiratory rate
  - Decrease in renal and, to a lesser extent, hepatic function

➤ **Basic rules for treatment of geriatric patients**
  - Because of their low rates of side effects and interactions with other drugs, herbal preparations can be safely and effectively combined with obligatory synthetic drugs, with a few exceptions such as St. John's wort, which should be monitored more closely.
  - A lower dose may be needed due to the slower metabolism of geriatric patients.

➤ **Value of herbal medicine:** Because of the high rate of acceptance by geriatric patients, herbal remedies can be a very helpful treatment alternative in this patient group.

➤ **Cost:** In some cases, herbal preparations are less costly than pharmaceutical drugs, despite the fact that insurance plans do not generally pay for them.

Pregnant and Nursing Mothers

➤ **Pharmacokinetic considerations**
  - Drug therapy is always a problematic issue in pregnant and nursing mothers because of the potential risk of damage to the fetus or infant.
  - Furthermore, it is almost impossible to completely rule out the possibility that a given drug may have harmful effects.

➤ **Basic rules for treatment of pregnant and nursing mothers**
  - Herbal remedies have a long history of being used to treat pregnant and nursing mothers.
  - Warnings indicated on product labels should be interpreted carefully.

- Herbal remedies or preparations that specifically are labeled with the statements, "Don't use during pregnancy," or "Don't use during breast-feeding" should not be used during those times unless under the guidance of an experienced herbalist or physician with training in herbal medicine.
- Other commercial herbal preparations or herb teas may not be specifically labeled "Don't use during pregnancy or nursing," but that does not imply that they are necessarily safe to use during these times. Bulk herb for teas are not often labeled, and some manufacturers may not be experienced or knowledgeable enough to label their products appropriately.
- In some cases, herbs or herb products have been used safely for centuries, and sometimes during pregnancy or nursing, but that does not mean they are safe. Harmful effects are sometimes subtle and not noticed, and may be apparent after continued use over time. In general herbs and herb products are less likely to be problematic during pregnancy and nursing with occasional use, and it is best to avoid chronic use of most herbs during these times.
- Virtually no herbs have high-quality research demonstrating lack of side effects during pregnancy or nursing, rather the use is based on centuries of apparently safe use. The other side to this argument is that just because an herb hasn't been proven safe by modern scientific standards doesn't mean that it is probably harmful. Many foods in common use have not been thoroughly tested to demonstrate safety with long-term use.
- Herbal medicines that bear warnings such as "Contraindicated during pregnancy " or "Contraindicated in nursing mothers" clearly should not be used by pregnant or nursing mothers. For a complete list of known contraindications for herbs during pregnancy and nursing, refer to *Botanical Safety Handbook* by McGuffin et al. (see References, p. 478).

Allergy Sufferers

➤ Certain medicinal plants contain allergens that may cause allergic reactions of variable severity (even, in rare cases, anaphylactic shock) in individuals with a corresponding predisposition. Medicinal plants are capable of triggering type I (immediate) and type IV (delayed) allergic reactions.

➤ The allergenic potency of medicinal plants varies in accordance with the type of the plant and the composition of its constituents.

➤ Cross-sensitivities are a frequent problem.

◉ *Note:* Allergy to a given plant does not necessarily mean that the patient will be hypersensitive to pharmaceutical preparations made from this plant.

➤ **Type I allergies**

- *Pathophysiology*: Antibodies of the IgE type start a chain reaction that triggers the release of different mediators (e. g., histamine).
- *Clinical features*
  - *Allergic symptoms* including allergic conjunctivitis, rhinitis, itching, urticaria, Quincke's edema and allergic asthma as well as cramplike epigastric complaints accompanied by diarrhea may develop with seconds to minutes after exposure. In secondary reactions, they may develop within 4 to 6 hours after exposure.

2.2 Special Patient Groups

- - *Anaphylactic shock* usually does not occur unless the allergens are injected intravenously.
  - *Herbal drugs known to trigger type I allergies*
    - Essential oils derived from fennel, ginger, garlic, coriander, caraway seed, lovage, balm, pepper, sage, mustard, and various citrus plants are important triggers. Because of their ability to cause mucosal irritation, they may also enhance other allergies. Inhalation of dust of iris root, poke root, mustard, horseradish, castor oil, or linseed may cause rhinitis.
    - Herbal remedies do not play a major role in pollen allergies.

➤ **Type IV allergies**
- *Pathophysiology:* Mediators of inflammation are released by sensitized T lymphocytes.
- *Clinical features:* Contact eczema with itching, skin redness, swelling, and scaling develops at the site of exposure within 48 to 72 hours.
- *Herbal drugs known to trigger type IV allergies:* Low-molecular-weight secondary plant chemicals such as coumarins (from parsley family members like angelica, clovers like red clover, etc.) and terpenes (from many plant families such as ginkgo), as well as flavones and sesquiterpene lactones (from composite plants such as feverfew or arnica).

Intensive Care Patients

➤ Because of their rapid onset of action and superior dosability, synthetic drugs are preferentially used in intensive care medicine. Nonetheless, certain herbal drugs are suitable for adjuvant therapy, such as ginger tea or capsules to help alleviate nausea.

➤ Early and effective treatment with herbal remedies with known immunomodulating effects such as echinacea can reduce the required dose of antibiotics and improve wound healing. Standard herbal treatments for various indications are described in Section Four (p. 290 ff.).

➤ Herbal treatment measures are selected in accordance with the type and severity of the disease and the individual needs of the patient. Standard herbal treatments for various indications are described in Section Four (p. 290 ff.). A few basic rules for the use of herbal remedies are presented below.

Preparation of Teas

➤ **Preparatory measures**
  - *Tea mixtures:* Shake the container holding the tea mixture prior to use to ensure the uniform distribution of all components.
  - *Herbal teas containing essential oils:* The herbs (fruit or seeds such as fennel) should not be chopped or crushed until immediately prior to use.
  - ◉ *Note:* The caking of hygroscopic preparations such as water-soluble (instant) teas makes it impossible to measure the preparation accurately. Therefore, the spoon used to remove the tea granules or powder should be completely dry and the container should be immediately recapped. In North America, instant tea powders are mostly available only for Chinese herbs, and most extract powders are in capsule or tablet form for ease of use.

➤ **Tea preparation**
  - *Infusion:* Pour boiling water onto the required amount of the herb, cover, and allow to steep for 10 to 15 minutes, then strain. A dose of 1 teaspoon herb per cup (150 mL) of water is generally recommended.
  - *Decoction:* Pour cold water onto the required amount of the herb, bring to a boil, then cover and allow to simmer for 10 to 15 minutes. Remove from heat and allow to stand for a few moments, in some cases up to 10 minutes if a slightly stronger preparation is desired, then strain. Several days of tea can be stored safely in the refrigerator, then warmed at the time of consumption. A dose of 1 teaspoon herb preparation per cup (150 mL) of water is generally recommended.
  - *Maceration (cold extract):* Pour cold water onto the comminuted herb. A dose of 1 teaspoon herb per cup (150 mL) of water is generally recommended. The herb–water mixture is allowed to stand at room temperature for 5 to 8 hours, stirred occasionally, then strained. Because of the rapid spread of bacteria and molds, teas prepared by maceration may be briefly boiled before consumption, though the use of sanitary utensils and refrigeration of the tea mixture for up to 3 days in the refrigerator makes this mostly unnecessary. Make sure utensils are clean.

➤ **Combined forms of preparation**
  - Recommended for the preparation of tea mixtures containing certain constituents that should preferably be extracted with cold water and others that are best extracted with boiling water.
  - A dose of 1 teaspoon tea mixture per cup of water is generally recommended. Half the required amount of water is poured onto the full dose of the tea mixture, which is then left to steep for 5 to 8 hours and finally strained. The other half of the water is later boiled and poured onto the herbs caught in the tea strainer, then added to the cold extract.

➤ **General tips**
  - Medicinal teas should be prepared in a non-metallic receptacle such as a glass coffeepot or teapot. Teapots with a lid are preferable.
  - The tea should be stirred occasionally while steeping, then pressed against the tea strainer when finished.

2.3 Basics of Administering Herbal Preparations

- Teas for colds and flu should be sweetened with honey, whereas those for gastrointestinal, liver, and biliary complaints are ideally taken unsweetened. Use only as much sweetener for these herbs as is necessary to take them regularly, because tasting the bitter enhances the therapeutic action. Diabetics should use a sugar substitute.
- Special tea cups with a tight-fitting lid should be used to reduce the loss of volatile constituents by evaporation.

➤ **Dosage**
- *Adults:* 1 teaspoon of herb per 150 mL (5 ounces) of water.
- *Children up to 10 years of age:* 1 teaspoon of herb per 250 mL (8 ounces) of water.
- *Children up to 1 year of age:* 1/2 teaspoon of herb per 250 mL of water.
- Daily dose: 2 to 3 cups per day, sipped slowly.

◉ *Note:* General dosage recommendations are provided in this section. The specific instructions for use of a given product are found on the product label. Certain tea preparations should not be administered to children. The patient or guardian should always read the product label and, if uncertain, ask a pharmacist or herbalist. Certain medicinal teas can produce side effects when overdosed.

➤ **Duration of use**
- Medicinal teas should generally be taken for 4 weeks. Afterwards, the patient should discontinue the tea for 4 weeks or switch to another tea with similar effects.
  - *Exceptions:* St. John's wort or hawthorn teas, which must be used for at least 3 months. Many "tonic" teas recommended by a licensed traditional Chinese medicine practitioner are taken for several months or more, depending on the patient's response, although the formula is often changed regularly.

Preparation of Wraps and Fomentations

➤ Herbal compresses, wraps, and fomentations are popular in Europe and other countries where herbal preparations are used as part of a traditional healing system. Applying herbs or herbal teas externally in this way is safe when a few cautions are observed. Local anti-inflammatory effects and stimulation of circulation and enhanced tissue repair can be expected because of constituents such as the gingerols from ginger, which are absorbed transdermally.

➤ **Definition:** Wraps are made by winding multiple layers of cloth around an affected body part. The prepared herbs are placed in the innermost cloth, which serves as the carrier. When using fomentations, poultices, and compresses, the cloth bearing the herbal preparation is placed in direct contact with the affected body part.

➤ **Materials:** Natural materials such as cotton, linen, flannel, or wool (e.g., used sheets, kitchen towels, diapers, handkerchiefs, gauze compresses, and towels as well as sheets made of terry cloth, flannel, or moleskin) should be used (see Fig. **2**). The use of synthetic materials or mixed fabrics is not recommended.

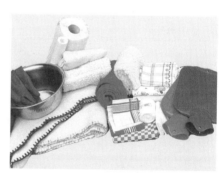

Fig. **2** Recommended wrapping materials. Adapted with permission from A. Sonn, *Wickel und Auflagen*, Thieme, Stuttgart, 1998.

- *Innermost layer:* Cotton or linen
- *Middle layer:* Cotton (e. g., terry cloth)
- *Outer layer:* Wool, moleskin or cotton (flat sheets, wool blankets, scarves)
- One or two hot water bottles
- Fixing material (e. g., adhesive tape, Velcro strips, or safety pins)

➤ **Procedure**
- *Preparatory steps:* Spread the wrapping materials on a table or countertop and prepare the herbs (additive) as recommended on the product label (Fig. **3**). When the preparation is in place, the patient should be allowed to rest without unnecessary distractions.

➤ **Technique**
- The temperature of the wrap is selected in accordance with the type of herb used as the additive. It is also important to monitor each patient in accordance with their age, general health condition, and body temperature.
- The sheet or packet with the herbal remedy is placed on the body or affected body part and covered with a layer of fabric. The body or body part is then wrapped in a second, outer layer. The patient should be covered with a

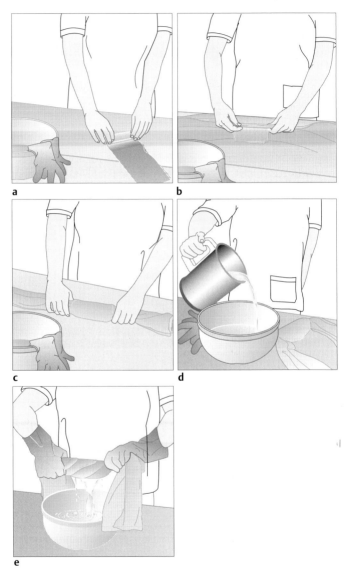

Fig. **3** Preparation of wraps and fomentations. Adapted with permission from A. Sonn, *Wickel und Auflagen*, Thieme, Stuttgart, 1998.

warm blanket. Special attention should be paid to keeping the feet warm (place a hot water bottle under the feet, if necessary).

– To prevent skin burns or irritation, a protective cloth should be placed between the skin and the hot water bottle.

– *Duration of effect:* The wrapping materials should be applied quickly but calmly. The amount of time the wrap should be left on depends on the type of wrap used (see Section Four, p. 291 ff.). The patient in the wraps should be monitored carefully.

– *Resting period:* After the wraps or fomentations have been removed, the patient should be allowed to rest for 15 to 20 minutes.

◉ *Note:* The herbs used as the additive can be discarded in the normal household garbage container, or composted along with kitchen food scraps or yard trimmings. Used herbs should never be reused or consumed.

Footbaths

➤ **Materials:** Wash basin or vessel large enough for the feet to fit in comfortably, warm water, and the herbs to be used as the additive.

➤ **Procedure**

– *Preparation:* Fill the basin or vessel with water heated to the appropriate temperature, then add the selected herbal additive (e. g., a tea infusion, essential oil, sea salt, or mustard flour). The ankle bone should be immersed in the water.

Technique

– The patient should wear comfortable clothing and sit in a relaxed position. If the patient is cold, a light blanket can be placed around the knees.

– *Soaking time:* The feet should be soaked for 5 to 20 minutes, depending on which type of herb was used as the additive.

– Afterwards, the feet should be dried with a towel but not rinsed unless mustard flour was used. Leaving mustard flour on the feet can cause skin necrosis. This can be prevented by rinsing the feet with lukewarm water after the footbath.

– *Resting period*
  • After the footbath, the patient should put on warm socks and rest for half an hour. If preferred, the footbath can be taken at night before retiring.
  • Invigorating footbaths should be taken around noon, and the patient should remain mobile afterwards.

Inhalation

➤ **General remarks:** Inhalation is mainly used to treat diseases of the airways. This is most easily achieved with steam inhalation.

➤ **Materials:** Heat-proof vessel, towel, herbal additive.

➤ **Procedure**

– *Preparation:* Prepare a hot tea infusion or add essential oil to hot water and pour into the vessel. Herbal tea infusions, essential oils, or salt-water solutions can constitute the herbal additive.

Technique

– The patient's head should be held at a comfortable distance above the steam. The hair should be covered with a towel to ensure that the vapors are trapped between the head and the vessel. The hot vapors should be inhaled for 10 to 15 minutes.

2.4 Working Techniques

Body washes

➤ **General comments:** The effects of body washes vary in accordance with the washing technique, the selected water temperature and the reason for using the herbal additive (e. g., to reduce fever, to stop itching, or to reduce sweating).

➤ **Materials:** Wash basin, towels (at least two), wash cloths, herbal additive (tea infusion, essential oil, or bath salts).

➤ **Procedure**
  – *Preparation:* Fill the basin with water heated to the desired temperature and place the additive into it. If essential oils are used, it is important to add a natural emulsifying agent such as milk, cream, or honey.

  Technique
  – Whole-body washes should always begin with the head and end with the feet.
  – To achieve a relaxing effect, the patient should be washed in circular motions proceeding in the direction of hair growth and moving away from the center of the body.
  – To achieve an invigorating effect, the circular motions should be directed against the direction of hair growth and toward the center of the body. This procedure stimulates receptors in the hair bulbs and increases central lymph and blood volume, both generating a slight arousal reaction.
  – The patient's skin should not be allowed to cool off during or immediately after the washing procedure.

  ◎ *Note:* The additive should be an herb the patient likes to smell and to which the patient is not allergic.

Adonis (*Adonis vernalis* L.) _____

➤ **Synonyms:** False hellebore; Adonisröschen (Ger.)
➤ **General comments:** The aerial plant parts of *Adonis vernalis* L. are used in medicine.
➤ **Pharmacology**
  – *Herb:* Adonis (Adonidis herba).
  – *Important constituents:* Flavonoids and steroid cardiac glycosides.
  – *Pharmacological properties:* Steroid glycosides have a positive inotropic action.
➤ **Indications**
  – Heart failure (NYHA classes I–II)
  – Cardiac arrhythmia
  – Nervous heart disorders
➤ **Contraindications:** Pregnant or nursing mothers, children under 12 years of age, and individuals hypersensitive to digitaloid drugs should not use adonis.
➤ **Dosage and duration of use**
  – *Daily dose:* Mean 0.5 g, maximum 3 g.
➤ **Adverse effects:** Vomiting, diarrhea, headache, loss of appetite, gynecomastia. Signs of overdose range from mild cardiac arrhythmias to life-threatening ventricular tachycardia, atrial tachycardia with AV block, stupor, confusion, hallucinations, impaired vision, depression, and/or psychoses. Adonis poisoning is rare since the oral absorption rate is low.
➤ **Herb–drug interactions:** Comparable to those of other digitaloid pharmaceutical drugs such as foxglove.
➤ **Summary assessment:** Owing to its low and irreproducible absorption behavior and the lack of adequate data on the drug, adonis is used only in combination with other digitaloid drugs.
✿ **Literature**
  – Monographs: DAB 1998; Commission E
  – Scientific publications: see p. 478
  – Loew D: Phytotherapie bei Herzinsuffizienz. Z Phytother 18 (1997), 92–96.

Angelica (*Angelica archangelica* L.) _____

➤ **Synonyms:** European angelica; Engelwurz (Ger.)
➤ **General comments:** Angelica has an aromatic odor and a sweetish taste.
➤ **Pharmacology**
  – *Herb:* Angelica root (Angelicae radix).
  – *Important constituents:* Essential oils (β-phellandrene, α-pinene), furanocoumarins (bergapten, xanthotoxin, imperatorin, isoimperatorin, angelicin, archangelicin), and caffeic acid derivatives (chlorogenic acid).
  – *Pharmacological properties:* Angelica root extracts act as calcium antagonists in vitro.
➤ **Indications**
  – Lack of appetite, anorexia
  – Dyspeptic complaints
➤ **Contraindications:** Pregnancy.
➤ **Dosage and duration of use:** 2 or 3 weeks, or longer under recommendation by an experienced health-care provider.

➤ **Adverse effects:** Sunbathing or intense exposure to UV light should be avoided when using Angelica root, since the furanocouramins in the drug may induce photodermatosis in susceptible individuals.

➤ **Herb–drug interactions:** None known.

✿ **Literature**
  – Monographs: Commission E
  – Scientific publications: see p. 478 Scientific publications: see p. 478

Aniseed (*Pimpinella anisum* L.)

➤ **Synonyms:** Anise; Anis (Ger.)

➤ **General comments:** The essential oil extracted from the mature and dried fruit is used in medicine.

➤ **Pharmacology**
  – *Herb:* Aniseed (Anisi fructus).
  – *Important constituents:* Essential oil (2–6%) consisting mainly of *trans*-anethole (ca. 94%) as well as apigenin-7-*O*-glucoside and luteolin-7-*O*-glucoside.
  – *Pharmacological properties:* Aniseed has expectorant, weakly spasmolytic and antibacterial action. Aniseed oil has antibacterial and antiviral activity.

➤ **Indications**
  – Fever, colds, and flu
  – Cough, runny nose, bronchitis
  – Inflammations of the mouth and throat
  – Dyspeptic complaints
  – Lack of appetite
  – Acute pharyngitis

➤ **Contraindications:** Hypersensitivity to aniseed or anethole; pregnancy.

➤ **Dosage and duration of use**
  – *Internal administration*
    • *Daily dose:* 3 g dried seeds.
    • *Tea:* One cup in the morning and/or evening (expectorant). For gastrointestinal complaints: 1 tablespoon daily (adults), 1 teaspoon in bottle (infants).
  – *When used as a liniment*, apply the oil every 30 to 60 minutes (acute) or 1 to 3 times a day (chronic).

➤ **Adverse effects:** Occasional allergic reactions of the skin, respiratory tract and gastrointestinal tract. Health hazards in conjunction with proper administration of the designated therapeutic doses of the drug are not known. In very rare cases, sensitization can occur after repeated contact.

➤ **Herb–drug interactions:** None known.

➤ ***Common misconceptions:*** Claims of estrogenic action have never been proven.

➤ **Summary assessment:** The information presented here is based on empirical experience. No recent studies are available. The carminative action of aniseed is weaker than that of fennel or caraway, but it is a better expectorant than fennel

✿ **Literature**
  – Monographs: ESCOP, Commission E
  – Reichling J, Merkel B: Elicitor-Induced Formation of Coumarin Derivatives of Pimpinella anisum. Planta Med 59 (1993), 187.

Arnica (*Arnica montana* L.)

➤ **General comments:** Medicinal arnica oil is extracted from fresh or dried arnica flowers.

➤ **Pharmacology**
  - *Herb:* Arnica flower (Arnicae flos).
  - *Important constituents*
    • *A. montana:* Sesquiterpene lactones of the pseudoguaianolide type (mainly esters of helenalin and 11α,13-dihydrohelenalin), essential oil (0.2–0.35%), and flavonoids (0.4–0.6%).
    • *A. chamissonis ssp. foliosa:* Sesquiterpene lactones of the pseudoguaian-olide type (0.2–1.5%), helenalin derivatives, arnifolins, and chamissonolides.
  - *Pharmacological properties:* The sesquiterpenes (e. g. helenalin) have anti-microbial action in vitro and antiphlogistic action in animals. Helenalin inhibits the activation of the transcription factor NF-κB, which is a main mediator of the immune response. Topical arnica has antiphlogistic, analgesic, and antiseptic action (due to the sesquiterpene lactones). The essential oil and flavonoid compounds may contribute to these effects.

➤ **Indications**
  - Thrombophlebitis
  - Furunculosis and inflammations resulting from insect bites
  - Inflammation of the skin
  - Inflammation of the mouth and throat
  - Rheumatic muscle and joint complaints
  - Contusions

➤ **Contraindications:** Known allergy to arnica or other composite plants.
  ◉ *Warning:* Arnica tincture should not be applied to open wounds or used undiluted.

➤ **Dosage and duration of use**
  - *External use*
    • *1 : 10 tincture* (DAB): One part arnica flower to 10 parts ethanol 70% (v/v) (dry-weight basis).
    • *Fomentations:* Dilute arnica tincture at a ratio of 1 to 3–10 parts water.
    • *Mouth wash:* Dilute tincture at a ratio of 1 : 10, since the tincture is unstable if diluted at a ratio of 1 : 100.
    • *Ointment:* Mix (generally 10–20%, but no more than 25%) arnica tincture in a neutral ointment base. The ointment should contain no more than 15% arnica oil.
    • *Oil:* One part drug extract to 5 parts slightly warmed, vegetable oil, such as olive oil.
  - *Internal use:* Not recommended. Concentrated tincture can cause irritation of the gastrointestinal mucosa accompanied by nausea, vomiting, diarrhea and bleeding, and in high enough doses can lead to respiratory stimulation, paralysis of the heart, and death.

➤ **Adverse effects:** Health hazards in conjunction with external administration of the designated therapeutic doses of arnica are minor. Frequent use of the undiluted tincture can lead to sensitization (allergic skin rashes, itching, blistering, ulcers/superficial gangrene). The external application of very high concentrations of the drug can cause primary toxic blister formation and necrosis.

➤ **Herb–drug interactions:** None known.

⊙ *Important:* Arnica flower should not be used by persons allergic to the plant. When selecting the remedy, the individual preferences of the patients should be taken into consideration.

➤ ***Common misconceptions:*** Not all varieties of arnica trigger contact allergies. Ointments made using the Spanish species of *Arnica montana* contain very low concentrations of the allergy-causing substance helenalin.

➤ **Summary assessment:** Arnica is an effective remedy, especially for contusions and strained muscles.

✿ **Literature**

- Monographs: DAB 1998, ESCOP, Commission E
- Scientific publications: see p. 478; Hörmann HP, Kortin HC: Allergic acute contact dermatitis due to Arnica tincture self-medication. Phytomedicine 4 (1995), 315–317; Lyss G, Schmidt TJ, Merfort I, Pahl HL: Helenalin an anti-inflammatory sesquiterpene lactone from Arnica selectively inhibits transcription factor NF-κB. Biol Chem, 378 (1997), 951–961; Willuhn G, Leven W: Qualität von Arnikazubereitungen. Deutsche Apotheker Ztg 135 (1995), 1939–1942.

Artichoke (*Cynara scolymus* L.)

➤ **General comments:** The dried whole or chopped basal leaves and the fresh or dried herb of *Cynara scolymus* L. are used in medicine.

➤ **Pharmacology**

- *Herb:* Artichoke leaf (Cynarae folium).
- *Important constituents:* Caffeic acid derivatives, ca. 1 % (chlorogenic acid, neochlorogenic acid, cryptochlorogenic acid, cynarin), flavonoids, 0.5 % (cynaroside, scolymoside, cynarotrioside, luteolin), and sesquiterpene lactones, 4 % (cynaropicrin, 47–83 %, dehydrocynaropicrin, grossheimin, and cynaratriol).
- *Pharmacological properties:* Sesquiterpene lactones (bitter principles), hydroxycinnamic acid and flavonoids have choleretic, hepatoprotective, antidyspeptic, and antilipemic effects. The herb was shown to reduce cholesterol levels in rats (luteolin inhibits cholesterol synthesis), as well as to increase choleresis and reduce symptoms of dyspepsia, compared with controls, in randomized double-blind studies with healthy human volunteers. In a small trial ($n = 44$), artichoke extract reduced total cholesterol in volunteers with baseline values above 220 mg/dL, compared with controls.

➤ **Indications**

- Lack of appetite
- Meteorism
- Liver and gallbladder complaints
- Hyperlipoproteinemia (high-dose, standardized extracts)

➤ **Contraindications:** Allergy to composite plants; biliary tract obstruction; gallstones.

➤ **Dosage and duration of use:** The fresh leaves, fresh expressed plant juice, and dry extracts are used in medicinal preparations.

- *Daily dose:* 6 g drug.

➤ **Adverse effects:** There are no known health hazards or side effects in conjunction with proper administration of the designated therapeutic doses of the herb.

➤ **Herb–drug interactions:** None known.
➤ **Summary assessment:** Clinical studies of the antidyspeptic effect of artichoke have been performed. The antilipemic effect is still being investigated.
✿ **Literature**
  – Monographs: BHP 96; Brazil 3; ESCOP. Commission E
  – Scientific publications: see p. 478; Petrowicz O, Gebhardt R, Donner M, Schwandt P, Kraft K: Effects of artichoke leaf extract on lipoprotein metabolism in vitro and in vivo. Atherosclerosis 129 (1997), 147; Fintelmann V: Antidyspeptische und lipidsenkende Wirkung von Artischockenblätterextrakt. Z Phytother 17 (1996), Beilage ZFA; Gebhardt R: Antioxidative and protective properties of extracts from leaves of the artichoke (Cynara scolymus L.) against hydroperoxide-induced oxidative stress in cultured rat hepatocytes. Toxicol Appl Pharmacol, 144(1997), 279–286; Wasielewski S: Artischockenblätterextrakt: Prävention der Arteriosklerose. Deutsche Apotheker Ztg 137 (1997), 2065–2067.

Asian Ginseng (*Panax ginseng* C.H. Meyer)

➤ **Pharmacology**
  – *Herb:* Asian ginseng root (Ginseng radix). The herb consists of the dried primary roots (tap roots), secondary roots, and hair roots of four- to seven-year-old *Panax ginseng* C. H. M. plants and preparations of the same.
  – *Important constituents:* Triterpene saponins (0.8–6%) such as gingenosides; panaxans; panaxynol, essential oil.
  – *Pharmacological properties:* Asian ginseng induces an unspecific increase in the endogenous defenses of animals to exogenous noxae and physical, chemical and biological stressors, that is, it has an adaptogenic or antistress effect. Stress models demonstrated that Asian ginseng increased the animals' ability to cope with psychological and physical pressure. In addition, ginseng increases, shortens the recovery phase, and enhances coordination and memory in humans.
➤ **Indications**
  – Exhaustion, convalescence
  – Decreased mental and physical performance and concentration
  – Fatigue and debility
➤ **Contraindications:** A contraindication in people with hypertension, especially with concomitant caffeine consumption is frequently given in North America; however, little clinical or research evidence exists to confirm this.
➤ **Dosage and duration of use:**
  – *Tea:* Boil 3 g of the finely cut dried roots for at least 30 or 45 minutes and steep for another 15 minutes. Strain and drink or store in refrigerator for use during the day. If only larger root pieces and whole roots are available, the patient should crush or cut the roots into coarse pieces before use; precrushed roots may also be available.
  – *Daily dose:* Dry extract: 1–2 g. For a usual 5 : 1 extract, the dose would be about 1 g, equivalent to 2 "0" caps or usually 2 tablets/day. Standardized extract (5–10% ginsenosides, typically 200 mg per unit); 1–2 capsules or tablets twice daily. Tea: one cup, 3 to 4 times a day. Treatment should be continued for 3 months followed by a break, after which treatment can be re-initiated.

➤ **Adverse effects:** Insomnia, hypertension, and edema have been reported as symptoms of overdose.

➤ **Herb–drug interactions:** The concurrent use of beverages and substances containing caffeine should be avoided.

➤ **Summary assessment:** Asian ginseng is an herbal drug with reliable effectiveness in the specified indications. Clinical studies on the efficacy of Asian ginseng are available. Use of teas from whole roots chopped or ground at home are acceptable; other use should be restricted to standardized preparations. As recent studies show, some products are substandard, despite their labeling.

✿ **Literature**

– Monographs: DAB 1998; ESCOP, Commission E

– Scientific publications: see p. 478; Blasius H: Phytotherapie: Adaptogene Wirkung von Ginseng. Deutsche Apotheker Ztg 135 (1995), 2136–2138; Pfister-Hotz G: Phytotherapie in der Geriatrie. Z Phytother 18 (1997), 165–162.

Birch (*Betula pendula* Roth.)

➤ **General comments:** Two birch species are used in medicine, *Betula pendula* and *Betula pubescens*. Various medicinal preparations are made from the leaves of these two species.

➤ **Pharmacology**
  – *Drug:* Birch leaf (Betulae folium).
  – *Important constituents:* Flavonoids, triterpene saponins, essential oil, and phenyl-carboxylic acids.
  – *Pharmacological properties:* The chemical substances in birch leaf increase the urinary volume and enhance the flow of urine in the urinary tract, resulting in the increased elimination of water (aquaresis).

➤ **Indications**
  – Rheumatic diseases (supportive treatment)
  – Used as a diuretic to flush bacteria out of the lower urinary tract and to flush out renal gravel.

➤ **Contraindications:** The drug is not recommended in patients with cardiac or renal edema.
  – Steep 1–2 tablespoons of the drug in 150 mL of hot water.
    • *Dosage:* One cup, between meals, 3 to 4 times a day. An adequate intake of fluids is essential.

➤ **Adverse effects:** Health hazards in conjunction with proper administration of the designated therapeutic doses of the drug are not known.

➤ **Herb–drug interactions:** None known.

➤ *Common misconceptions:* Birch leaf does not irritate the renal parenchyma.

➤ **Summary assessment:** Birch leaf is an effective herbal aquaretic. It can be usefully combined with other aquaretics.

✿ **Literature**
  – Monographs: ESCOP, Commission E
  – Scientific publications: see p. 478

Bitter Orange (*Citrus aurantium sinensis* [L.] Osbeck)

➤ **General comments:** Both fresh and dried orange peel as well as the oil distilled from the peel are used in medicine.

➤ **Pharmacology**
  – *Herb:* Orange peel (Aurantii pericarpium). The herb consists of the fresh or dried peel of *Citrus aurantium* (L.) O., without the spongy white layer (albedo layer), and preparations of the same.
  – *Important constituents:* Ca. 1.5 % essential oil ((+)-limonene, 90 %). Expressed orange oil also contains lipophilic flavonoids and furanocoumarins.
  – *Pharmacological properties:* Orange peel increases gastric juice production through reflex mechanisms.

➤ **Indications**
  – Lack of appetite
  – Dyspeptic complaints

➤ **Contraindications:** None known.

➤ **Dosage and duration of use**
  – *Mean daily dose:* 12 g.
  – *Daily dose:* 10–15 g of the herb.

➤ **Adverse effects:** There are no known health hazards or side effects in conjunction with proper administration of the designated therapeutic doses of the herb. The essential oil has a slight potential for sensitization after skin contact.
➤ **Herb–drug interactions:** None known.
➤ **Summary assessment:** Orange peel has relatively weak effects, but can be usefully combined with other herbal preparations.
✿ **Literature**
  – Monographs: Commission E, Mar 31
  – Scientific publications: see p. 478; Hausen B: Allergiepflanzen, Pflanzenallergene. ecomed Verlagsgesellsch. mbH, Landsberg 1988; Ihrig M: Qualitätskontrolle von süßem Orangenschalenöl. PZ 140 (1995), 2350–2353; Kern W, List PH, Hörhammer L (Ed): Hagers Handbuch der Pharmazeutischen Praxis. 4. Aufl., Bde. 1–8, Springer Verlag Berlin, Heidelberg, New York 1992–1994.

Bittersweet (*Solanum dulcamara* L.)

➤ **Synonyms:** Bitter nightshade; Bittersüß (Ger.)
➤ **General comments:** The stems, which have especially high concentrations of the active principles, are selected for medicinal use.
➤ **Pharmacology**
  – *Herb:* Bittersweet stems (Dulcamarae stipites). The herb consists of the dried stems of 2- to 3-year-old *Solanum dulcamara* L. plants, collected in the spring before the start of leafing or in the late fall after the leaves have shed, and preparations of the same.
  – *Important constituents:* Steroid alkaloid glycosides (0.07–0.4 %) and steroid saponins.
  – *Pharmacological properties:* Saponins enhance the absorption of steroid alkaloid glycosides. They stimulate phagocytosis and have hemolytic, cytotoxic, antiviral, anticholinergic, and local anesthetic effects. The constituent solasodine has a cortisone-like effect in individuals with rheumatic polyarthritis and Bekhterev's arthritis, and it has a desensitizing effect.
➤ **Indications**
  – Eczema, boils, acne
  – Warts
  – For supportive treatment of chronic eczema
➤ **Contraindications:** Pregnancy and breast feeding.
➤ **Dosage and duration of use:** No dose or duration of use specified for external use.
  – *Decoction:* Add 1–2 g of the herb to 250 mL of water.
  – *External use only:* Apply compresses soaked in bittersweet decoction several times a day.
➤ **Adverse effects:** There are no known health hazards or side effects in conjunction with proper administration of the designated therapeutic doses of the herb. Toxic effects are not to be expected when doses less than approximately 25 g per day are used.
➤ **Herb–drug interactions:** None known.
➤ **Summary assessment:** In recent years, bittersweet has become increasingly popular for treatment of chronic eczema, but further study is necessary to validate its efficacy in this indication.
✿ **Literature**
  – Monographs: Commission E

Black Cohosh (*Actaea racemosa* L. Nutt.)

➤ **Synonym:** *Cimicifuga racemosa* Nutt.
➤ **General comments:** The herb grows in the United States and Canada, where it was used by the aboriginal population to treat snake bites and to facilitate labor.
➤ **Pharmacology**
  – *Herb:* Black cohosh (Cimicifugae rhizoma). The herb consists of the dried rhizomes of *Actaea racemosa* L. and preparations of the same. Unstandardized liquid and standardized powdered extracts in capsules and tablets are widely available.
  – *Important constituents:* Triterpene glycosides (actein, cimifugoside), flavonoids (formononetin), and resins (cimifugin); also other phytoestrogens, which are chemically unidentified.
  – *Pharmacological properties:* The extract did not increase the weight of the uterus in ovariectomized animals. The phytoestrogens in the rhizome of *Actaea racemosa* bind to the estrogen receptors, and have selective estrogen receptor modulator properties. In one double-blind placebo-controlled clinical study, black cohosh extract was shown to improve the symptoms of menopause, especially hot flushes.
➤ **Indications**
  – Menopausal complaints
  – Premenstrual syndrome (PMS)
  – Menstrual cramps
➤ **Contraindications**
  – Pregnancy and breast feeding
  – Hormone-dependent tumors
➤ **Dosage and duration of use**
  – *Daily dose:* 3 g herb.
  – *Tincture (1 : 10):* 10 drops on a cube of sugar, 3 times a day. Allow to dissolve slowly in the mouth.
  – *Standardized extract products* (containing 200 mg extract), 1 tablet or capsule twice daily.
  – Black cohosh root should not be used for more than 6 months without the supervision of a qualified health care practitioner.
➤ **Adverse effects:** Can occasionally upset the stomach.
➤ **Herb–drug interactions:** None known.
➤ **Summary assessment:** Black cohosh is a well-tolerated herbal remedy that is becoming increasingly popular, especially for treatment of menopausal complaints.
✿ **Literature**
  – Monographs: ESCOP, Commission E
  – Scientific publications: see p. 478; Einer-Jensen N, Zhao J, Andersen KP, Kristoffersen K: Cimicifuga and Melbrosia lack oestrogenic effects in mice and rats. Maturitas 25 (1995), 149–153; Gruenwald J: Standardized Black Cohosh (Cimicifuga) Extract Clinical Monograph. Quarterly Review of Natural Medicine 4 (1998), 117–125; Jarry H et al: Treatment of Menopausal Symptoms with Extracts of Cimicifuga Racemosa, In vivo and in vitro Evidence for Estrogenic Activity. Loew D et al. (Ed.): Phytopharmaka in Forschung und klinischer Anwendung. Darmstadt, 1995, S 99–112; Liske E:

Therapeutic Efficacy and Safety of Cimicifuga racemosa for Gynecologic Disorders. Advances in Therapy 15, 1 (1998), 45–53.

Buckthorn (*Rhamnus cathartica* L.)

➤ **Synonyms:** Common buckthorn, European buckthorn; Kreuzdorn (Ger.)
➤ **General comments:** The buckthorn bush is widely distributed throughout Europe. Its fruit is used as a laxative.
➤ **Pharmacology**
  – *Herb:* Buckthorn fruit (Rhamni cathartici fructus). The herb consists of the fresh or dried ripe drupes of *Rhamnus cathartica* L. and preparations of the same.
  – *Important constituents:* Anthracene derivatives (2–7%) (anthranoids), tannins (3–4%), and flavonoids (1–2%).
  – *Pharmacological properties:* Anthranoid compounds are antiabsorptive and hydragogue laxatives. Hence, the herb softens the stools and increases the volume of the bowel contents.
➤ **Indications:** Constipation.
➤ **Contraindications:** Bowel obstruction, acute intestinal inflammations, appendicitis, abdominal pain of unknown origin. Pregnant or nursing mothers should not use buckthorn fruit unless directed by a physician. Use is contraindicated in children under 12 years of age.
➤ **Dosage and duration of use**
  – *Tea:* Steep 4 g (ca. 1 teaspoon) of the chopped herb in 1 cup of boiled water for 10 to 15 minutes. Alternatively, place the herb in cold water, boil for 2 to 3 minutes, then strain immediately.
    • *Dosage:* One cup in the morning and at night.
  – *Daily dose:* 2–5 g.
  – As a rule, the minimum dose required to soften the stools should be used, and continuous use of the herb should be restricted to only a few days.
➤ **Adverse effects:** The laxative effect of the herb can lead to cramplike gastrointestinal complaints. Long-term use can result in the loss of electrolytes, particularly potassium ions, thereby leading to problems such as hyperaldosteronism and decreased bowel motility. Arrhythmias, nephropathies, edemas, and accelerated bone degeneration are rare side effects. Consumption of large quantities of buckthorn fruit can lead to diarrhea with vomiting and kidney irritation.
➤ **Herb–drug interactions:** Owing to its laxative effect, buckthorn fruit can impair the absorption of pharmaceutical drugs or herbal preparations containing potentially toxic or life-sparing constituents such as cardiac glycosides (i. e., *Digitalis* spp.) if taken concomitantly.
  ◎ *Warning:* Chronic use or abuse of the herb can increase the potency of cardiac glycosides and diuretics owing to the resulting potassium deficiency.
➤ **Summary assessment:** Buckthorn fruit and other herbs containing anthranoids should not be used to treat chronic constipation.
✿ **Literature**
  – Monographs: DAB 1998; Commission E
  – Scientific publications: see p. 478; Anon: Abwehr von Arzneimittelrisiken, Stufe II. Deutsche Apotheker Ztg 136 (1996), 2353–2354; Anon: Anwendungseinschränkungen für Anthranoid-haltige Abführmittel angeordnet. PUZ 25 (1996), 341–342.

Butcher's Broom (*Ruscus aculeatus* L.)

➤ **General comments:** Butcher's broom is native to almost all parts of Europe, West Asia and North Africa and has been used in medicine since ancient times.
➤ **Pharmacology**
  – *Herb:* Butcher's broom rhizome (Rusci aculeati rhizoma). The herb consists of the dried rhizomes and roots of *Ruscus aculeatus* L. and preparations of the same.
  – *Important constituents:* Steroid saponins (4–6%) (ruscin, ruscoside, aglycon of neoruscogenin, ruscogenin) and benzofuranes.
  – *Pharmacological properties:* Butcher's broom is antiexudative, antiphlogistic, and venotonic.
➤ **Indications**
  – Hemorrhoids
  – Varicose veins
➤ **Contraindications:** None known.
➤ **Dosage and duration of use**
  – *External use:* Daily dose: 7–11 mg total ruscogenins.
  – *Internal use:* Daily dose: 100–200 mg total ruscogenins.
➤ **Adverse effects:** None known. Rare cases of diarrhea and lymphocellular colitis have been reported.
➤ **Herb–drug interactions:** None known.
➤ **Summary assessment:** The indications specified for butcher's broom have not been substantiated in controlled clinical studies, but are based on many years of empirical experience.
➤ **Literature**
  – Monographs: ESCOP, Commission E
  – Scientific publications: see p. 478; Adamek B, Drozdzik M, Samochowiec L, Wojcicki J: Clinical effect of buckwheat herb, Ruscus extract and troxerutin on retinopathy and lipids in diabetic patients. Phytotherapy Res 10 (1996), 659–662; Dunaouau CH et al: Triterpenes and sterols from Ruscus aculeatus. Planta Med 62 (1997), 189–190.

Calamus (*Acorus calamus* L.)

➤ **Synonyms:** Acorus, sweetflag; Kalmus (Ger.)
➤ **General comments:** Calamus is a very common plant, the rhizome of which is used in medicine.
➤ **Pharmacology**
  – *Herb:* Calamus rhizome (Calami rhizoma). The herb consists of the dried, coarsely chopped (and usually peeled) rhizome of *Acorus calamus* (L.). Calamus oil is distilled from the same plant.
  – *Important constituents:* Essential oil (1.7–9.3 %), α- and γ-asarone, β-gurjunene, α-calacorene, and acorone (the content of cis-isoasarone and, especially, β-asarone depends on the degree of ploidy of the plant).
  – *Pharmacological properties:* Calamus inhibits platelet aggregation in vitro and has vermicidal and insecticidal properties. In animal studies, the herb demonstrated spasmolytic and sedative effects, reduced spontaneous stomach activity, and lowered the ulcer index (reduced the production of gastric juices and acids). Calamus also has stomachic action due to the presence of bitter principles and the spasmolytic effect of its essential oil. Calamus induces hyperemia when applied externally.
➤ **Indications**
  – *Internal use:* Dyspeptic complaints.
  – *External use:* To induce local hyperemia and treat exhaustion. Used as a bath additive, it stimulates the circulation in the arms and legs.
➤ **Contraindications:** Should not be used by pregnant or nursing mothers or by children under 6 years of age.
➤ **Dosage and duration of use**
  – *Tea:* Steep 1–1.5 g (ca. 2 teaspoons) of the herb in ca. 150 mL of boiled water for 3 to 5 minutes.
    • *Dosage:* One cup with each meal.
  – *Bath additive:* Use 250–500 g of the herb to prepare an infusion and add to bath water.
➤ **Adverse effects:** There are no known health hazards or side effects in humans in conjunction with proper administration of the designated therapeutic doses of calamus of European origin (the essential oil of the European herb contains 15 % β-asarone) Alcoholic extracts of calamus will contain considerably more β-asarone and should not be used for more than a few days.
  ◎ *Warning:* Long-term use of the herb is not recommended since malignancies were found to develop in rats.
➤ **Herb–drug interactions:** None known.
➤ **Summary assessment:** Calamus has not been systematically evaluated, and prolonged use of the herb is not recommended. In Germany, no official risk-to-benefit assessment of calamus root has yet been published in any monograph. The use of Indian calamus is not permitted owing to its high β-asarone content.
✿ **Literature**
  – Monographs: None available.
  – Scientific publications: see p. 478; Schneider K, Jurenitsch, J: Kalmus als Arzneidroge: Nutzen oder Risiko. Pharmazie 47 (1992), 79–85; Steinegger E, Hänsel R: Pharmakognosie. 5. Aufl., Springer Verlag, Heidelberg 1992.

Camphor Tree (*Cinnamomum camphora* L. Sieb.)

➤ **General comments:** Medicinal camphor is the product of steam distillation of wood chips obtained from the camphor tree.

➤ **Pharmacology**
  – *Herb:* Camphor (Cinnamomi camphorae aetheroleum)
    • The herb consists of either natural or synthetic camphor. Natural $R(+)$ camphor is obtained by steam distilling the wood of the camphor tree, the product of which is then purified by sublimation.
    • Camphor is applied locally in liquid (camphor spirit) or semisolid form (liniment or ointment). The liquid form is used for inhalation therapy.
  – *Important constituents:* D-(+)-camphor and (1*R*,4*R*)-1,7,7-trimethyl-bicyclo-[2,2,1]-heptan-2-one. Synthetic camphor is designated DL-camphor.
  – *Pharmacological properties:* Used externally, camphor induces hyperemia and bronchosecretolysis.

➤ **Indications**
  – Cardiac arrhythmias
  – Coughs and bronchitis
  – Low blood pressure
  – Nervous heart disorders
  – Rheumatic complaints

➤ **Contraindications:** Camphor should not be applied to the face, especially the nose, of infants and small children. It is not recommended for internal use.

➤ **Dosage and duration of use**
  – *Semisolid forms* (ointments, liniments) generally contain 10–20 % camphor (maximum camphor content 25 %); preparations for infants and small children should contain no more than 5 %.
  – *Camphor spirit* containing 9.5–10.5 % camphor (DAB 10): Apply to skin several times a day.

➤ **Adverse effects:** Skin irritation; poisoning due to excessive drug absorption and/or inhalation (especially in children) can induce states of intoxication, delirium, convulsions, and respiration regulation disorders. Oily camphor liniments can induce contact eczema.

➤ **Herb–drug interactions:** None known.

✿ **Literature**
  – Monographs: DAB 1998; Commission E
  – Scientific publications: see p. 478; Bruchhausen F von, Ebel S, Frahm AW, Hackenthal E (Eds): Hagers Handbuch der Pharmazeutischen Praxis. 5. Aufl., Bde 7–9 (Stoffe), Springer Verlag Berlin, Heidelberg, New York 1993; Roth L, Daunderer M, Kormann K: Giftpflanzen, Pflanzengifte. 4. Aufl., Ecomed Fachverlag Landsberg/Lech 1993.

Caraway (*Carum carvi* L.):
Caraway Oil (Carvi aetheroleum)

➤ **General comments:** Caraway is a well-known culinary herb, the fruits of which are also used in medicine (e. g., as a carminative).

➤ **Pharmacology**
  – *Herb:* Caraway oil (Carvi aetheroleum). The herb consists of the essential oil distilled from the ripe seedlike fruit of *Carum carvi* L.

- *Important constituents:* D-(+)-carvone (45–65%) and D-(+)-limonene (30–40%).
- *Pharmacological properties:* Carvone demonstrated antimicrobial action against *Bacillus subtilis, Pseudomonas aeruginosa, Candida albicans,* and *Aspergillus niger.* It was also reported to have a moderate effect on dermatophytes. Caraway oil has spasmolytic effects in animals.

➤ **Indications:** Dyspeptic complaints.

➤ **Contraindications:** None known.

➤ **Dosage and duration of use**
  - *Dosage:* 1 to 2 drops of caraway oil on sugar.
  - *Daily dose:* 3 to 6 drops.

➤ **Adverse effects:** There are no known health hazards or side effects in conjunction with proper administration of the designated therapeutic doses of the herb. Long-term, high-dose administration of caraway oil (e. g., in caraway liqueur) can cause kidney and liver damage.

➤ **Herb–drug interactions:** None known.

➤ **Summary assessment:** Caraway oil has a marked carminative effect (see also Caraway Seeds (Carvi fructus).

Caraway Fruit (Carvi fructus)

➤ **Pharmacology**
  - *Herb:* Caraway fruit (Carvi fructus). The herb consists of the ripe, dried, seedlike fruit of *Carum carvi* L.
  - *Important constituents:* Essential oil (3–7%), fatty oil (10–18%) containing petroselinic acid (40–50%), oleic acid (29–30%), and polysaccharides (13%).
  - *Pharmacological properties:* See Caraway Oil.

➤ **Indications:** Dyspeptic complaints.

➤ **Contraindications:** None known.

➤ **Dosage and duration of use**
  - *Tea:* Steep 1 to 2 teaspoons (ca. 1.5 g) of the herb, crushed immediately prior to use, in 150 mL of hot water for 10 to 15 minutes in a covered vessel.
    - One dose equals 1–5 g herb.
  - *Daily dose:* 1.5–6 g herb.

➤ **Adverse effects:** There are no known health hazards or side effects in conjunction with proper administration of the designated therapeutic doses of the herb. Long-term, high-dose administration of caraway oil (e. g., in caraway liqueur) can cause kidney and liver damage.

➤ **Herb–drug interactions:** None known.

➤ **Summary assessment:** Caraway is a stronger carminative than either anise or fennel. Caraway seeds should be crushed immediately prior to use to prevent unnecessary loss of the highly volatile essential oil.

✿ **Literature**
  - Monographs: DAB 1998; ESCOP, Commission E
  - Scientific publications: see p. 478.

Cayenne (*Capsicum annuum* L.)

➤ **Synonyms:** Red pepper, hot pepper; Paprika (Ger.)

➤ **General comments:** The cayenne plant is native to Central America. Its hot and spicy fruit is best known as a spice, but is also used in medicine.

➤ **Pharmacology**
- *Herb:* Cayenne fruit (Capsici fructus). The herb consists of the ripe, dried fruit (without calyx) of *Capsicum annuum* L. or *Capsicum fructescens* L.
- *Important constituents:* Capsaicinoids (mainly capsaicin, 32–38%), dihydrocapsaicin (18–52%), carotinoids (0.3–0.8%), and flavonoids.
- *Pharmacological properties:* Capsaicinoids are potent inducers of local hyperemia. Topical application of the herb initially induces erythema accompanied by sensations of pain and heat, followed by a phase of insensitivity (reversible or irreversible deactivation of afferent fibers). The antinociceptor and antiphlogistic effects of the herb can persist for several hours to several weeks.

➤ **Indications**
- Muscular tension
- Rheumatic diseases

➤ **Contraindications:** Skin diseases or inflammation, broken skin.
   ◉ *Important:* Cayenne should not come into contact with the mucous membranes.

➤ **Dosage and duration of use**
- *Tincture (1:10):* Apply a few drops to the affected area of the skin and rub in thoroughly. Repeat several times daily.
- *Semisolid preparations* should contain no more than 50 mg of capsaicin in 100 g of a neutral base.
- Despite official warnings in the monograph of using Cayenne for more than three consecutive days, to prevent the occurrence of side effects, in North America the use of prescription pharmaceutical preparations for shingles and rheumatism for extended periods has caused no problems.

➤ **Adverse effects:** Cayenne can cause blistering and ulcer formation above and beyond the desired hyperemic effect.

➤ **Herb–drug interactions:** None known.

➤ **Summary assessment:** Cayenne can be usefully combined with other anti-inflammatory herbal preparations.

✿ **Literature**
- Monographs: DAB 1998; Commission E
- Scientific publications: see p. 478; Anon: Behandlung chronischer Schmerzen: Capsaicin—Lichtblick für Schmerzpatienten. Deutsche Apotheker Ztg 137 (1997), 1027–1028; Anon: Phytotherapie: Pflanzliche Antirheumatika—was bringen sie? Deutsche Apotheker Ztg 136 (1996), 4012–4015; Kreymeier J: Rheumatherapie mit Phytopharmaka. Deutsche Apotheker Ztg 137 (1997), 611–613.

Chamomile (*Matricaria recutita* L. Rauschert) _____

➤ **Synonyms:** German chamomile; Kamille (Ger.)

➤ **General comments:** Chamomile is widely distributed throughout Europe and is a favorite of people who like to pick their own herbs. When collecting chamomile, it is important to remember that the receptacle of true (German) chamomile is hollow and conical. The flower heads are used in medicine.

➤ **Pharmacology**
- *Herb:* Chamomile flower (Matricariae flos). The herb consists of the fresh or dried flower heads of *Matricaria recutita* L., which is also called *Chamomilla recutita* (L.) R., and preparations of the same.

– *Important constituents:* Essential oil (0.4–1.5 %) containing mainly α-bisab-olol (5–70 %), bisabolol oxides A and B (5–60 %), β-*trans*-farnesene (7–45 %), and chamazulene (1–35 %) derived from matricin, a nonvolatile proazulene, by steam distillation. Flavonoids and mucilage are also present.
– *Pharmacological properties:* The essential oil has antiphlogistic and spasmo-lytic effects and promotes wound healing. The compound α-bisabolol in-hibits fungal and bacterial growth.

➤ **Indications**
– Colds and fever
– Inflammation of the skin
– Coughs and bronchitis
– Decreased resistance to infections
– Inflammations of the mouth and throat
– Mild nervousness or insomnia (not rated by the Commission E)

➤ **Contraindications:** Chamomile flower should not be used in compresses ap-plied in the eye region to prevent pollen and other flower particles from get-ting in the eyes.

➤ **Dosage and duration of use**
– *Tea:* Pour 1 cup of hot water onto 1 tablespoon (3 g) of the herb, cover, and steep for 5 to 10 minutes (1 teaspoon = 1 g herb).
  • *Dosage:* One cup, freshly prepared, between meals, 3 to 4 times a day.
– *Bath additive:* Steep 50 g of the herb in 1 liter of hot water, then add to bath water.
– *Steam bath:* Pour hot water onto ca. 6 g of the herb.
– *Mouthwash and gargle:* Rinse the mouth or gargle with the fresh tea infu-sion several times a day.

➤ **Adverse effects:** There are no known health hazards or side effects in conjunc-tion with proper administration of the designated therapeutic doses of the herb. The herb has a slight potential for sensitization.

➤ **Herb–drug interactions:** None known.

➤ **Summary assessment:** Chamomile is a well-known, well-tolerated, thor-oughly investigated herb with a relatively wide therapeutic range. Only distil-lates and alcohol preparations of the herb contain therapeutically effective concentrations of the essential oil.

✿ **Literature**
– Monographs: DAB 1998; ESCOP; Commission E
– Scientific publications: see p. 478; Ammon HPT, Sabieraj J, Kaul R: Kamille – Mechanismus der antiphlogistischen Wirkung von Kamillenextrakten und -inhaltsstoffen. Deutsche Apotheker Ztg 136 (1996), 1821–1834; Mil-ler T, Wittstock U, Lindequist U, Teuscher E: Effects of some components of the essential oil of chamomile, Chamomilla recutita, on Histamine release from mast cells. Planta Med 62 (1997), 60–61.

Chaste Tree (*Vitex agnus-castus* L.)

➤ **General comments:** Chaste tree has been used as an herbal remedy since an-cient times. Its natural habitat ranges from the Mediterranean region to Wes-tern Asia.

➤ **Pharmacology**
– *Herb:* Chaste tree fruit (Agni casti fructus). The herb consists of the ripe, dried fruit of *Vitex agnus-castus* L. and preparations of the same.

– *Important constituents:* Iridoids (agnuside, aucubin), flavonoids, and essential oil (0.8–1.6 %).
– *Pharmacological properties:* Chaste tree fruit has dopaminergic effects and inhibits lactation. It suppresses the release of prolactin and reduces the symptoms of premenstrual syndrome. In animals, the extract was found to inhibit lactation, normalize stress-induced hyperprolactinemia, and exert dopaminergic effects. Clinical studies demonstrated a positive effect on symptoms associated with hyperprolactinemia such as mastalgia and other symptoms of PMS.

▶ **Indications**
– Menopausal complaints
– Premenstrual syndrome (PMS)

▶ **Contraindications:** Pregnancy and breast feeding

▶ **Dosage and duration of use**
– *Daily dose:* 30–40 mg of the herb, usually in the form of 1–2 mL of an aqueous-alcohol extract, first thing in the morning.

▶ **Adverse effects:** Exanthema (skin eruptions) is an occasional side effect.

▶ **Herb–drug interactions:** None known.

▶ **Summary assessment:** Chaste tree fruit is an effective remedy for premenstrual syndrome, especially for relieving mastalgia, as has been demonstrated in clinical studies.

✿ **Literature**
– Monographs: ESCOP, Commission E
– Scientific publications: see p. 478; Jarry H et al: In vitro prolactin but not LH and FSH release is inhibited by compounds in extracts of Agnus castus, direct evidence for a dopaminergic principle by the dopamine receptor assay. Exp Clin Endocrinol 102 (1994), 448–454; Loew D, Gorkow C, Schrödter A et al: Zur dosisabhängigen Verträglichkeit eines Agnus-castus-Spezialextraktes. Z Phytother 17 (1996), 237–243; Winterhoff H: Arzneipflanzen mit endokriner Wirksamkeit. Z Phytother 14 (1993), 83–94.

Clove (*Syzygium aromaticum* L. Merr. et L.M. Perry)

▶ **Pharmacology**
– *Herb:* Clove (Caryophylli flos). The herb consists of the hand-picked and dried flower buds of *Syzygium aromaticum* (L.) Merr. et L.M. Perry.
– *Important constituents:* Essential oil (15–21 %), consisting of 70–90 % eugenol plus eugenyl acetate, eugenol acetate (17 %), and β-caryophyllene (5–12 %), as well as flavonoids and tannins (10 %).
– *Pharmacological properties:* Caryophylli flos is said to have bactericidal, fungicidal, virustatic, antioxidant, hepatoprotective, local anesthetic, and spasmolytic effects, but only a few of these effects have been proven experimentally. The only confirmed data apply to the essential oil.

▶ **Indications**
– Inflammations of the mouth and throat
– Used in dental medicine as a topical pain reliever

▶ **Contraindications:** None known.

▶ **Dosage and duration of use**
– *As a mouthwash/gargle:* Rinse the mouth or gargle several times a day with an aqueous solution containing 1–5 % of the essential oil.

– *For dental complaints:* Apply the undiluted essential oil as a topical pain reliever.

➤ **Adverse effects:** Allergic reactions to eugenol can occur as a rare side effect. The concentrated essential oil can irritate the mucous membranes.

➤ **Herb–drug interactions:** None known.

➤ **Summary assessment:** Clove is an herb with demonstrated effectiveness. The medicinal uses for the herb are a consequence of the therapeutic action of clove oil. No clinical studies are available. Clove is safe enough for unrestricted over-the-counter use.

❀ **Literature**
– Monographs: DAB 10; Commission E
– Scientific publications: see p. 478; Cai L, Wu CHD: Compounds from Syzygium aromaticum possessing growth inhibitory activity against oral pathogenes. J Nat Prod 59 (1996), 987–990: Debelmas AM, Rochat J: Plant Med Phytother 1 (1967), 23; Tanaka T, Orii Y, Nonaka GI et al: Syziginins A and B, two ellegitannins from Syzygium aromaticum. Phytochemistry 43 (1996), 1345–1348.

Coffee (*Coffea arabica* L.)

➤ **Pharmacology**
– *Herb:* Coffee bean (*Coffeae semen*). The herb consists of the dried, husked beans of *Coffea arabica* (L.) and other *Coffea* species.
– Coffee charcoal (Coffeae carbo), the ground, blackish-brown to charcoal roasted outer seed parts of the dried green seeds of *Coffea arabica* L. s.l., *Coffea liberica* B. et H., *Coffea canephore* P. et F., and other coffee species.
– *Important constituents:* Purine alkaloids (caffeine, 0.6–2.2%), theobromine, theophylline, caffeic and ferulic acid esters of quinic acid (chlorogenic acid, 5–8%), trigonelline, no–diterpene glycoside esters (atractyloside), and diterpenes (diterpene alcohol fatty acid esters kahweol and cafestol). Roasted coffee beans contain many aroma substances due to the pyrolysis of carbohydrates, proteins, fats, and amino acids.
– *Pharmacological properties:* The stimulatory effect of caffeine sets in within a few minutes after administration. Most of the effects specified for coffee are attributable to the action of caffeine.
  • *Effects of caffeine:* Caffeine has positive inotropic effects and, when administered in high doses, exerts a positive chronotropic effect on the heart and stimulates the central nervous system. It relaxes the smooth muscles of the blood vessels (except in the brain, where it causes vasoconstriction) and bronchi. Caffeine has short-term diuretic effects, stimulates the secretion of gastric juices, and increases the release of catecholamines.
  • *Cardiovascular effects:* Individuals who normally do not drink coffee exhibit an average 10 mmHg increase in systolic blood pressure within 1 hour of administration of 250 mg of caffeine. Habitual coffee drinkers are tolerant to this dose.
  • An average dose of 5 to 6 cups of coffee per day (made by steeping the herb in boiling water for 10 minutes) for 9 weeks significantly increases the total cholesterol and LDL cholesterol levels in serum. The use of filter paper can reduce this effect by 80%.

> **Indications**
>   – Migraine headaches
>   – Decreased performance
> **Contraindications:** None known.
> **Dosage and duration of use:** Daily dose: 15 g of the herb.
> **Adverse effects:** Doses of up to 500 mg of caffeine (= 5 cups of coffee) per day are toxicologically safe for healthy adults who are habitual coffee drinkers. Patients with cardiovascular lability, kidney diseases, hyperthyroidism, a predisposition to convulsions, and certain psychiatric disorders (e. g., panic attacks) should use the herb cautiously.
>   – Side effects (attributable to coffee's chlorogenic acid content) include gastric hyperacidity, gastric irritation, diarrhea, and reduced appetite. Vomiting and abdominal cramps are signs of poisoning. Pregnant and nursing mothers should avoid caffeine. The maximum safe daily dose should not exceed 300 mg (equivalent to 3 cups of coffee).
>   – Caffeine can cause mental and physical dependence. Signs of withdrawal include headaches and sleep disorders.
>   ◉ *Important:* The prolonged administration of more than 1.5 g of caffeine per day is often observed to lead to unspecific symptoms such as restlessness, irritability, insomnia, palpitation, dizziness, vomiting, diarrhea, lack of appetite, and headaches. These effects can even occur with chronic use of as little as 300–500 mg/day in sensitive individuals.
> **Herb–drug interactions:** None known.
> **Summary assessment:** Ubiquitously used herbal preparation, OTC preparation, to increase mental performance. Clinically for headaches etc.
> ✿ **Literature**
>   – Monographs: Commission E (Coffee carbon)
>   – Scientific publications: see p. 478; Dieudonne S, Forero ME, Llano I: Lipid analysis of Coffea arabica Linn. beans and their possible hypercholesterolemic effects. Int J Food Sci Nutr, 159 (1997), 135–139; Mensink RP, Lebbink WJ, Lobbezoo IE, Weusten-Van der Wouw MP, Zock PL, Katan MB: Diterpene composition of oils from Arabica and Robusta coffee beans and their effects on serum lipids in man. J Intern Med, 237 (1995), 543–550; Ratnayake WM, Pelletier G, Hollywood R, Malcolm S, Stavric B: Investigation of the effect of coffee lipids on serum chloestrol in hamsters. Food Chem Toxicol, 33 (1995), 195–201; Anon: Kaffee erhöht den Cholesterinspiegel. Aga 19 (1991), 10682; Anon: Coffein-Entzugssyndrom bei Kaffeetrinkern. Deutsche Apotheker Ztg 133 (1993), 441; Bättig K: Kaffee in wissenschaftlicher Sicht. Z Phytother 9 (1988), 95; Butz S: Nurses-Health-Studie: Kaffee – kein Risikofaktor für koronare Herzkrankheit? Deutsche Apotheker Ztg 136 (1996), 1680–1682; Garattini S: Caffeine, Coffee and Health. Garattini S. Monographs of the Mario Negri Institute for Pharmacological Research, Milan. Raven Press, New York 1993; Lewin L: Gifte und Vergiftungen. 6th ed (reprint), Haug Verlag, Heidelberg 1992; Silnermann K et al: Entzugssymptome nach regelmäßigen Kaffeegenuß. New Engl J Med 327 (1992), 1109.

Condurango (*Marsdenia condurango* Reichb. F.)

➤ **Synonyms:** Marsdenia, eagle-vine bark; Kondurango (Ger.)
➤ **General comments:** The condurango tree grows in forests on the slopes of the Andes mountains. Its bark is used as a bitter.
➤ **Pharmacology**
  – *Herb:* Condurango bark (Condurango cortex). The herb consists of dried bark from the trunk and branches of *Marsdenia condurango* R. fil.
  – *Important constituents:* Pregnane glycosides, pregn-5-ene glycosides (including condurangin, 2 %), and caffeic acid derivatives (0.7–2.1 %).
  – *Pharmacological properties:* Like other bitters, condurangin increases the flow of saliva and gastric juices through reflex mechanisms. There is a lack of clinical data on the effects of the herb in humans.
➤ **Indications**
  – Loss of appetite
  – Dyspeptic complaints
➤ **Contraindications:** None known.
➤ **Dosage and duration of use**
  – *Daily dose:* 2–4 g of the herb.
  – Add the herb to cold water and wait for 3 to 4 hours. Drink the cold extract.
  – *Dosage:* One cup of the tea or one liqueur glassful of condurango wine 30 minutes before meals.
➤ **Adverse effects:** There are no known health hazards or side effects in conjunction with proper administration of the designated therapeutic doses of the herb.
➤ **Herb–drug interactions:** None known.
➤ **Summary assessment:** Condurango is a well-tolerated bitter herb that is becoming more popular in Europe today. It can usefully be combined with other bitter herbs.
✿ **Literature**
  – Monographs: Commission E

Coriander (*Coriandrum sativum* L.)

➤ **General comments:** The fruits of the coriander plant are used as a kitchen herb (bread, baked goods, etc.) and medicinal herb (e. g., for dyspeptic complaints).
➤ **Pharmacology**
  – *Herb:* Coriander (Coriandri fructus). The herb consists of the ripe, dried fruits of *Coriandrum sativum* L., var. *vulgare* A. and *microcarpum*.
  – *Important constituents:* 0.4–1.7 % essential oil (D-(+)-linalool/coriandrol (60–75 %) and 13–21 % fatty oil (oleic acid, linolenic acid).
  – *Pharmacological properties:* The essential oil stimulates the secretion of gastric juices and has carminative and mild spasmolytic effects.
➤ **Indications**
  – Lack of appetite
  – Dyspeptic complaints
➤ **Contraindications:** None known
➤ **Dosage and duration of use**
  – *Daily dose:* 3 g of the crushed herb.
  – Pour 150 mL of water onto 1 g of the fresh herb, crushed immediately prior to use, then cover and steep for 10 minutes.

- *Dosage:* One cup, between meals, 3 times a day.

➤ **Adverse effects:** There are no known health hazards or side effects in conjunction with proper administration of the designated therapeutic doses of the herb. Coriander has a slight potential for sensitization.

➤ **Herb–drug interactions:** None known.

➤ **Summary assessment:** Coriander is an old and familiar herbal remedy that should be used in combination with other antidyspeptic preparations. Clinical studies of the herb are not available.

✿ **Literature**
  – Monographs: Commission E

Cowslip (*Primula veris*) _____

➤ **See Primula**

Dandelion (*Taraxacum officinale* Weber)

➤ **General comments:** Dandelion is a widely distributed plant that has many uses in folk medicine. The whole plant is used in medicine.

➤ **Pharmacology**
   – *Herb:* Dandelion root and herb (Taraxaci radix cum herba). The herb consists of whole-plant material from *Taraxacum officinale* G. H. Weber ex Wigger s.l., collected at the time of flowering, and preparations of the same.
   – *Important constituents:* Sesquiterpene lactones (tannins), triterpenes (taraxasterol, γ-sitosterol, taraxerol, taraxol), flavonoids (luteolin-7-*O*-glucoside), and inulin (2–40 %).
   – *Pharmacological properties:* The tannins contained in dandelion root and herb have cholagogic and secretagogic action. In animals, dandelion root was found to have a saluretic effect attributable to its high concentrations of minerals.

➤ **Indications**
   – Lack of appetite
   – Dyspeptic complaints
   – Urinary tract infections

➤ **Contraindications:** Biliary tract obstruction, empyema of the gallbladder, and intestinal obstruction. Patients with gallbladder problems should not use dandelion unless instructed by a qualified health care provider owing to the risk of colic.

➤ **Dosage and duration of use**
   – *Tea:* Add 3–4 g (1 tablespoon) of the finely chopped herb to 150 mL of water, bring to a boil and steep for 15 minutes.
      • *Dosage:* One cup of the tea in the morning and at night.

➤ **Adverse effects:** Because dandelion acts as a secretagogue, it can cause complaints related to gastric hyperacidity. The herb has a weak potential for sensitization.

➤ **Herb–drug interactions:** None known.

➤ **Summary assessment:** Dandelion is a popular herbal medicament, but further scientific research is required to characterize its effects.

✿ **Literature**
   – Monographs: ESCOP; Commission E
   – Scientific publications: see p. 478; Budzianowski J: Coumarins, caffeoyltartaric acids and their artifactual esters from Taraxacum officinale: Planta Med 63 (1997), 288.

Devil's Claw (*Harpagophytum procumbens* Burch. D. C.)

➤ **General comments:** Devil's claw grows in the Kalahari Desert region of southern Africa. The plant has gained significance as an herbal medicament in recent years.

➤ **Pharmacology**
   – *Herb:* Devil's claw (Harpagophyti radix). The herb consists of the secondary storage roots of *Harpagophytum procumbens* (B.) D. C. and preparations of the same.
   – *Important constituents:* Iridoids (0.5–3 %) and iridoid glycosides such as harpagoside (0.5–0.6 %), harpagide, and procumbide. Phenylethanol

derivatives such as acteoside, verbascoside, and isoacteoside are also present.

– *Pharmacological properties:* Devil's claw stimulates the secretion of gastric juices and the production of bile (harpagoside). In animals, it has anti-inflammatory, analgesic, and antiarthritic effects, and harpagoside was found to inhibit the biosynthesis of certain prostaglandins that cause inflammation.

➤ **Indications**
– Lack of appetite
– Dyspeptic complaints
– Supportive treatment of degenerative connective tissue diseases

➤ **Contraindications:** Gastric and duodenal ulcers.

➤ **Dosage and duration of use**
– *Daily dose:* 1.5 g herb for lack of appetite; otherwise 4.5 g herb.
– *Tea:* Steep 1 teaspoon (4.5 g) of the finely chopped herb in 300 mL of boiled water for 8 hours. Divide into 3 portions to be taken throughout the day.
– *Tincture for external use:* Dilute 1 tablespoon with 250 mL of water and use for gargling or compresses.

➤ **Adverse effects:** Allergic reactions can occur in isolated cases.

➤ **Herb–drug interactions:** None known.

➤ **Summary assessment:** Preparations made of devil's claw are suitable for physician-supervised self-treatment. Devil's claw is an effective herbal remedy that is especially well suited for adjuvant treatment of rheumatic diseases. Used in this capacity, it can reduce the frequency and dose of synthetic antirheumatic drugs. Some recent controlled clinical trials suggest efficacy and safety.

✿ **Literature**
– Monographs: BHP 83; BHP 96; ESCOP; HAB 1; Commission E, Mar 31
– Scientific publications: see p. 478; Chantre P, Cappelaere A, Leblan D, et al. Efficacy and tolerance of *Harpagophytum procumbens* versus diacerhein in treatment of osteoarthritis. Phytomedicine 7(3), (2000), 177–183; Baghdikian L, et al. An analytical study, anti-inflammatory and analgesic effects of *Harpagophytum procumbens* and *Harpagophytum zeyheri*. Planta Med 63 (1997), 171–176.

Dwarf Pine (*Pinus mugo* spp.) ⎯⎯⎯⎯⎯⎯⎯⎯⎯⎯⎯⎯⎯⎯⎯⎯⎯

➤ See Pine.

Echinacea:
Paleflowered Echinacea (*Echinacea pallida* Nutt.)

- ➤ **Synonyms:** Pale coneflower; Blasse Kegelblume (Ger.)
- ➤ **General comments:** Paleflowered Echinacea is native to the United States. The root is used in medicine.
- ➤ **Pharmacology**
  - *Herb:* White Echinacea root (Echinaceae pallidae radix). The herb consists of the fresh or dried roots of *Echinacea pallida* (N.) N., collected during the fall, and preparations of the same.
  - *Important constituents:* Polysaccharides (immunostimulatory effects, rhamnoarabinogalactans), essential oil (0.2–2%), caffeic acid derivatives (echinacoside, 1%), and alkylamides (0.1%).
  - *Pharmacological properties:* Immunostimulatory, antibacterial, virustatic. Alcohol extracts of Paleflowered Echinacea root were found to stimulate phagocytosis in animals, and the rate of in vitro phagocytosis in granulocytes increased by 23% after injection. In mice, the proliferation of splenic cells increased greatly, and the production of cytokines and antibodies increased. Clinical studies demonstrated that bacterial and viral infections of the upper respiratory tract may improve more rapidly when treated with the herb.
- ➤ **Indications:** For supportive treatment of colds or flulike infections.
- ➤ **Contraindications:** Hypersensitivity to any of the compounds in Paleflowered Echinacea root in particular, or to composite plants in general. Parenteral administration of echinacea as used in Europe is contraindicated during pregnancy and in general discouraged.
  - ◎ *Warning:* Paleflowered Echinacea root should be used under the advice of a qualified health practitioner by individuals with progressive systemic diseases such as tuberculosis, leukosis, connective tissue diseases, multiple sclerosis, or other autoimmune diseases such as HIV infection.
- ➤ **Dosage and duration of use:** Continuous oral use of the tincture (1 : 5) or oral preparations for more than 2 weeks is not recommended.
- ➤ **Adverse effects:** There are no known health hazards or side effects in conjunction with proper internal or external administration of the designated therapeutic doses of the herb. Skin rashes and itching have been observed in isolated cases. Facial swelling, difficulty in breathing, dizziness and reduction of blood pressure are rare side effects.
- ➤ **Herb–drug interactions:** None known.
- ➤ **Summary assessment:** Paleflowered Echinacea root is less commonly used than the purple, the experimental and clinical investigation of the herb is not yet complete.
- ✿ **Literature**
  - Monographs: ESCOP; Commission E
  - Scientific publications: see p. 478; Beuscher N et al: Immunmodulierende Eigenschaften von Wurzelextrakten verschiedener Echinacea-Arten. Z Phytother 16 (1995), 157–166.

Purple Echinacea (*Echinacea purpurea* L. Moench).

- ➤ **Synonyms:** Purple coneflower; Purpurfarbene Kegelblume (Ger.)
- ➤ **General comments:** Purple Echinacea is native to the United States, where the native Americans utilized its immunity-enhancing properties. The aerial parts of the plant collected at the time of flowering are used in medicine.

> **Pharmacology**
  - *Herb:* Purple Echinacea (Echinaceae purpureae herba). The herb consists of the fresh aerial parts of *Echinacea purpurea* (L.) Moench, collected at the time of flowering.
  - *Important constituents:* Polysaccharides (with immunostimulatory effects; 4-O-methylglucuronylarabinoxylans, alkyl amides, acid rhamnoarabino-galactans), cichoric acid, and essential oil (0.08–0.32%).
  - *Pharmacological properties:* Purple Echinacea promotes wound healing. Parenteral and oral doses increase the phagocytosic capacity of granulocytes and macrophages; medium doses increase the production of T lymphocytes. Low doses of the expressed juice lead to induction of TNF-α, interleukin-1 and interleukin-6. The herb has shown antiviral properties in animal studies. Human studies show reduction and shortening of symptoms of viral syndromes, in particular the common cold, but other studies show no effect. Still not proven conclusively with human studies.

> **Indications**
  - Colds and fever
  - Urinary tract infections
  - Coughs and bronchitis
  - Decreased resistance to infections
  - Runny nose
  - Wounds and burns (external use)

> **Contraindications:** Hypersensitivity to any of the compounds in Purple Echinacea in particular or to composite plants in general.

  ⊙ *Warning:* Purple Echinacea should be used by individuals with progressive systemic diseases such as tuberculosis, leukosis, connective tissue disease, multiple sclerosis or other autoimmune diseases such as HIV infection under the advice of a qualified health practitioner.

> **Dosage and duration of use**
  - Take as recommended by the manufacturer.
  - *Daily dose:* 6–9 mL of the expressed juice; should not be used continuously for more than 2 weeks.

> **Adverse effects:** Skin rashes and itching have been observed in isolated cases. Facial swelling, difficulty in breathing, dizziness, and reduction of blood pressure are rare side effects. Parenteral administration of Purple Echinacea, as used in Europe, is contraindicated during pregnancy and in general discouraged.

> **Herb–drug interactions:** None known.

> **Summary assessment:** Purple Echinacea is a commonly used herb, the effectiveness of which has been demonstrated in a growing number of studies. A preventive effect with respect to flulike infections has not been proven.

✿ **Literature**
  - Monographs: ESCOP; Commission E
  - Scientific publications: see p. 478; Melchert D, Linde K, Worku F et al: Immunomodulation with Echinacea—a systematic review of controlled clinical trials, Phytomedicine 1 (1994), 245–254; Mose J R: Med Welt 34 (1983), 51; Parnham MJ: Benfit-risk assessment of the squeezed sap of the purple coneflower (Echinacea purpurea) for long-term oral immunostimulation. Phytomedicine 3 (1996), 95–102.

Eleutherococcus (*Eleutherococcus senticosus* Rupr. Maxim)

➤ **Synonyms:** Siberian ginseng
➤ **General comments:** Siberian ginseng is a shrub with effects largely similar to those of ginseng, but is native to Siberia. The root is used in medicine.
➤ **Pharmacology**
   – *Herb:* Siberian ginseng root (Eleutherococci radix). The herb consists of the dried roots and/or rhizomes, and sometimes the dried prickly stems of *Eleutherococcus senticosus* R. e. M. and preparations of the same.
   – *Important constituents:* Triterpene saponins (0.12%), steroid glycoside eleutheroside A, hydroxycoumarins (isofraxidin, eleutheroside B1), phenylacrylic acid derivatives (eleutheroside B), lignans (sesamin, 0.23%, eleutheroside D, and the 4,4,´-di-*O*-glucoside of syringaresinol, 0.1%), and polysaccharides.
   – *Pharmacological properties:* The fluid extract of Eleutherococcus root has immunostimulatory, immunomodulatory, and antiviral effects due to its polysaccharide content. Eleutheroside B and other components were found to increase the stress tolerance of animals in many stress models (immobilization test, swim test, cold stress, etc.). The fluid extract increased the number of lymphocytes, especially T lymphocytes, and killer cells in healthy volunteers. Eleutheroside B has a testosterone-like effect.
➤ **Indications**
   – Decreased resistance to infections
   – Decreased performance
   – Prevention or supportive treatment of jet lag or altitude sickness
➤ **Contraindications:** None known.
➤ Dosage and duration of use:
   – *Daily dose:* 2–3 g herb.
   – *Fluid extract (1 : 1):* 3 to 5 drops in a glass of water several times a day.
➤ **Adverse effects:** There are no known health hazards or side effects in conjunction with proper administration of the designated therapeutic doses of the herb.
➤ **Herb–drug interactions:** None known.
➤ **Summary assessment:** Data on the effects of *Eleutherococcus* in human volunteers are available for the specified indications. The herb probably has many more potential uses.
✿ **Literature**
   – Monographs: DAB 1998 ESCOP
   – Scientific publications: see p. 478

English Ivy (*Hedera helix* L.)

➤ **General comments:** The young, tender leaves and shoots are used in medicine.
➤ **Pharmacology**
   – *Herb:* Ivy leaf (Hederae helicis folium). The herb consists of the dried foliage leaves of *Hedera helix* L. and preparations of the same.
   – *Important constituents:* Ca. 5% triterpene saponins (mainly hederacoside C, which is broken down into (-hederin) and alkaloids (emetine).
   – *Pharmacological properties:* Saponins have anti-inflammatory, antiviral, antibacterial, antimycotic, and anthelmintic effects in animals. They also have secretolytic/expectorant, antitussive, and spasmolytic action.
➤ **Indications:** Coughs and bronchitis
➤ **Contraindications:** None known.

➢ **Dosage and duration of use:** Only commercial ivy preparations should be taken according to the manufacturer's instructions.
➢ **Adverse effects:** Health hazards in conjunction with proper administration of the designated therapeutic doses of the drug are not known.
➢ **Herb–drug interactions:** None known.
➢ **Summary assessment:** Use should be restricted to commercially manufactured products. Recent clinical studies with positive effects in bronchitis are available.
✿ **Literature**
  – Monographs: ESCOP; Commission E
  – Scientific publications: see p. 478; Gladtke E: Zur Wirksamkeit eines Efeublätterpräparates (Prospan). Intern Praxis 32 (1992), 187; Trute A, Gross J, Mutschler E, Nahrstedt A: In vitro antispasmodic compounds of the dry extract obtained from Hedera helix. Planta Med 63 (1997), 125–129; Trute A, Nahrstedt A: Identification and quantitative analysis of phenolic dry extracts of Hedera helix. Planta Med 63 (1997), 177–179.

English Lavender (*Lavandula angustifolia* Mill.)

➢ **General comments:** English lavender flowers are widely used in folk medicine. The oil and the flowers are used in modern herbal medicine.
➢ **Pharmacology**
  – *Herb:* English lavender flower (Lavandulae flos). The herb consists of the dried flowers of *Lavandula angustifolia* M., collected just before full maturity, and preparations of the same.
  – Important constituents: Essential oil (1–3 %) consisting mainly of (–)-linalool (20–50 %) and linalyl acetate (30–40 %).
  – *Pharmacological properties:* In animal studies, lavender was found to have a neurodepressant effect (reduces the sleep induction phase and prolongs the duration of sleep) and to reduce motor activity. In humans, English lavender taken by inhalation was shown to take action in the limbic cortex (similarly to nitrazepam).
➢ **Indications**
  – Lack of appetite
  – Dyspeptic complaints
  – Circulatory disorders
  – Nervous complaints and insomnia
➢ **Contraindications:** None known.
➢ **Dosage and duration of use.**
  – *Tea:* Steep 1 to 2 teaspoons (1–2 g) lavender flower in 1 cup (150 mL) of hot water for 10 minutes.
  – *Daily dose:* 3–5 g of the herb, equivalent to 3 cups per day.
  – *Bath additive:* Steep 100 g of lavender flower in 2 liters of hot water, or add 100 g of lavender flower to 2 liters of cold water and bring to a boil. Strain, then add the concentrated infusion to the bath water.
  – *Infusion for external use:* Add a handful of lavender flower to 1 liter of water and boil for 10 minutes, then add another liter of water.
  – *Lavender oil:* Take 1 to 4 drops on a suitable medium, e. g., a cube of sugar.
➢ **Adverse effects:** There are no known health hazards or side effects in conjunction with proper administration of the designated therapeutic doses of the herb. The essential oil has a weak potential for sensitization.

➤ **Herb–drug interactions:** None known.
➤ **Summary assessment:** English lavender is a popular herb in empirical folk medicine, but it has not been adequately evaluated in pharmacological or clinical studies. English lavender combines well with other calming and sleep-promoting herbal preparations.

✿ **Literature**
  – Monographs: DAB 1998; Commission E
  – Scientific publications: see p. 478; Buchbauer G, Jirovetz L, Jäger W et al: Aromatherapy: Evidence for Sedative Effects of the Essential Oil of Lavender after Inhalation. Z Naturforsch 46c (1991), 1067–1072; Hausen B; Allgeriepflanzen, Pflanzenallergie. ecomed Verlagsgesellsch. mbH, Landsberg 1988.

English Plantain (*Plantago lanceolata* L.)

➤ **Synonyms:** Ribwort; Spitzwegerich (Ger.)
➤ **General comments:** English plantain has been used in many indications since antiquity. It is distributed in cool to moderate zones throughout the world.
➤ **Pharmacology**
  – *Herb:* English plantain leaftherb (Plantaginis lanceolatae folium/herba). The herb consists of the fresh or dried aerial parts of *Plantago lanceolata* L., collected at the time of flowering, and preparations of the same.
  – *Important constituents:* Iridoids (2–3%), including aucubin, rhinanthin, and catalpol, as well as mucilage (2–6%), flavonoids, and tannins (6%).
  – *Pharmacological properties:* Fluid extracts and expressed juices from the fresh leaves have bactericidal effects due to their content of aucubigenin (hydrolyzed aucubin) and an antimicrobial saponin. English plantain preparations have a short shelf-life, because aucubigenin is unstable. Aqueous English plantain extracts promote wound healing and accelerate blood coagulation. Aucubin is assumed to protect the liver and soothe the mucous membranes when inflamed. The tannins have astringent effects.
➤ **Indications**
  – Colds and fever
  – Skin inflammations
  – Coughs and bronchitis
  – Inflammations of the mouth and throat
  – Runny nose
➤ **Contraindications:** None known.
➤ **Dosage and duration of use**
  – *Tea:* Pour boiling water onto 2–4 g of the chopped herb, or place the dose in cold water and bring to a boil. Steep for 10 minutes, then strain. 2 teaspoons = ca. 3 g herb.
  ◎ *Important:* The enzyme that hydrolyzes aucubin is inactivated upon heating.
    • *Dosage:* One cup, several times a day.
  – *Daily dose:* 3–6 g herb.
  – For inflammations of the mouth and throat, gargle with the tea infusion several times a day.
➤ **Adverse effects:** There are no known health hazards or side effects in conjunction with proper administration of the designated therapeutic doses of the herb.

➤ **Herb–drug interactions:** None known.
➤ **Summary assessment:** The internal and external uses of plantain are generally regarded as safe and effective. Plantain is also a popular remedy in pediatric medicine (cough syrups).
✿ **Literature**
  – Monographs: DAB 1998, ESCOP; Commission E
  – Scientific publications: see p. 478; Murai M et al: Phenylethanoids in the herb of Planatago lanceolata and inhibitory effects on arachidonic acid-induced mouse ear edema. Planta Med 61 (1995), 479–480.

Eucalyptus Leaf (Eucalypti folium)

➤ **Pharmacology**
  – *Herb:* Eucalyptus leaf (Eucalypti folium). The herb consists of the dried mature leaves of older *Eucalyptus globulus* L. B. trees.
  – *Important constituents:* 1–3% essential oil (1,8-cineole, 45–75%, α-pinene, β-pinene, pinocarvone), and flavonoids (rutin, hyperoside, quercetin).
  – *Pharmacological properties:* Eucalyptus leaf has secretomotor, expectorant, astringent, and weakly spasmolytic action. The drug has anti-inflammatory and antiproliferative effects in animals.
➤ **Indications:** Coughs and bronchitis.
➤ **Contraindications:** See Eucalyptus Oil, internal use.
➤ **Dosage and duration of use**
  – *Tea:* Pour 150 mL boiling water onto 1.5–2 g of the finely chopped drug; cover and steep for 5 to 10 minutes.
  – *Daily dose:* 4–6 g dried leaves. One dose equals 1.5 g dried leaves.
➤ **Adverse effects:** Nausea, vomiting, and diarrhea can occur as rare side effects. No cases of overdose have been reported.
➤ **Herb–drug interactions:** None known.
➤ **Summary assessment:** Eucalyptus leaf is weaker than eucalyptus oil and should be combined with equal parts of other expectorants such as thyme and anise seed.
✿ **Literature**
  – Monographs: DAB 1998; Commission E
  – Scientific publications: see p. 478; Fenaroli's Handbook of Flavor Ingredients, Vol. 1, 2 nd Ed., CRC Press 1975; Osawa K et al: Macrocarpals H, I, and J from the leaves of Eucalyptus globulus. J Nat Prod 59 (1996), 824–827.

Eucalyptus Oil (*Eucalyptus globulus* L. B.)

➤ **General comments:** Eucalyptus oil is obtained by steam distilling and purifying the essential oil extracted from the fresh leaves or branch tips of *Eucalyptus globulus* L. B.
➤ **Pharmacology**
  – *Important constituents:* 80% (of the rectified essential oil) consists of 1,8-cineole; *p*-cymene and α-pinene are also present.
  – *Pharmacological properties:* Some of the properties listed below refer to isolated cineole. Eucalyptus oils have antibacterial and fungicidal effects in vitro. Eucalyptus oil inhibits prostaglandin synthesis and has weak hyperemic effects when applied topically. The drug also has expectorant,

secretomotor, antitussive, and surface-active surfactant-like effects and improves lung compliance.

➤ **Indications**
  – Coughs and bronchitis
  – Rheumatic complaints

➤ **Contraindications**
  – *Internal use:* Eucalyptus oil should not be used by children under 12 years of age or during the first trimester of pregnancy. It also should not be used by patients with inflammations of the gastrointestinal or biliary tract or severe liver diseases.
  – *External use:* Eucalyptus oil should not be applied to the face of infants and small children since it can cause laryngospasm, bronchospasm, asthma-like attacks and/or respiratory arrest.

➤ **Dosage and duration of use**
  – *Internal use:* Daily dose: 0.3–0.6 g drug (0.2 g = 10 drops). Take 3 to 6 drops in 150 mL warm water several times a day. Inhalation: Add 2 to 3 drops to boiling water and inhale the vapors.
  – *External use:* Oily and semisolid forms with 5–20% essential oil content. Aqueous ethanol preparations with 5–10% essential oil content. Liniment: Rub a few drops of 20% eucalyptus liniment onto the affected area of the skin.

➤ **Adverse effects:** Nausea, vomiting and diarrhea are rare side effects.

◉ *Warning:* Overdose can result in life-threatening poisoning (only a few drops can cause severe poisoning in children, and 4 to 5 mL can cause lethal poisoning in adults). Signs include a drop in blood pressure, circulatory disorders, collapse, and respiratory paralysis.

➤ **Herb–drug interactions:** Eucalyptus oil accelerates the decomposition of pharmaceutical drugs, thereby weakening or shortening their effectiveness.

➤ **Summary assessment:** Preliminary studies (see Literature) show that eucalyptus oil might be effective as an inhalant in steams to reduce inflammation and congestion in sinus conditions related to the common cold, asthma, and respiratory allergies.

✿ **Literature**
  – Monographs: DAB 10; ESCOP; Commission E
  – Scientific publications: see p. 478; Juergens UR, Stober M, Vetter H: Inhibition of cytokine production and arachidonic acid metabolism by eucalyptol (1,8-cineole) in human blood monocytes in vitro. Eur J Med Res, 3(11) (1998), 508–510; Riechelmann H, Brommer C, Hinni M, Martin C: Response of human ciliated respiratory cells to a mixture of menthol, eucalyptus oil and pine needle oil. Arzneimittelforschung 47(9) (1997), 1035–1039; Gräfe AK: Besonderheiten der Arzneimitteltherapie im Säuglings- und Kindesalter. PZ 140 (1995), 2659–2667.

European Elder (*Sambucus nigra* L.) _____

➤ **General comments:** Elder flowers and fruit (berries) are used in medicine.

➤ **Pharmacology**
  – *Herb*
    • Elder flower (Sambuci flos). The herb consists of the dried and sifted flower heads of *Sambucus nigra* L. and preparations of the same.

- Elder berry (Sambuci fructus). The herbal preparations are syrups and powdered extracts in capsules and tablets.
- *Important constituents:* Flavonoids (3 %), including rutin, isoquercitrin, quercetin, and hyperoside, essential oil (0.03 – 0.14 %), and caffeic acid derivatives (ca. 3 %).
- *Pharmacological properties:* Elder flower was found to increase bronchial secretion in animals. The essential oil and flavonoids play a role in its sudorific (sweat-producing) action, but no scientific investigations are available on this subject. Elder fruit is used for easing the symptoms of colds and flu. Some research in human cell cultures demonstrates antiviral and immunomodulating effects. Two small clinical trials showed shortening of recovery time in patients with influenza. Elder berry is not officially recommended in a German monograph.

➤ **Indications**
- Fever and colds, mild cases of flu
- Coughs and bronchitis (supportive)
- Antiviral and immunomodulating effects as demonstrated in some small clinical trials

➤ **Contraindications:** None known.

➤ **Dosage and duration of use**
- *Tea:* Steep 2 teaspoons (3 – 4 g) of elder flower in 150 mL of boiled water for 5 minutes.
  - *Dosage:* One to two cups of the tea, as hot as possible, several times a day (especially in the second half of the day).
- *Daily dose:* 10 – 15 g drug.
- *Fruit and syrups:* Infuse 1 teaspoon in 1 cup of freshly boiled water for 30 minutes, and drink 1 cup 2 or 3 times daily. For syrups, 2 to 3 teaspoons daily.

➤ **Adverse effects:** There are no known health hazards or side effects in conjunction with proper administration of the designated therapeutic doses of the herb.

➤ **Herb–drug interactions:** None known.

➤ **Summary assessment:** Elder flower is a widely used household remedy with long traditional use in the specified indications. Use of elder berry is more common in North America.

✿ **Literature**
- Monographs: Commission E
- Scientific publications: see p. 478

European Golden Rod (*Solidago virgaurea* L.)

➤ **Pharmacology**
- *Herb:* European golden rod (Solidaginis virgaureae herba). The herb consists of the aerial parts of *Solidago virgaurea* (L.).
- *Important constituents:* Triterpene saponins (0.2 – 0.3 %), essential oil (0.4 – 0.5 %; less than 0.2 % in the stored drug), polysaccharides (6 – 8 %), 1.1 – 2 % flavonoids (rutin, 0.8 %), phenol glycosides (0.2 – 1.0 %), and caffeic acid derivatives (0.2 – 0.4 %).
- *Pharmacological properties:* European golden rod has diuretic and analgesic action (due to the content of phenol glycosides). The essential oil and

saponins have antimicrobial, weakly spasmolytic, antiexudative, and aquaretic effects.

➤ **Indications**
  – Used for irrigation therapy, to flush the kidneys of patients with urinary tract infections and to eliminate renal or urinary calculi.
  – For prevention of urinary calculi and renal gravel.

➤ **Contraindications:** Irrigation therapy is not recommended in patients with cardiac or renal edema.

➤ **Dosage and duration of use**
  – *Tea:* Steep 1 to 2 teaspoons (3–5 g) of the dried herb in ca. 150 mL of boiled water for 15 minutes.
    • *Dosage:* One cup, between meals, 2 to 4 times a day.
  – *Daily dose:* 6–12 g chopped drug for infusions or other internally used galenicals.
  ◉ *Important:* An ample supply of fluids is essential.

➤ **Adverse effects:** No known health hazards.

➤ **Herb–drug interactions:** None known.

◉ *Warning:* Patients with chronic renal disease should not use European golden rod unless instructed by a physician or qualified health care provider.

➤ **Summary assessment:** The indications for European goldenrod are based on the pharmacological properties of its constituents and therapeutic experience. European goldenrod combines well with other aquaretic and urinary disinfectant drugs.

➤ **Literature**
  – Monographs: DAB 1998; ESCOP; Commission E
  – Scientific publications: see p. 478; Bader G, Wray, V, Hiller, K: The main saponins from the arial parts and the roots of Solidago virgaurea subsp. virgaurea. Planta Med 61 (1995), 158–161; Hiller K, Bader G: Goldruten-Kraut–Portrait einer Arzneipflanze. Z Phytother 17 (1996), 123–130.

Fennel (*Foeniculum vulgare* Miller)

➤ **General comments:** The oil and seedlike fruit of *Foeniculum vulgare* Miller are used in medicine.

➤ **Pharmacology**
  – *Herb*
    • Fennel oil (Foeniculi aetheroleum) is the essential oil obtained by steam distilling the dried ripe fruit of common fennel (*Foeniculum vulgare*) or sweet fennel (*Foeniculum dulce*).
    • Fennel seed/fruit (Foeniculi fructus) is the dried ripe fruit of *Foeniculum vulgare* M. var. *vulgare*.
  – *Important constituents*
    • Common fennel: *trans*-Anethole (50–75 %), fenchone (12–33 %), and estragole (2–5 %).
    • Sweet fennel: *trans*-Anethole (80–90 %), fenchone (1–10 %), and estragole (3–10 %).
    • Both varieties contain flavonoids, rutin, and fatty oil (9–21 %).

➤ **Pharmacological properties**
  – Anethole promotes smooth-muscle motility in the digestive tracts; higher doses have antispasmodic effects. A dose-dependent reduction of the density of respiratory fluid (bronchosecretolysis) occurs. Fenchone has antimicrobial and fungicidal effects in vitro.
  – Fennel seed has a spasmolytic effect on the smooth muscles and accelerates the vibration rate of the ciliary epithelium of the bronchial mucosa (secretomotor action). When used in vitro, fennel is antimicrobial, gastric motility-enhancing, antiexudative, and presumably antiproliferative.

➤ **Indications**
  – Dyspeptic complaints
  – Coughs and bronchitis
  – Catarrh of the upper respiratory tract in children (fennel honey or syrup)

➤ **Contraindications:** Fennel oil should not be used by pregnant mothers or small children.

➤ **Dosage and duration of use**
  – *Fennel honey* (contains 0.5 g fennel oil per kg) or fennel syrup:
    • *Daily dose:* 10–20 g. The sugar content must be taken into account when used by diabetic patients.
  – *Fennel oil*
    • *Dosage:* 2–5 drops, diluted in water or chamomile tea, after each meal.
    • *Daily dose:* 0.1–0.6 mL. Should not be used for more than 2 weeks.
  – *Fennel seed tea:* Steep 2–5 g of the herb, crushed or ground immediately prior to use, in 150 mL of boiled water for 10 to 15 minutes.
    • *Dosage:* One cup between meals, 2 to 4 times a day.
    • *Daily dose:* 5–7 g crushed fruits.
  – *Fennel syrup:* Fennel tincture: 0.8 mL (30 drops) to 2 mL, 3 times a day.
    • *Daily dose:* 10–20 g. Should not be used for more than 2 weeks without consulting an experienced practitioner.

➤ **Adverse effects:** No known health hazards. Allergic reactions can occur as a very rare side effect. Cross-reactions with celery allergies are also possible.

➤ **Herb–drug interactions:** None known.

➤ **Summary assessment:** Fennel is a herb used worldwide with empirically demonstrated effects.

✿ **Literature**
  – Monographs
    • Fennel oil: DAB 1998; Commission E
    • Fennel seed: ESCOP; Commission E
  – Scientific publications: see p. 478; Hiller K: Pharmazeutische Bewertung ausgewählter Teedrogen. Deutsche Apotheker Ztg 135 (1995), 1425–1440; Massoud H: Study on the essential oil in seeds of some fennel cultivars under Egyptian environmental conditions. Planta Med 58 (1992), A681; Parzinger R: Fenchel. Deutsche Apotheker Ztg 136 (1996), 529–530; Albert-Puleo M: J Ethnopharmacol 2 (1980), 337; Betts TJ: J Pharm Pharmacol 20 (1968), 61–64, 469–472; Czygan FC: Z Phytother 8 (1987), 82; El-Khrisy EAM et al: Fitoterapia 51 (1980), 273; Forster HB et al: Planta Med 40 (1980), 309; Harborne JB, Williams CE: Phytochemistry 11 (1972), 1741–1750; Harries N et al: J Clin Pharm 2 (1978), 171; Rothbacher H, Kraus A: Pharmazie 25 (1970), 566; Trenkle K: PA 27 (1972), 319–324.

Flax (*Linum usitatissimum* L.)

➤ **Synonyms:** Flaxseed; Leinsamen (Ger.)

➤ **General comments:** There are many species of flax. Some are used to make fabrics, whereas others are used to produce flaxseed oil, a valuable foodstuff and medicinal product.

➤ **Pharmacology**
  – *Herb:* Flaxseed (Lini semen). The herb consists of the ripe, dried seeds of *Linum usitatissimum* and preparations of the same.
  – *Important constituents:* 3–10 % mucilage (arabinoxylans, galactans, rhamnogalacturonans), cyanogenetic glycosides (0.05–0.1 %), and 10–45 % fatty oil (linolenic acid, 40–70 %; linoleic acid, 10–25 %; oleic acid, 13–30 %).
  – *Pharmacological properties:* Linseed has laxative action due to its fiber and mucilage components. Linseed lowers the cholesterol concentration in the liver of animals. Prussic acid is not produced from the cyanogenetic acids.

➤ **Indications**
  – Constipation
  – Gastritis
  – Enteritis
  – Skin irritations

➤ **Contraindications:** Bowel obstruction, esophageal stenosis or narrowing of the gastrointestinal tract and acute inflammatory diseases of the bowel, esophagus, or cardia.

➤ **Dosage and duration of use**
  – *Internal use*
    • *Constipation:* One tablespoon of whole or crushed flaxseed, 2 to 3 times a day, in two 6-ounce glasses of water (at least 150 mL).
    • *Gastritis, enteritis:* Flaxseed gruel prepared using 2 to 3 tablespoons of ground or chopped flaxseed.
  – *External use (poultices):* For inflammatory skin diseases, prepare a gruel made by mixing 125 g of flaxseed meal with 1 cup of water and wrap in a suitable cloth. Apply a hot, wet poultice to the affected area of the skin twice daily.

➤ **Adverse effects:** Bowel obstruction can occur when large quantities of flax-seed are used to treat constipation without an adequate intake of fluids. The cyanogenetic glycosides do not pose a health risk. Some commercial flaxseeds have been identified in the past that contain levels of cadmium beyond recommended government limits. This should be considered during chronic use of flaxseed.

➤ **Herb–drug interactions:** Flaxseed can impair the absorption of pharmaceutical drugs or herbal preparations containing very potent constituents such as cardiac glycosides (i. e. *Digitalis* spp.) if taken concomitantly.

➤ **Summary assessment:** Flaxseed is an herbal laxative that is also suitable for treatment of chronic constipation. It has a very low rate of side effects and does not interfere with the physiology of the bowels.

✿ **Literature**
  – Monographs: ESCOP; Commission E
  – Scientific publications: see p. 478.

Frangula (*Rhamnus frangula L.*)

➤ **Synonyms:** Alder buckthorn, black alder; Faulbaum (Ger.)
➤ **Pharmacology**
  – *Herb:* Frangula bark (Frangulae cortex). The herb consists of the dried bark of branches and twigs of *Rhamnus frangula* L. (Frangula alnus Miller)
  – ◉ *Important:* Since fresh Frangula bark can induce nausea, the drug must be stored for one year before use.
  – *Important constituents:* Anthraquinone derivatives (4–6%), including anthranoids, glucofrangulin A and B, and frangulins A, B and C.
  – *Pharmacological properties:* Anthraquinones promote the active secretion of electrolytes and water into the intestinal lumen while simultaneously inhibiting their absorption from the intestine. The liquefaction of the bowel contents leads to an increase in intestinal filling pressure. Stimulation of intestinal peristalsis also occurs.

➤ **Indications:** For short term treatment of occasional constipation.
➤ **Contraindications:** Bowel obstruction, acute inflammation of the bowels, appendicitis. Frangula bark should not be used by children under 10 years of age or by pregnant or nursing mothers.

➤ **Dosage and duration of use**
  – *Tea:* Steep 2 g of the finely chopped dried bark in 150 mL of boiled water for 15 minutes.
    • *Dosage:* One cup in the morning and evening. Sweeten with honey and add orange peel to taste if desired.
  – An aqueous suspension containing 0.6 g of the powdered drug normally produces a bowel movement within 6 to 24 hours.
  – *Daily dose of glucofrangulins:* 20–30 mg, calculated based on the content of glucofrangulin A.
  – The smallest dose required to produce soft stools should be used.
  – *Duration of treatment:* No more than 1 to 2 weeks.

➤ **Adverse effects:** Vomiting and cramplike gastrointestinal complaints.
◉ *Warning:* Prolonged use leads to the loss of electrolytes, especially potassium ions, which can result in hyperaldosteronism, inhibit intestinal motility and, in rare cases, cause cardiac arrhythmia, nephropathy, muscle weakness, edema, muscle weakness and accelerated bone degeneration.

➤ **Herb–drug interactions:** Because of the loss of calcium, the drug can increase the effects of cardiac glycosides if taken concurrently.

➤ **Summary assessment:** Frangula bark should be taken only for short periods of time to alleviate constipation or to empty the bowels prior to X-ray examinations. In North America, cascara sagrada (*Rhamnus purshianus*) is more commonly used in this way.

✿ **Literature**
   – Monographs: DAB 10; ESCOP; Commission E
   – Scientific publications: see p. 478; Anon: Abwehr von Arzneimittelrisiken, Stufe II. Deutsche Apotheker Ztg. 136 (1996), 3253–3254.

Fumitory (*Fumaria officinalis L.*)

➤ **Synonyms:** Earthsmoke; Erdrauch (Ger.)

➤ **General comments:** The dried herb and fresh aerial parts collected at the time of flowering are used in medicine.

➤ **Pharmacology**
   – *Herb:* Fumitory herb (Fumariae herba). The herb consists of the dried aerial parts of *Fumaria officinalis* L. collected at the time of flowering.
   – *Important constituents:* Isoquinoline alkaloids (1.25 %), including (–)-scoulerin, protopine/fumarine, fumaricin, (+)-fumarilin, fumaretin, and fumarofin. Flavonoids (rutin), fumaric acid, and hydroxycinnamic acid derivatives (caffeoylmalic acid) are also present.
   – *Pharmacological properties:* Mild spasmolytic action in the biliary tract and gastrointestinal tract.

➤ **Indications**
   – Liver and gallbladder complaints
   – Cholelithiasis
   – Cholecystitis
   – Diseases of the liver
   – Other diseases of the gallbladder/biliary tract

➤ **Contraindications**: None known.

➤ **Dosage and duration of use**
   – *Tea:* Steep 2–3 g of the dried herb in 150 mL of boiled water for 10 minutes.
      • *Dosage*: One cup of the warm tea 30 minutes before meals.
   – *Tincture:* 1 : 5. Dose: 2–4 ml, 3 times daily.
   – *Expressed juice:* 2 to 3 teaspoons (2.4–3.5 g drug) a day, to be taken as a cold infusion (maceration) or hot infusion.
   – *Freshly triturated plant material:* 1 teaspoon, 3 times a day.
   – *Daily dose:* 6 g dried herb.

➤ **Adverse effects:** No known health hazards.

➤ **Herb–drug interactions:** None known.

➤ **Summary assessment:** Mild herbal preparation, mainly used in supportive program for liver and gallbladder problems.

✿ **Literature**
   – *Monographs:* BHP 96; DAB 1998; EB 6; HAB 1; Commission E, Mar 31; PF X
   – Scientific publications: see p. 478; Duke JA: Die amphochloeretische Wirkung der Fumaria officinalis. Z Allg Med 34 (1985), 1819; Hahn R, Nahrstedt A: High Content of Hydroxycinnamic Acids Esterified with (+)-D-Malic-Acid in the Upper Parts of Fumaria officinalis. Planta Med 59 (1993),

189; Roth L, Daunderer M, Kormann K: Giftpflanzen, Pflanzengifte. 4. Aufl., Ecomed Fachverlag Landsberg/Lech 1993; Willaman JJ, Hui-Li L: Lloydia 33 (1970), 1.

Garlic (*Allium sativum* L.) _____

➤ **General comments:** Garlic is an ancient culinary and medicinal herb, the bulbs of which are used in medicine.

➤ **Pharmacology**
– *Herb:* Garlic (Allii sativi bulbus). The herb consists of the fresh or dried bulbs of *Allium sativum* L., which consist of a main bulb and several daughter bulbs.
– *Important constituents:* Alliins (ca. 1 %), propenylalliin (ca. 0.2 %), methylalliin, and alliaceous oils (allicin and ajoene).
– *Pharmacological properties:* Garlic is antimicrobial, antilipemic, vasodilatory, antioxidant, and fibrinolytic, and inhibits platelet aggregation. Clinical studies demonstrated that the herb inhibits platelet aggregation, increases the bleeding and coagulation times, lowers serum lipids in some individuals, and enhances fibrinolytic activity.

➤ **Indications:** The following indications are recommended in the monographs:
– Prevention of arteriosclerosis
– Hypertension
– There has been some convincing experience, but no rating by the Commission E, in the following indications:
• For minor infections
• For supporting therapy of gastric ulcers because of a strong anti-*Helicobacter* activity

➤ **Contraindications:** None known.

➤ **Dosage and duration of use**
– *Daily dose:* 4 g fresh garlic, that is, 1 to 2 fresh garlic bulbs per day or the corresponding dose of a commercial preparation. Garlic must be crushed to release allicin immediately before it is used in any way.

➤ **Adverse effects:** There are no known health hazards or side effects in conjunction with proper administration of the designated therapeutic doses of the herb. Consumption of large quantities of garlic can irritate the stomach.

➤ **Herb–drug interactions:** There is a slight possibility of interaction with blood-thinning medications such as dicoumarol.
Warning: Avoid use of garlic for approximately 1 week before and after major surgery.

➤ **Summary assessment:** Garlic is an ancient medicinal herb, the uses of which have been investigated in a number of studies. The antihypertensive and lipid-lowering effects are rather weak. There is still need for further research on the herb.

✿ **Literature**
– Monographs: ESCOP; Commission E
– Scientific publications: see p. 478; Ide N et al: Aged garlic extract and its constituents inhibit Cu++ -induced oxidative modification of low density lipoproteins. Planta Med 63 (1997), 263–264; Koch HP, Lawson LD: Garlic – The Science and Therapeutic Application of Allium sativum L. and Related Species, Williams & Wilkins, Baltimore, 1996; Orekov AN, Gruenwald J: Effects of Garlic on Atherosclerosis. Nutrition 13 (1997), 656–663.

Ginger (*Zingiber officinale* Roscoe) _____

➤ **General comments:** The plant is indigenous to the Southeast Asian region. The rhizome is used in medicine.

> **Pharmacology**
> – *Herb:* Ginger root (Zingiberis rhizoma). The herb consists of the peeled fresh or dried rhizomes of *Zingiber officinalis* R. and preparations of the same.
> – *Important constituents:* Essential oil (2.5–3.0 %) containing α-zingiberene, ar-curcumene, β-bisabolene, neral, geranial, (E)-α-farnesene, and zingiberol. Gingerols, diarylheptanoids (gingerenones A and B), and starch (50 %) are also present.
> – *Pharmacological properties:* Ginger has antiemetic action, stimulates the flow of saliva and gastric juices, and increases intestinal peristalsis. It also has known antibacterial, antifungal, molluscacidal, nematocidal, and antiplatelet effects.

> **Indications**
> – Lack of appetite
> – Travel sickness
> – Dyspeptic complaints
> – External use as a compress for contusion and arthritis pain

> **Contraindications**
> – Morning sickness of pregnancy

> **Dosage and duration of use**
> – *Internal use:* Daily dose: 2–4 g dried or fresh rhizome.
>   • *Tea:* Simmer 0.5–1 g of the dried or fresh, sliced or coarsely powdered rhizome in a covered pot for 15 minutes, then pass through a tea strainer (1 teaspoon = ca. 3 g drug).
>   • *As an antiemetic:* Take 2 g of the freshly powdered rhizome in fluids.
> – One dose equals 0.3–1.5 g herb.
> – *External use:* A compress of warm ginger tea for contusions and arthritis pain (see p. 309).

> **Adverse effects:** There are no known health hazards or side effects in conjunction with proper administration of the designated therapeutic doses of the herb.

◉ *Warning:* Owing to its cholagogic activity, patients with gallstones should not use ginger before consulting a qualified health care provider.

> **Herb–drug interactions:** None known.

> **Summary assessment:** Ginger is a well-investigated herb with demonstrated effectiveness in the specified indications. The majority of clinical trials performed showed a benefit for postoperative nausea, motion sickness, and morning sickness, but a few studies showed no effect.

✿ **Literature**
> – Monographs: DAB 1998; ESCOP; Commission E
> – Scientific publications: see p. 478; Kawai T et al: Anti-emetic principles of Magnolia obovata bark and Zingiber officinale rhizome. Planta Med 60 (1994), 17; Kikuzaki H, Tsai SM, Nakatani N: Gingerdiol related compounds from the rhizomes of Zingiber officinale. Phytochemistry 31 (1992), 1783–1786.

Ginkgo (*Ginkgo biloba* L.) _____

> **Synonyms:** Japanese temple tree, maidenhair tree; Ginkgobaum (Ger.)
> **Pharmacology**
> – *Herb:* Ginkgo leaf (Ginkgo bilobae folium). The herb consists of the dried leaves of *Ginkgo biloba* L. and preparations of the same.

- *Important constituents:* Flavonoids (0.5–1.8 %), including quercetin bio-sides, monosides, and triosides, isorhamnetins, and 3´-O-methyl myris-ticins as well as biflavonoids (0.4–1.9 %), proanthocyanidins (8–12 %), di-terpenes (0.06–0.23 %; ginkgolides A, B, C), and sesquiterpenes (bilobalide, 0.04–0.2 %).
- *Pharmacological properties:* Ginkgo has antioxidant and membrane-stabi-lizing activity and improves the circulation. In addition, it increases cere-bral tolerance to hypoxia, reduces the age-related reduction of muscarin-ergic choline receptors and α_2-adrenoceptors, and increases the hip-pocampal absorption of choline. In animals, bilobalide and ginkgolides were found to improve the flow capacity of the blood by lowering viscosity, inactivating toxic oxygen radicals and improving the circulation in cerebral and peripheral arteries. The herb inhibits the development and promotes the elimination of cerebral edema, improves the utilization of ATP and glu-cose, and stabilizes the cell membranes. Clinical, controlled double-blind studies in humans have confirmed the results of animal experiments (gink-go was found to improve the memory capacity and microcirculation and reduce the viscosity of plasma).

➤ **Indications**
- Several small studies found a moderate benefit when using Ginko for ver-tigo (dizziness) and tinnitus of vascular and involutional origin.
- Circulatory disorders (peripheral artery occlusion, especially intermittent claudication, for which some controlled studies reported a benefit).
- Memory enhancement in younger people or people with no preexisting memory impairment has been suggested, with both positive and negative recent clinical trials, but this remains controversial.
- For symptomatic treatment of cerebro-organic impairment of mental per-formance. (Controlled studies showed modest, but statistically significant positive results for cerebral insufficiency. Several reports have indicated modest benefit in controlled studies for Alzheimer's and non-Alzheimer's dementia.)

➤ **Contraindications:** Hypersensitivity to ginkgo preparations.

➤ **Dosage and duration of use**
- *For decreased mental performance:* Oral daily dose: 120–240 mg of a spe-cially formulated, standardized *Ginkgo biloba* extract (GBE; 24 % flavone glycosides, 6 % terpenoids), divided into 2 to 3 portions, to be taken for a period of at least 12 weeks. Thereafter, treatment should be continued after a positive assessment result.
- *For peripheral artery occlusion, vertigo, and tinnitus:* 120–160 mg GBE per day. Used for 6 to 8 weeks for treatment of vertigo and tinnitus; longer use is only justified if some improvement can be registered. According to some studies use for at least 3 months is necessary for full effect.

➤ **Adverse effects:** Mild gastrointestinal complaints, headaches, and allergic re-actions are very rare side effects.

➤ **Herb–drug interactions:** May potentiate anticoagulant activity of aspirin, warfarin, heparin, and other similar drugs.

◎ *Warning:* Caution may be indicated during the perioperative period (see Herb–drug interactions).

➤ **Summary assessment:** Ginkgo is an herb with a number of positive and well-designed clinical trials, especially for improving symptoms of dementia in the elderly. Also improvement of walking performance in intermittent claudication has been shown. Despite some positive trials, memory enhancement in healthy persons remains controversial. Treatment should not be initiated before consulting a qualified health care provider.

✿ **Literature**

– Monographs, ESCOP; Commission E (the positive assessment in the monograph applies only to a specially formulated, standardized GBE; see p. 72).

– Scientific publications: see p. 478; Caesar W: Alles über Ginkgo. Deutsche Apotheker Ztg 134 (1994), 4363; Deutsches Institut für medizinische Dokumentation und Information (Ed): ICD-10. Internationale und statistische Klassifikation der Krankheiten und verwandter Gesundheitsprobleme. 10. Revision. Bd 1. Urban & Schwarzenberg, München Wien Baltimore 1994; Dingermann T: Phytopharmaka im Alter: Crataegus, Ginkgo, Hypericum und Kava-Kava. PZ 140 (1995), 2017–2024; Hopfenmüller W: Nachweis der therapeutischen Wirksamkeit eines Ginkgo biloba-Spezialextraktes. Metaanalyse von 11 klinischen Studien bei Patienten mit Hirnleistungsstörungen im Alter. Arzneim Forsch/Drug Res 44 (1994), 1005–1013; Joyeux M et al: Comparative antilipoperoxidant, antinecrotic and scavenging properties of terpenes and biflavones from Ginkgo and some flavonoids. Planta Med 61 (1995), 126–129; Kanowski S et al: Proof of efficacy of the ginkgo biloba special extract Egb 761 in outpatients suffering from primary degenerative dementia of the Alzheimer type and multi-infarct dementia. Pharmacopsychiatry 4 (1995), 149–158; Pfister-Hotz G: Phytotherapie in der Geriatrie. Z Phytother 18 (1997), 165–162.

Hawthorn (*Crataegus laevigata* (Poiret) D. C.) _____

➤ **General comments:** Many species of hawthorn are distributed throughout the moderate zones of the Northern Hemisphere. The use of its leaves and flowers as a remedy for heart disorders dates back to the nineteenth century.

➤ **Pharmacology**
  – *Herb:* Hawthorn leaf and flower (Crataegi folium cum flore). The herb consists of the leaves and flowers of *Crataegus laevigata* DC. or, less frequently, of other hawthorn species.
  – *Important constituents:* Flavonoids (1.8 %) such as hyperoside (0.28 %), rutin (0.17 %), and vitexin (0.2 %), and oligomeric procyanidins (2–3 %).
  – *Pharmacological properties:* The procyanidins and flavonoids in hawthorn determine its therapeutic action. These substances effect an increase in coronary blood flow and dilate the blood vessels, thereby enhancing myocardial circulation and perfusion. The herb has positive inotropic, chronotropic and dromotropic effects, and improves the tolerance to hypoxia. The cardiotropic effects of *Crataegus* are attributed to an increase in the membrane permeability to calcium ions and an increase in the intracellular cyclic AMP concentration. Altogether, this makes the heart work more economically.

➤ **Indications**
  – Supportive treatment for heart failure (NYHA class I–II)
  – As a strengthening tonic for prevention of heart irregularities and congestive heart failure

➤ **Contraindications:** None known.

➤ **Dosage and duration of use**
  – *Daily dose:* 3.5–19.8 mg flavonoids, calculated as hyperoside (DAB 10), or 160–900 mg extract (4 : 1 to 7 : 1 with ethanol 45 % v/v or methanol 70 % v/v), corresponding to 30–168.7 mg oligomeric procyanidins, calculated as epicatechol. Hawthorn leaf/flower can be used for unlimited periods.

➤ **Adverse effects:** There are no known health hazards or side effects in conjunction with proper administration of the designated therapeutic doses of the herb.

➤ **Herb–drug interactions:** None known.

➤ **Summary assessment:** Clinical studies demonstrating the efficacy of hawthorn leaf/flower in NYHA class I–II heart failure are available.

✿ **Literature**
  – Monographs: DAB 1998; ESCOP; Commission E
  – Scientific publications: see p. 478; Bahorun T, Gressier B, Trotin F et al: Oxygen species scavenging activity of phenolic activities, fresh plant organs and pharmaceutical preparations. Arzneim Forsch 46 (1996), 1086–1089; Kaul R: Pflanzliche Procyanidine. Vorkommen, Klassifikation und pharmakologische Wirkungen. PUZ 25 (1996), 175–185; Tauchert M, Loew D: Crataegi folium cum flore bei Herzinsuffizienz. In: Loew, D., Rietbrock, N. (Ed): Phytopharmaka in Forschung und klinischer Anwendung. Steinkopf Verlag, Darmstadt (1995), 137–144.

Heartsease (*Viola tricolor* L.)

➤ **Synonyms:** Wild pansy; Wildes Stiefmütterchen (Ger.)
➤ **General comments:** Heartsease is distributed throughout all the temperate regions of Eurasia. The herb has been used as a remedy for skin ailments since the middle ages.
➤ **Pharmacology**
   – *Herb:* Heartsease (Violae tricoloris herba). The herb consists of the dried aerial parts of *Viola tricolor* L., collected at the time of flowering, and preparations of the same. The subspecies *vulgaris* (K.) O and *arvensis* (M.) G. are the main herb sources.
   – *Important constituents:* Flavonoids, 0.2–0.4 % (rutin, 23 %), phenolcarboxylic acids such as salicylic acid (0.06–0.3 %) and violutoside, mucilage (10 %), and tannins (2–5 %).
   – *Pharmacological properties:* Mucilage has soothing properties. In animal experiments, eczema was found to improve after long-term oral administration of the herb.
➤ **Indications:** Skin inflammations.
➤ **Contraindications:** None known.
➤ **Dosage and duration of use:** Steep 1 teaspoon of the finely chopped herb in 1 cup of hot water for 5 minutes. Soak gauze compresses in the infusion and apply to the affected area of the skin.
➤ **Adverse effects:** There are no known health hazards or side effects in conjunction with proper administration of the designated therapeutic doses of the herb.
➤ **Herb–drug interactions:** None known.
➤ **Summary assessment:** Wild pansy is most commonly used to treat milk crust and mild seborrheic skin conditions. Industrial wild pansy preparations are not available.
✿ **Literature**
   – Monographs: Commission E
   – Scientific publications: see p. 478

Hops (*Humulus lupulus* L.)

➤ **General comments:** The hop plant has a very bitter taste and is an important ingredient in beer brewing. The cones of the hop plant are used in medicine.
➤ **Pharmacology**
   – *Herb:* Hops/hop cones (Lupuli flos). The herb consists of the whole, dried female inflorescences of *Humulus lupulus* L. and preparations of the same.
   – *Important constituents:* 10 % acylphloroglucinols (α-bitter acids, humulone, β-bitter acids, lupulone), 0.3–1.0 % essential oil (myrcene, 27–62 %), humulene, 2-methylbut-3-en-2-ol), tannins, and flavonoids (isoxanthohumol).
   – *Pharmacological properties:* Hops can have sedative effects; the drug promotes the induction of sleep. The efficacy of the drug depends on the quality of the individual extract. In animals, 2-methyl-3-buten-2-ol was found to produce lasting, profound anesthetic sleep. The bitter acids in hops have antibacterial/antimycotic action and stimulate the secretion of gastric juices.
➤ **Indications:** Nervous tension and insomnia.

➤ **Contraindications:** None known.
➤ **Dosage and duration of use**
  – One dose equals 0.5 g herb.
  – Single dose when used as a sleep aid is 1–2 g herb.
  – Single dose when used for nervous tension is 2 to 3 cups of the tea during the daytime and before retiring. Infuse 1–2 g of the dried strobiles in a cup of boiled water for 20 minutes.
  – *Tincture:* One dose equals 1–2 mL.
➤ **Adverse effects:** There are no known health hazards or side effects in conjunction with proper administration of the designated therapeutic doses of the drug.
◉ *Important:* Contact with fresh hops can cause sensitization (hop-pickers' disease).
➤ **Herb–drug interactions:** None known.
➤ **Summary assessment:** The soporific (sleep-inducing) effect of hops is weaker than that of valerian root extract. Hence, hops should preferably be taken in combination with other soporific preparations.
✿ **Literature**
  – Monographs: DAB 10; ESCOP; Commission E
  – Scientific publications: see p. 478; Orth-Wagner S, Ressin WJ, Friedrich I: Phytosedativum gegen Schlafstörungen. Z Phytother 16 (1995), 147–156; Stevens JF, Ivancic M, Hsu VL, Deinzer ML: Prenylflavonoids from Humulus lupulus. Phytochemistry 44 (1997), 1575–1585.

Horehound (*Marrubium vulgare* L.)

➤ **Synonyms:** White horehound; Andorn (Ger.)
➤ **Pharmacology**
  – *Herb:* Horehound herb (Marrubii herba). The herb consists of the fresh or dried aerial parts of *Marrubium vulgare* L. and preparations of the same.
  – *Important constituents:* Diterpene bitter principles (0.1–1.0 % marrubiin and ca. 0.1 % premarrubiin), caffeic acid derivatives (chlorogenic acid, cryptochlorogenic acid), flavonoids (luteolin-7-lactate, apigenin-7-lactate), and essential oil (0.05–0.6 %), including camphene, *p*-cymene, and fenchen.
  – *Pharmacological properties:* Marrubinic acid increases the flow of bile in animals. It relaxes the sphincter of Oddi, demonstrating an antispasmodic effect, which might help explain its traditional use for easing coughs. The essential oil constituents, diterpene bitters, tannins, and flavonoids (bitter principles) enhance the secretion of gastric juices.
➤ **Indications**
  – Lack of appetite
  – Dyspeptic complaints
  – Coughs and bronchitis
  – Inflammations of the mouth and throat
➤ **Contraindications:** None known.
➤ **Dosage and duration of use**
  – *1 : 1 fluid extract* containing ethanol 20 % (v/v) (BHP 83).
    • *Dosage:* 2–44 mL, three times daily.
  – *Liquid extracts* (ca. 1 : 6), cough lozenges, and syrups are commonly found and used. Dosage according to manufacturer's recommendations.

➤ **Adverse effects:** There are no known health hazards or side effects in conjunction with proper administration of the designated therapeutic doses of the herb.

➤ **Herb–drug interactions:** None known.

➤ **Summary assessment:** Marrubium is a seldom-used herb, partly because of its very bitter taste, except in over-the-counter cough syrups and lozenges, which contain sweetener. No systematic data on its efficacy are currently available.

✿ **Literature**
  – Monographs: Commission E
  – Scientific publications: see p. 478; Roth L, Daunderer M, Kormann K: Giftpflanzen, Pflanzengifte. 4. Aufl., Ecomed Fachverlag Landsberg/Lech 1993.

Horse Chestnut (*Aesculus hippocastanum* L.)

➤ **General comments:** The horse chestnut tree was originally native to Southeastern Europe and the Near East, but has naturalized throughout Europe. The seeds are used in herbal medicine.

➤ **Pharmacology**
  – *Herb:* Horse chestnut seed (Hippocastani semen). The herb consists of the dried seeds of *Aesculus hippocastanum* L. and preparations of the same.
  – *Important constituents:* Aescin is the most important constituent. Triterpene saponins (3–5 %) and flavonoids are also present.
  – *Pharmacological properties:* Horse chestnut extract was found to be antiexudative and reduce capillary wall permeability, leading to an overall antiedematous effect. Clinical data on the venotonic effects are available. In humans, the herb significantly reduces transcapillary filtration. Oral application was found to significantly improve the symptoms of chronic venous insufficiency in double-blind studies. It was found to significantly reduce leg edemas, similarly to the results of compression treatments.

➤ **Indications**
  – Complaints associated with chronic venous insufficiency
  – Posttraumatic or postoperative soft-tissue swelling

➤ **Contraindications:** None known.

➤ **Dosage and duration of use:** Daily dose should be equivalent to 100 mg of aescin.

➤ **Adverse effects:** Inflammation of the mucous membranes in the gastrointestinal tract can occur as a rare side effect after internal use.

➤ **Herb–drug interactions:** None known.

◉ *Important:* Ointments containing aescin should not be rubbed vigorously onto the skin, but applied gently. They might otherwise cause or worsen phlebitis.

◉ *Important:* High-dose horse-chestnut formulations should not be used in the last two trimesters of pregnancy or when nursing a baby unless absolutely necessary.

➤ **Summary assessment:** Horse chestnut seed is an effective and clinically well-researched herbal medicament. Individuals with chronic venous insufficiency should not abstain from compression treatments.

✿ **Literature**
  – Monographs: DAB 1998; ESCOP; Commission E
  – Scientific publications: see p. 478; Daub B: Chronische Veneninsuffizienz: Roßkastanienextrakt oder Kompressionsstrumpf – gleiche Wirkung. Deutsche Apotheker Ztg 136 (1996), 946.

Horsetail (*Equisetum arvense* L.)

➤ **General comments:** Horsetail (field horsetail) is a widespread plant known for its high silicic acid content.

➤ **Pharmacology**
- *Herb:* Horsetail herb (Equiseti herb). The herb consists of the dried, sterile green stems of *Equisetum arvense* L., collected during the summer months.
- *Important constituents:* Flavonoids (0.6–0.9%), caffeic acid esters (1%), and silicic acid (5–7.7%).
- *Pharmacological properties:* Horsetail herb has aquaretic and spasmolytic effects in animals. Its wound-healing properties are probably attributable to its content of flavonoids and silicic acid.

➤ **Indications**
- Urinary tract infections
- Renal or urinary calculi
- Wounds and burns

➤ **Contraindications:** Horsetail should not be used for diuresis in patients with cardiac or renal edema.

➤ **Dosage and duration of use**
- *Internal use:* Boil 2–3 g of the herb in 150–200 mL of water for 5 minutes, then steep for 10 to 15 minutes.
  - *Dosage:* One cup, between meals, several times a day.
  - *Daily dose:* 6 g herb. An adequate intake of fluids is essential (i. e. about two 6-ounce glasses of water).
- *External use:* For compresses, boil 10 g herb in 1 liter of water for 5 minutes, then steep for 10 to 15 minutes.

➤ **Adverse effects:** There are no known health hazards or side effects in conjunction with proper administration of the designated therapeutic doses of the herb.

➤ **Herb–drug interactions:** None known.

➤ **Summary assessment:** When used internally, horsetail should be combined with other aquaretic preparations.

✿ **Literature**
- Monographs: DAB 1998; Commission E
- Scientific publications: see p. 478; Beckert C et al: Styrylpyrone biosynthesis in Equisetum arvense L. Phytochemistry 44 (1997), 275–283.

Iceland Moss (*Cetraria islandica* L. acharius)

▶ **Synonyms:** Cetrariae lichen, Fucus islandicus; Isländisches Moos (Ger.)
▶ **General comments:** Iceland moss is a lichen that is widespread in the alpine and arctic regions of the Northern Hemisphere. The thallus, or plant body, is used in medicine.
▶ **Pharmacology**
  - *Herb:* Iceland moss (*Lichen islandicus*). The herb consists of the dried thallus of *Cetraria islandica* (L.) A. s.l. and preparations of the same.
  - *Important constituents:* Mucilage containing glucans (50%), lichenin, and isolichenin. Lichen acids (3–4.5%) and other substances and compounds with antibacterial effects are also present.
  - The herb has soothing and coating effects due to its content of polysaccharides. Lichenic acids stimulate the appetite and the secretion of saliva. The extract also has weak antibiotic effects.
▶ **Indications**
  - Lack of appetite
  - Dyspeptic complaints
  - Coughs and bronchitis
  - Inflammations of the mouth and throat
▶ **Contraindications:** None known.
▶ **Dosage and duration of use**
  - *Tea:* Steep 1.5–2.5 g (1 to 2 teaspoons) of the finely chopped herb in boiled water for 10 minutes. Sweeten if desired.
  - *Daily dose:* 4–6 g herb. One dose equals 1.5 g herb, equivalent to 1 cup of tea.
  - To obtain preparations that are less bitter, pour hot water onto the herb and discard the water immediately, then pour hot water onto the herb again and steep.
▶ **Adverse effects:** There are no known health hazards or side effects in conjunction with proper administration of the designated therapeutic doses of the herb.
▶ **Herb–drug interactions:** None known.
▶ **Summary assessment:** Iceland moss is a popular remedy in folk medicine, but only a few scientific studies on the herb have been conducted so far.
✿ **Literature**
  - Monographs: DAB 1998; ESCOP; Commission E
  - Scientific publications: see p. 478; Pengsuparp T et al: Mechanistic evaluation of new plant-derived compounds that inhibit HIV-1 reverse transcriptase. J Nat Prod 58 (1995), 1024–1031; Wunderer H: Zentral und peripher wirksame Antitussiva: eine kritische Übersicht. PZ 142 (1997), 847–852.

Java Tea (*Orthosiphon aristatus* Miquel)

▶ **Synonyms:** Orthosiphon.
▶ **General comments:** Java tea is native to Southeast Asia. The inhabitants of the region have used its leaves as a remedy for bladder and kidney disorders for decades.
▶ **Pharmacology**

- *Herb:* Java tea leaf (Orthosiphonis folium). The herb consists of the foliage leaves and stem tips of *Orthosiphon aristatus* or *Orthosiphon spicatus* (T.) B. (syn. *Orthosiphon stamineus* B.), collected shortly before the time of flowering, and preparations of the same.
- *Important constituents:* Essential oil (0.02–0.6%) containing mainly β-caryophyllene, α-humulene, and caryophyllene epoxide. Flavonoids (eupatorin), triterpene saponins (up to 4.5%), and potassium salts are also present.
- *Pharmacological properties:* The essential oil has antimicrobial and antiphlogistic effects. In animal and human studies, the herb was found to have an aquaretic effect (due to the combined effects of saponins and flavonoids).

➤ **Indications**
   - Urinary tract infections
   - Renal or urinary calculi
➤ **Contraindications:** Irrigation therapy is not recommended if cardiac or renal edema is present.
➤ **Dosage and duration of use**
   - *Tea:* Steep 2 g of the herb in 150 mL of hot water for 15 minutes.
     - *Dosage:* One cup, several times a day.
   - *Daily dose:* 6–12 g of the herb.
   - ◉ *Important:* An adequate intake of fluids (at least 2 liters per day) is essential.
➤ **Adverse effects:** There are no known health hazards or side effects in conjunction with proper administration of the designated therapeutic doses of the herb.
➤ **Herb–drug interactions:** None known.
➤ **Summary assessment:** Java tea leaf combines well with other aquaretic and urinary antiseptic herbal preparations.
➤ **Literature**
   - Monographs: DAB 10; ESCOP; Commission E
   - Scientific publications: see p. 478

Juniper (*Juniperus communis* L.)

➤ **General comments:** The juniper tree or bush is distributed throughout the Northern Hemisphere. Its berrylike fruit (cones) have been used for aquaresis and wound healing since ancient times.
➤ **Pharmacology**
   - *Herb:* Juniper berry (Juniperi fructus). The herb consists of the ripe, fresh or dried berrylike fruit of *Juniperus communis* L. and preparations of the same.
   - *Important constituents:* Essential oil (0.8–2%, depending on the site of herb origin), monoterpene hydrocarbons (α-pinenes, terpinen-4-ol), diterpenes oligomeric proanthocyanidins of the catechin type, monosaccharides (invert sugar, 20–30%), and flavonoids.
   - *Pharmacological properties:* Because of its essential oils (especially terpinen-4-ol), juniper berry has an aquaretic effect. In animals, it was shown to have mild antihypertensive and antiexudative effects.
➤ **Indications**
   - *Internal use*
     - Lack of appetite

- Dyspeptic complaints
- For aquaresis in unspecific inflammations of the lower urinary tract
  - ◉ *Important:* The cause of urinary tract infection must always be clarified by a physician.
- *External use:* Essential oil as a bath additive for supportive treatment of rheumatic diseases (see p. 286).

▶ **Contraindications**
- *Internal use:* Pregnancy, inflammatory kidney diseases.
- *External use:* Extensive skin injuries, acute skin diseases, severe febrile and infectious diseases, heart failure and hypertension.

▶ **Dosage and duration of use**
- *Infusion:* Steep 1 teaspoon of crushed, dried juniper berries in 1 cup (150 mL) of boiled water for 10 minutes.
  - *Dosage:* One cup, 3 times a day.
- *Tincture:* Steep 20 g of the herb in 80 g of ethanol 70 % for 8 days.
  - *Dosage:* 20 to 30 drops, 2 to 3 times a day.
- *Daily dose:* 2–10 g (maximum dose) of the herb, corresponding to 20–100 mg of the essential oil.
- When used internally, the duration of treatment should be restricted to a maximum of 6 weeks owing to the potential for tissue irritation by pinenes.

▶ **Adverse effects:** Overdose or long-term internal use can cause kidney irritation and/or damage.

▶ **Herb–drug interactions:** None known.

▶ **Summary assessment:** Juniper is an effective herbal medicament in the specified indications. It combines well with other aquaretic and urinary antiseptic preparations.

✿ **Literature**
- Monographs: DAB 1998; ESCOP; Commission E
- Scientific publications: see p. 478; Schilcher H, Heil BM: Nierentoxizität von Wacholderbeerzubereitungen. Z Phytother 15 (1994), 205–213; Schmidt M: Wacholderzubereitungen. Muß die Monographie umgeschrieben werden? Deutsche Apotheker Ztg 135 (1995), 1260–1264.

Kava (*Piper methysticum* G. Forster)

➢ **Synonyms:** Kava-kava, intoxicating pepper.

➢ **General comments:** Kava is indigenous to the islands of the South Pacific. The native Polynesians use the rhizome to make a mildly intoxicating beverage. Kava rhizome extract has anxiolytic and sedative effects.

➢ **Pharmacology**

– *Herb:* Kava rhizome (Piperis methystici rhizoma). The herb consists of the peeled, cut and dried rhizomes (usually with the root parts removed) of *Piper methysticum* G. F. and preparations of the same.

– *Important constituents:* Kava lactones (kava pyrones, 5–12 %) consisting mainly of (+)-kavain (1.8 %), (+)-methysticin (1.2 %), desmethoxyyangonin (1 %), and yangonin (1 %).

– *Pharmacological properties:* Kava pyrones have sedative and central muscle relaxant effects. Anticonvulsive, neuroprotective, narcosis-enhancing, central muscle relaxant, spasmolytic, analgesic, and local anesthetic effects were observed in animals. The herb has anxiolytic and soporific effects in humans.

➢ **Indications:** Nervous tension, states of tension and anxiety.

➢ **Contraindications:** Pregnancy, breast feeding, and endogenous depression (increased risk of suicide). The herb should not be taken for more than 3 months without the advice of a qualified health care practitioner.

➢ **Dosage and duration of use**

– *Daily dose:* 60–120 mg of herb preparations.

➢ **Adverse effects:** The prolonged use of high doses of kava can, in rare cases, lead to gastrointestinal complaints, oculomotor equilibrium disorders, pupil dilation, and insufficiency of accommodation. Slight morning fatigue can occur in the initial phase of treatment. Disorders of complex movement with otherwise unimpaired consciousness are initial signs of overdose, followed by fatigue and a tendency to fall asleep. Kava increases the action of substances that affect the central nervous system, e. g., alcohol, barbiturates, and other psychoactive drugs. A few studies yielded some indication of hepatotoxicity in relation to administration of kava. Though this information is limited to date and still awaits scientific evaluation, it is recommended to consider the following when using kava products.

◉ *Warning:* Kava should not be taken on a daily basis for more than 4 weeks.

◉ *Warning:* Use of kava should be discontinued if symptoms of jaundice appear.

◉ *Warning:* Patients with a history of liver problems or who suspect possible liver problems or who are taking pharmaceutical drugs should use kava only with the advice of a professional health care provider.

◉ *Warning:* See p. 212 for cautions in the use of kava in disorders of the nervous system.

➢ **Herb–drug interactions:** Kava should not be used by anyone who has liver problems, is taking any drugs with known adverse effects on the liver, such as NSAIDS, or is a regular consumer of alcohol.

➢ **Summary assessment:** Kava is an effective herb in the specified indications (herbal tranquilizer). It has a low incidence of side effects and its effects have been relatively well investigated.

✿ Literature

- Monographs: ESCOP; Commission E
- Scientific publications: see p. 478; Gleitz J et al: Kavain inhibits non-stereo-specifically veratridine-activated Na+ channels. Planta Med 62 (1996), 580–581; Hänsel R: Kava-Kava (Piper methysticum G. Forster) in der modernen Arzneimittelforschung. Portrait einer Arzneipflanze. Z Phytother 17 (1996), 180–195; Volz HP: Die anxiolytische Wirksamkeit von Kava-Spezialextrakt WS 1490 unter Langzeittherapie – eine randomisierte Doppelblindstudie. Z Phytother Abstraktband, (1995), 9.

Lemon Balm (*Melissa officinalis* L.)

➤ **Synonyms:** Balm; Melisse (Ger.).
➤ **General comments:** Balm is native in the eastern Mediterranean and Western Asian regions. Lemon balm plants in Central Europe are either cultivated or naturalized. The plant has been used as a medicinal herb since ancient times.
➤ **Pharmacology**
  – *Herb:* Lemon balm leaf (Melissae folium). The herb consists of the fresh or dried foliage leaves of *Melissa officinalis* L. and preparations of the same.
  – *Important constituents:* Essential oil (0.02–0.8%) containing geranial/α-citral and neral/β-citral (40–75% in total).
  – *Pharmacological properties:* Lemon balm has antiviral and antioxidant effects in vitro. Choleretic, calming, and carminative effects have been observed in animals.
➤ **Indications**
  – General nervousness and sleeplessness
  – Herpes labialis (external application)
➤ **Contraindications:** None known.
➤ **Dosage and duration of use**
  – *Tea:* Steep 1.5–4.5 g of the herb in 1 cup of hot water for 10 minutes.
    • *Dosage:* One cup, several times a day.
  – *Daily dose:* 1.5–4.5 g of the herb.
➤ **Adverse effects:** None following proper administration of the designated therapeutic doses.
➤ **Herb–drug interactions:** None known.
➤ **Summary assessment:** Lemon balm is a popular herbal medicament that combines well with other herbs with a similar therapeutic range. Clinical studies on the herb (oral application as monodrug) are not available.
✿ **Literature**
  – Monographs: DAB 1998; ESCOP; Commission E
  – Scientific publications: see p. 478; Hermann EC jr, Kucera LS: Antiviral substances in plants of the mint family (Labiatae): II. Nontanninic polyphenols of Melissa officinalis. Proc Soc Exp Bio Med 124 (1995), 869; Mohrig A. Melissenextrakt bei Herpes simplex – die Alternative zu Nucleosid-Analoga. Deutsche Apotheker Ztg 136 (1996), 4575–4580; Orth-Wagner S. Ressin WJ, Friedrich I: Phytosedativum gegen Schlafstörungen. Z Phytother 16 (1995), 147–156; Schultze W, König WA, Hilker A, Richter R: Melissenöle. Deutsche Apotheker Ztg 135 (1995), 557–577; Walz A: Melisse hilft heilen. Deutsche Apotheker Ztg 136 (1996) 26.

Lesser Centaury (*Centaurium erythraea*)

➤ **Synonyms:** Broad-leaved centaury, common centaury; Tausendgüldenkraut (Ger.)
➤ **General comments:** The dried aerial parts of *Centaurium erythraea* Rafn collected at the time of flowering are used in medicine.
➤ **Pharmacology**
  – *Herb:* Centaury herb (Centaurii herba).
  – *Important constituents:* Iridoids and bitter principles, mainly swertiamarin (75%), gentiopicrin, and sweroside.

– *Pharmacological properties:* Reflex stimulation of saliva and gastric juice secretion. The herb also has antiphlogistic and antipyretic action in animals.

➤ **Indications**
  – Lack of appetite
  – Dyspeptic complaints

➤ **Contraindications:** Ulcers of the stomach and small intestine.

➤ **Dosage and duration of use**
  – *Tea:* Steep 2–3 g of the herb in 150 mL of boiled water for 15 minutes. Take $^1/_2$ hour before meals.
  – *Daily dose:* 6 g dried herb for tea.
  – *1 : 5 tincture:* 2–5 g per day.

➤ **Adverse effects:** There are no known health hazards or side effects in conjunction with proper administration of the designated therapeutic doses of the drug.

➤ **Herb–drug interactions:** None known.

➤ **Summary assessment:** Owing to its bitter principles, centaury can effectively stimulate the appetite and digestion.

✿ **Literature**
  – Monographs: DAB 1998; ESCOP; Commission E
  – Schimmer O, Mauthner H: Centaurium erythraea RAFN. Tausendgüldenkraut. Z Phytother 15 (1994), 299–304; Schimmer O, Mauthner H: Polymethoxylated xanthones from the herb of Centaurium erythraea with strong antimutagenic properties in Salmonella typhimurim. Planta Med 62 (1996), 561–564.

Licorice (*Glycyrrhiza glabra* L.)

➤ **General comments:** Licorice is a shrub native to the Mediterranean region that grows to heights of 1 to 1.5 meters. The root is used in medicine.

➤ **Pharmacology**
  – Herb
    • *Licorice root* (Liquiritiae radix). The herb consists of the dried, unpeeled roots and stolons of *Glycyrrhiza glabra* L. and preparations of the same.
    • *Licorice extract* (Succus liquiritiae). The herb consists of the liquid derived by boiling licorice root in hot water and thickening it by concentration under vacuum (licorice juice).
  – *Important constituents:* Triterpene saponins (3–15 %) such as glycyrrhizinic acid, aglycone 18β-glycyrrhetinic acid, and their salts classified as glycyrrhizin. Flavonoids (liquiritigenin) and isoflavonoids are also present.
  – Saponins have expectorant and secretolytic effects in animals; the flavonoid component has spasmolytic effects. 18β-Glycyrrhetinic acid inhibits prostaglandin synthesis, lipoxygenase, and cortisol metabolism, thereby exerting antiphlogistic and ulceroprotective effects. No clinical data on the efficacy of licorice preparations in respiratory tract disease are available.

➤ **Indications**
  – Gastritis
  – Coughing and bronchitis

➤ **Contraindications:** Chronic liver disease, cholestatic liver diseases, cirrhosis of the liver, severe renal failure, hypertension, hypokalemia, and pregnancy.

➤ **Dosage and duration of use**
  – *Tea:* Pour 150 mL of boiled water onto 2 – 4 g (1 teaspoon = ca. 3 g) of the finely chopped or coarsely powdered herb, or place the herb in cold water and bring to a boil. Steep for 10 to 15 minutes, then strain.
    • *Dosage:* One cup, after meals, 2 to 3 times a day.
  – *Succus liquiritiae:* 0.5 – 1 g herb for catarrhs of the upper respiratory tract; 1.5 – 3 g herb for peptic ulcers.
  – *Daily dose:* 5 – 15 g herb (equivalent to 200 – 600 mg glycyrrhizin).
➤ **Adverse effects:** Hypokalemia, hypernatremia, edema, hypertension, heart disorders and, in rare cases, myoglobinuria can occur after long-term, high-dose (50 mg/day or more) administration owing to the mineralocorticomimetic (aldosterone-like) effect of the saponins in the herb. Therefore, continuous use of licorice preparations should not exceed 6 weeks and the use of licorice fluid extract and commercial licorice products should be medically supervised.
  ◉ *Important:* These side effects do not occur with deglycyrrhinized succus preparations. These are commonly available as commercial preparations (capsules and tablets) under the name DGL (deglycyrrhinized licorice).
➤ **Herb–drug interactions:** Thiazide and loop diuretics can increase the mineralocorticoid effects of licorice.
➤ **Summary assessment:** Licorice is suitable for self-treatment if it used short term and all safety warnings are heeded. Licorice should be used in combination with other expectorant or secretolytic herbs.
➤ **Literature**
  – Monographs: DAB 1998; ESCOP; Commission E
  – Scientific publications: see p. 478; Khaksa G et al: Anti-inflammatory and anti-nociceptive activity of disodium glycyrrhetinic acid hemiphthalate. Planta Med 62 (1996), 326 – 328; Nose M et al: A comparision of the anti-hepatotoxica activity between glycyrrhizin and glycerrhetinic acid. Planta Med 60 (1994), 136.

Lily-of-the-valley (*Convallaria majalis* L.)

➤ **General comments:** The dried, cream-colored petals and flower heads are used in medicine. The plant was originally native to Europe, but was later introduced to North America and northern Asia.
➤ **Pharmacology**
  – *Herb:* Lily-of-the-valley herb (Convallariae herba). The herb consists of the aerial parts of *Convallaria majalis* L. or closely related species, collected during the time of flowering.
  – *Important constituents:* Steroid cardiac glycosides (cardenolides, 0.1 – 0.5 %). Depending on its site of origin, the herb may also contain convallatoxin (Western and Northwestern Europe) or convalloside (Northern and Eastern Europe) or convallatoxin and convallatoxol (Central Europe).
  – *Pharmacological properties:* The glycosides in Convallaria have effects similar to those of digitoxin and strophanthin. The herb increases the contractile force and velocity of the myocardium while extending the relaxation time. It also reduces the heart rate, slows stimulus conduction, and increases the excitability of ventricular muscles (positive inotropic, negative chronotropic, negative dromotropic, and positive bathmotropic effects). Lily-of-the-valley was found to have diuretic, natriuretic, and vasoconstrictive effects in animals.

▶ **Indications**
  – Heart failure (NYHA classes I and II)
  – Cardiac arrhythmias
  – Nervous heart disorders
▶ **Contraindications:** Hypokalemia, hypercalcemia
▶ **Dosage and duration of use:** All specifications refer to standardized lily-of-the-valley powder (DAB 8).
  – *Tincture (1 : 10):* Single dose, 2.0 g; daily dose, 6.0 g.
  – *Fluid extract (1 : 1):* Single dose, 0.2 g; daily dose, 0.6 g.
  – *Dry extract (4 : 1):* Single dose, 0.05 g; daily dose, 0.15 g.
▶ **Adverse effects**
  – Health hazards in conjunction with proper administration of the designated therapeutic doses of the herb are not known. Overdose can induce nausea, vomiting, headaches, stupor and cardiac arrhythmias and can impair color vision.
  – The risk of lily-of-the-valley poisoning following oral administration of the herb is relatively low because only small quantities of the glycosides are absorbed.
▶ **Herb–drug interactions:** Lily-of-the-valley increases the effects and side effects of quinidine, calcium salts, saluretics, laxatives, and glucocorticoids when used concomitantly.
◉ *Warning:* Lily-of-the-valley should be used only under medical supervision and according to the instructions of a qualified health care provider.
▶ **Summary assessment:** Lily-of-the-valley is a rarely used herbal remedy, but can be recommended for the indications specified above.
✿ **Literature**
  – Monographs: DAB 1998: Commission E
  – Scientific publications: see p. 478; Krenn L, Schlifelner, L, Stimpfl, T. Kopp, B: HPLC separation and quantitative determination of cardenolides in Herba Convallariae. Planta Med 58 (1992), A682; Laufke R: Planta Med 6 (1958), 237; Loew D: Phytotherapie bei Herzinsuffizienz. Z Phytother 18 (1997), 92–96.

Linden (*Tilia* spp.)

▶ **Synonyms:** Lime tree; Linde (Ger.).
▶ **General comments:** The linden tree is commonly used in the wood processing industry. Linden flower has been used in medicine since the eighteenth century.
▶ **Pharmacology**
  – *Herb:* Linden flower (Tiliae flos). The herb consists of the dried flowers of *Tilia cordata* M. and/or *Tilia platyphyllos* S. and preparations of the same.
  – *Important constituents:* Flavonoids (1 %) including astragalin, isoquercitrin, kaempferol 3-*O*-rhamnoside, quercetin, and tiliroside. Mucilage (10 %) containing arabinogalactans with a uronic acid component), essential oil (0.01–0.2 %), and tannins (2 %) are also present.
  – *Pharmacological properties:* Linden flower is reputed to have antitussive, astringent, diaphoretic, diuretic, and general immunostimulant effects, but there is a lack of scientific evidence to validate these uses. The tannins, glycosides, and essential oil in linden flower have antimicrobial effects in humans. The inhalation of steam enriched with linden flower extract was more effective in improving the symptoms of uncomplicated colds than the inhalation of steam alone (control group).

➤ **Indications:** Colds and associated cough.
➤ **Contraindications:** None known.
➤ **Dosage and duration of use**
  – *Daily dose:* 2 – 4 g of the herb.
  – *Tea:* Steep 2 g of the herb in 1 cup of boiled water for 5 to 10 minute (1 teaspoon = ca. 1.8 g herb). The tea should be drunk while as hot as possi ble and is best taken during the afternoon.
➤ **Adverse effects:** There are no known health hazards or side effects in conjunc tion with proper administration of the designated therapeutic doses of the herb
➤ **Herb–drug interactions:** None known
➤ **Summary assessment:** Linden flower is commonly used in folk medicine, bu hardly any scientific studies of its effects have been performed.
✿ **Literature**
  – Monographs: DAB 10; Commission E
  – Scientific publications: see p. 478

Lovage (*Levisticum officinale* Koch)

➤ **General comments:** Lovage is a widely used culinary herb. The rhizome is use in medicine.
➤ **Pharmacology**
  – *Herb:* Lovage root (Levistici radix). The herb consists of the dried rhizome and roots of *Levisticum officinale* K. and preparations of the same.
  – *Important constituents:* Essential oil (0.35 – 1.7 %) containing alkylphthali des, (*E*)- and (*Z*)-ligustilide, 3-butylphthalide, and ligusticum lactone Hydroxycoumarins (umbelliferone) and furanocoumarins (bergapter apterin) are also present.
  – *Pharmacological properties:* In animal studies, the essential oil was found t have spasmolytic, anticholinergic, antibacterial, and sedative effects on th smooth muscles. The herb has aquaretic action due to its content of turpen tine.
➤ **Indications**
  – Urinary tract infections
  – Renal or urinary calculi
➤ **Contraindications:** Irrigation therapy is not recommended for elimination o cardiac or renal edema.
➤ **Dosage and duration of use**
  – *Tea:* Steep 2 g of herb in 1 cup of boiled water.
    • *Dosage:* One cup, between meals, several times a day.
  – *Daily dose:* 4 – 8 g herb.
➤ **Adverse effects:** Lovage has a slight potential for sensitization. Because of it irritant effects, individuals with nephritis, lower urinary tract inflammation o decreased renal function should not use the essential oil. In fair-skinned indi viduals, lovage can cause increased sensitivity to ultraviolet light (phototoxi effect of furanocoumarins).
➤ **Herb–drug interactions:** None known.
➤ **Summary assessment:** Lovage should be used in combination with othe herbal urological remedies.
✿ **Literature**
  – Monographs: Commission E

Mallow (*Malva sylvestris* L.)

➤ **General comments:** Mallow can be found in the subtropics and temperate regions of both hemispheres today.

Mallow flower (Malvae flos)

➤ **Pharmacology**
  – *Herb:* Mallow flower (Malvae flos). The herb consists of the dried flowers of *Malva sylvestris* L. and/or *M. sylvestris* L. ssp. *mauritiana* (L.) A. e. G. and preparations of the same.
  – *Important constituents:* Mucilage (6–10%) containing rhamnogalacturonans and arabinogalactans; anthocyans (malvin), polysaccharides, and flavonoids.
  – *Pharmacological properties:* The herb has coating and soothing effects attributable to its high mucilage content.
➤ **Indications**
  – Coughs and bronchitis
  – Inflammations of the mouth and throat
➤ **Contraindications: None known.**
➤ **Dosage and duration of use**
  – *Tea:* Place 1.5–2 g of the finely chopped herb in cold water, bring to a boil and remove from heat, or pour boiling water onto the herb. Steep for 10 minutes, then strain.
    • *Dosage:* One cup, 2 to 3 times a day.
  – *Daily dose:* 5 g of the herb.
➤ **Adverse effects:** Health hazards in conjunction with proper administration of the designated therapeutic doses of the herb are not known.
➤ **Herb–drug interactions:** None known.
➤ **Summary assessment:** Mallow flower has demonstrated efficacy in the specified indications.
✿ **Literature**
  – Monographs: Commission E
  – Scientific publications: see p. 478; Classen B, Amelunxen F, Blaschek W: Malva sylvestris – Mikroskopische Untersuchungen zur Entstehung von Schleimbehältern. Deutsche Apotheker Ztg 134 (1994), 3597.

Mallow Leaf (Malvae folium)

➤ **Pharmacology**
  – *Herb:* Mallow leaf (Malvae folium). The herb consists of the dried foliage leaves of *Malva sylvestris* L. and/or *Malva neglecta* W. and preparations of the same.
  – *Important constituents:* Mucilage (6–8%) containing mainly rhamnogalacturonans and arabinogalactans, flavonoids (hypolaetin-3-*O*-glucoside, gossypetin-3-*O*-glucoside), and flavonoid sulfates such as gossypetin-8-*O*-β-D-glucuronide-3-sulfate and hypolaetin-8-O-glucoside-3′-sulfate.
  – *Pharmacological properties:* No data available.
➤ **Indications**
  – Coughs and bronchitis
  – Inflammations of the mouth and throat
➤ **Contraindications:** None known.

> **Dosage and duration of use**
> – *Tea:* Steep 3–5 g of the herb (ca. 2 teaspoons) in 150 mL of boiled water for 10 to 15 minutes, or place the herb in cold water and steep for 2 to 3 hours while stirring occasionally.
>   • *Dosage:* One cup, 1 to 2 times a day.
> – *Daily dose:* 5 g of the herb.
> **Adverse effects:** None known.
> **Herb–drug interactions:** None known,
> **Summary assessment:** Mallow leaf is a herbal medicament with demonstrated effects at the recommended therapeutic doses.
✿ **Literature**
> – Monographs: Commission E
> – Scientific publications: see p. 478; Classen B, Amelunxen F, Blaschek W: *Malva sylvestris* – Mikroskopische Untersuchungen zur Entstehung von Schleimbehältern. Deutsche Apotheker Ztg 134 (1994), 3597.

Marigold (*Calendula officinalis* L.)

> **Synonyms:** Calendula; Ringelblume (Ger.)
> **General comments:** This plant is widely distributed throughout the Northern Hemisphere and is a very popular remedy in folk medicine. Its flowers are used in herbal medicine.
> **Pharmacology**
> – *Herb:* Marigold flower (Calendulae flos). The herb consists of the ray flowers of the completely mature flower heads of *Calendula officinalis* L.
> – *Important constituents:* Triterpene saponins (2–10%), triterpene alcohols (4.8%), flavonoids (0.3–0.8%), hydroxycoumarins, carotinoids, essential oil (0.2%), and water-soluble polysaccharides (15%).
> – *Pharmacological properties:* Marigold flower is antimicrobial (essential oil, flavones), fungicidal, virucidal (influenza and herpes simplex viruses), antiphlogistic, vulnerary, and immunostimulant (polysaccharides). Extensive research data on the herb are available.
> **Indications**
> – Inflammations of the mouth and throat
> – Burns and wounds, including those that tend to heal poorly
> **Contraindications:** None known.
> **Dosage and duration of use**
> – *Tea:* Steep 1 to 2 teaspoons (2–3 g) of the herb in 150 mL of hot water for approximately 10 minutes. Use the warm tea as a mouthwash or gargle several times a day.
> – *Compresses:* Soak a linen compress in Marigold infusion. Apply fresh compresses several times a day.
> **Adverse effects:** There are no known health hazards or side effects in conjunction with proper administration of the designated therapeutic doses of the herb.
> **Herb–drug interactions:** None known.
> **Summary assessment:** Marigold flower is a reliable wound-healing agent. It is generally regarded as safe, even when used in children.

✿ Literature
- Monographs: DAB 1998; ESCOP; Commission E
- Scientific publications: see p. 478; Mennet-von Eiff M, Meier B: Phytothera-pie in der Dermatologie. Z Phytother 16 (1995), 201–210.

Marshmallow (*Althaea officinalis* L.)
Marshmallow Leaf (*Althaea officinalis* L.) _____

▶ **Pharmacology**
- *Herb:* Marshmallow leaf (Althaeae folium). The herb consists of the dried foliage leaves of *Althaea officinalis* L.
- *Important constituents:* 6–10% mucilage (colloidal polysaccharides and arabinogalactans)
- *Pharmacological properties:* Since mucilage has a coating effect, it soothes irritated mucous membranes. Anti-inflammatory and immunostimulatory effects have been shown in animals and in vitro.

▶ **Indications**
- Dry, unproductive cough
- Irritations of the mouth and throat

▶ **Contraindications:** None known.

▶ **Dosage and duration of use**
- *Tea:* Steep 1–2 g of the dried herb in hot water.
  - *Dosage:* One cup, several times a day.
- *Daily dose:* 5 g herb.

▶ **Adverse effects:** None known.

▶ **Herb–drug interactions:** None known.

▶ **Summary assessment:** See Marshmallow Root.

▶ **Literature**
- Monographs: Commission E
- Scientific publications: see p. 478; Hahn-Deinstrop E: Eibischwurzel Iden-tifizierung von Eibischwurzel-Extrakt und Gehaltsbestimmung in einem Instant-Tee. Deutsche Apotheker Ztg 135 (1995), 1147–1149; Wunderer H: Zentral und peripher wirksame Antitussiva: eine kritische Übersicht. PZ 142 (1997), 847–852.

Marshmallow Root (*Althaea officinalis* L.) _____

▶ **Pharmacology**
- *Herb:* Marshmallow root (Althaeae radix). The herb consists of the dried, chopped, peeled, or unpeeled roots of *Althaea officinalis* L.
- *Important constituents:* 10–20% mucilage (colloid-soluble polysaccha-rides, rhamnogalacturonans, arabinogalactans) and 30–38% starch.
- Pharmacological properties: See Marshmallow Leaf.

▶ **Indications**
- Inflammations of the mouth and throat and associated dry cough
- Mild gastritis

▶ **Contraindications:** None known.

▶ **Dosage and duration of use:** The chopped roots are used to make aqueous extracts and other galenicals for internal use.
- *Tea:* Add 6 g of the roots to 150 mL cold water and allow to steep for 90 minutes, stirring frequently.

- *Dosage:* One cup of the rewarmed tea, several times a day. The tea can also be used as a mouthwash.
➤ **Adverse effects:** None known.
➤ **Herb–drug interactions:** None known.
➤ **Summary assessment:** Marshmallow root is a well tolerated herb that is often used in pediatric medicine.

✿ **Literature**
 – Monographs: DAB 10; ESCOP; Commission E
 – Scientific publications: see p. 478; Hahn-Deinstrop E: Eibischwurzel: Identifizierung von Eibischwurzel-Extrakt und Gehaltsbestimmung in einem Instant-Tee. Deutsche Apotheker Ztg 135 (1995), 1147–1149.

Meadowsweet (*Filipendula ulmaria* L. Maxim)

➤ **Synonyms:** Queen-of-the-meadow, bridewort; Mädesüß (Ger.)
➤ **General comment:** The dried flowers are used in medicine. The meadowsweet is native to all parts of the Northern Hemisphere.
➤ **Pharmacology**
 – *Herb:* Meadowsweet flower (Spiraeae flos). The herb consists of the dried flowers of *Filipendula ulmaria* (L.) M. and preparations of the same.
 – *Important constituents:* Essential oil (0.2 %) containing salicylaldehyde and salicylic acid methyl ester, up to 5 % flavonoids (spiraeoside, quercetin-4′-glucoside, 3–4 %), and tannins (ellagitannins).
 – *Pharmacological properties:* Meadowsweet flower has antimicrobial, antipyretic, and aquaretic effects. In animal experiments, the herb was found to have a positive effect on the healing of peptic ulcers and to increase smooth-muscle tone. These effects are attributable to its flavonoid components.
➤ **Indications**
 – Colds and fever
 – Coughs and bronchitis
➤ **Contraindications:** Because meadowsweet contains salicylates, individuals with a known hypersensitivity to salicylates should not use it.
➤ **Dosage and duration of use**
 – *Tea:* Steep 1 teaspoon (ca. 1.4 g herb) of the herb in boiled water for 10 minutes.
 • *Dosage:* One cup, several times a day.
 – *Daily dose:* 2.5–3.5 g (flowers).
➤ **Adverse effects:** There are no known health hazards or side effects in conjunction with proper administration of the designated therapeutic doses of the herb. It can upset the stomach and cause nausea if overdosed.
➤ **Herb–drug interactions:** None known.
➤ **Summary assessment:** Meadowsweet is a well-known household remedy for colds and flu.

✿ **Literature**
 – Monographs: Belg IV; EB 6; HAB 1; Helv V; Commission E
 – Scientific publications: see p. 478; Barnaulov OD: Rastit Resur 14 (1987), 573; Haslam E et al: Ann Proc Phytochemistry Soc Eur 25 (1985), 252; Hörhammer L et al: Arch Pharm 61 (1956), 133; Valle MG et al: Planta Med 54 (1988), 181.

Milk Thistle (*Silybum marianum* L. Gaertn.)

➤ **Synonyms:** Marian thistle; Mariendistel (Ger.)
➤ **General comments:** The milk thistle is a native European medicinal plant that has been used since ancient times. It has striking deep green leaves with white spots along the veins.
➤ **Pharmacology**
  – *Herb:* Milk thistle fruit (Cardui mariae herba). The herb consists of the pappus-free, ripe fruit of *Silybum marianum* (L.) G.
  – *Important constituents:* Silymarin (flavonolignan mixture, 1.5–3%), primary components silybin A and B (combination of the two is called silibinin), iso-silybin A, isosilybin B, silychristin, silydianin, flavonoids (apigenin, chryso-eriol, eriodictyol, naringenin, quercetin, taxifolin), and fatty oil (20–30%).
  – *Pharmacological properties:* Silymarin and silibinin were found to have hepatoprotective effects in studies on liver damage. Silymarin stimulates RNA polymerase I in the nucleus of hepatocytes. This, in turn, increases the rate of ribosomal protein synthesis and enhances the regenerative capacity of the liver. Silymarin is an effective antidote for *Amanita* mushroom poisoning because it antagonizes the inhibition of RNA polymerase I by α-amanitine. The herb also has weak cholagogic properties.
➤ **Indications**
  – Dyspeptic complaints
  – Liver and gallbladder complaints
➤ **Contraindications:** None known.
➤ **Dosage and duration of use**
  – *Daily dose:* 200–400 mg silymarin based on the silibinin content (usually 80%) in a divided dose, around mealtimes.
➤ **Adverse effects:** None known.
➤ **Herb–drug interactions:** None known.
➤ **Summary assessment:** Milk thistle is used to treat dyspeptic complaints. It should be used in combination with other gallbladder remedies. The hepatoprotective effects should be confirmed in modern clinical trials.
✿ **Literature**
  – Monographs: DAB 1998; Commission E
  – Scientific publications: see p. 478; Lorenz D, Mennicke WH, Behrendt W: Untersuchungen zur Elimination von Silymarin bei cholecystektomierten Patienten. Planta Med 45 (1992), 216–233; Schulz HU, Schürer M, Krumbiegel G et al: Untersuchungen zum Freisetzungsverhalten und zur Bioäquivalenz von Silymarin-Präparaten. Arzneim Forsch/Drug Res 45 (1995), 61–64; Tuchweber B et al: J Med 4 (1973), 327.

European Mistletoe (*Viscum album* L.)

➤ **General comments:** The medicinal use of mistletoe dates back to the pre-Christian era. The plant grows mainly in Europe.

Mistletoe Herb (Visci herba)

➤ **Pharmacology:** Mistletoe herb consists of the leaves, fruit, and flowers on the fresh or dried young branches of *Viscum album* L. and preparations of the same.
  – *Important constituents:* Lectins (glycoproteins with an 11% carbohydrate fraction) and mistletoe lectin (ML) 1 (ML1, VAA-1, viscumin), ML2 and ML3

(VAA-2). These lectin fractions comprise a mixture of isolectins, 0.05–0.1 % polypeptides (viscotoxins A2, A3, B and Ps-1), 4–5 % mucilage (galacturonans, arabinogalactans), sugar alcohols (mannitol, quebrachitol, pinitol, viscumitol), and flavonoids (glycoside derivatives of quercetin, quercetin methyl ethers, isorhamnetin, sakuranetin, homoeriodictyol).

- *Pharmacological properties:* Mistletoe lectins have cytostatic, immunostimulatory, and antihypertensive effects. The herb significantly improves the symptoms of chronic joint disease by triggering cutivisceral reflexes and improves the quality of life of cancer patients.

➤ **Indications**
  - Rheumatism
  - Adjuvant tumor therapy
  - Hypertension
  - For prevention of arteriosclerosis

➤ **Contraindications:**
  - chronic-progressive infections such as tuberculosis, and conditions associated with high fever
  - Administration of mistletoe by the parenteral route can lead to protein hypersensitivity.

➤ **Dosage and duration of use**
  - *Tea* (for adjuvant treatment of hypertension or for prevention of arteriosclerosis): Pour 1 cup of cold water onto 2.5 g (1 teaspoon) of the finely chopped herb, allow to stand at room temperature for 12 hours, then strain.
    - *Dosage:* One to two cups per day.
  - *Fluid extract (1 : 1)*, prepared using diluted ethanol: 1–3 mL three times a day.
  - *Daily dose:* 10 g of the herb.
  - *Tincture (1 : 10):* 20 drops to 1 mL three times a day.

➤ **Adverse effects:** Mistletoe is not toxic when administered via the oral route. Parenteral administration of mistletoe extract can induce local skin reactions (mainly wheals, sometimes necrosis), chills, fever, headaches, anginal complaints, orthostatic circulatory disorders, and allergic reactions. Wheal formation and elevated body temperature are considered to be signs of the herb's immunostimulatory effects.

➤ **Summary assessment:** Studies on the efficacy of parenteral mistletoe preparations in cancer patients are currently in progress.

✿ **Literature**
  - Monographs: DAB 1998; Commission E
  - Scientific publications: see p. 478; Anon: Die Mistel. Deutsche Apotheke Ztg 136 (1996), 4330–4332; Beuth J, Lenartz D, Uhlenbruck G: Lektionoptimierter Mistelextrakt. Z Phytother 18 (1997), 85–91; Gabius HJ: Mytho Mistel: Anspruch und Wirklichkeit. PZ 140 (1995), 1029–1030; Hamache H: Mistel (Viscum album L.) – Forschung und therapeutische Anwendung Z Phytother 18 (1997), 34–35; Saenz MT, Ahumada MC, Garcia MD Extracts from Viscum and Crataegus are cytotoxic against larynx cancer cells. Z Naturforsch C 52 (1–2)(1997), 42–44; Schmidt S: Unkonventionelle Heilverfahren in der Tumortherapie. Z Phytother 17 (1996), 115–117 Timoshenko AV et al: Influence of the galactoside-specific lectin from Viscum album and its subunits on cell aggregation and selected intracellular parameters of rat thymocytes. Planta Med 61 (1995), 130–133.

Mullein (*Verbascum densiflorum* Bertol.) _____

➤ **Synonyms:** Dense-flowered mullein; Königskerze (Ger.)
➤ **General comments:** Mullein flowers and leaves have been used in a variety of traditional indications (e. g., as an expectorant) since ancient times. The flowers are used in modern herbal medicine.
➤ **Pharmacology**
  – *Herb:* Mullein flower (Verbasci flos). The herb consists of the flowers of *Verbascum densiflorum* B. or *Verbascum phlomoides* L. and preparations of the same.
  – *Important constituents:* Triterpene saponins, iridoids (aucubin, 6β-xylosylaucubin, catalpol), caffeic acid derivatives (verbascoside, acteoside), 0.5–4.0 % flavonoids (rutin, diosmin, quercetin-7-*O*-glucoside), and 3 % mucilage (arabinogalactans, xyloglucans).
  – *Pharmacological properties:* The expectorant and soothing properties of mullein are due to the action of its mucilage and saponin constituents.
➤ **Indications:** Dry, unproductive cough and chronic bronchitis.
➤ **Contraindications:** None known.
➤ **Dosage and duration of use**
  – *Tea:* Steep 1.5–2 g (3 to 4 teaspoons) of the flowers in 150 mL of boiled water for 10 to 15 minutes.
  – *Daily dose:* 3–4 g of the herb.
➤ **Adverse effects:** There are no known health hazards or side effects in conjunction with proper administration of the designated therapeutic doses of the herb.
➤ **Herb–drug interactions:** None known.
➤ **Summary assessment:** Mullein is an old and familiar herbal remedy that should be used in combination with other mucilage-containing herbs in preparations such as cough syrups.
✿ **Literature**
  – Monographs: Commission E
  – Scientific publications: see p. 478; Grzybek J, Szewczyk A: Verbascum-Arten – Königskerze oder Wollblume. Portrait einer Arzneipflanze. Z Phytother 17 (1996), 389–398.

Nasturium (*Tropaeolum majus* L.)

➤ **Synonyms:** Indian cress; Kapuzinerkresse (Ger.)
➤ **Pharmacology**
  - *Herb:* Nasturium herb (Tropaeoli herba). The herb consists of the aerial parts (seeds or foliage leaves) of *Tropaeolum majus* or therapeutically effective preparations of the same.
  - *Important constituents:* Glucosinolates (0.1 % in the fresh plant) including glucotropaeolin and benzyl isothiocyanate (released when the cells are destroyed), ascorbic acid (vitamin C, ca. 300 mg/100 g fresh plant), cucurbitacins (cucurbitacins B and E), and fatty oils (ca. 7.5 % in the seeds) including erucic acid (ca. 50 %), 11-*cis*-eicosenoic acid (25 %), and oleic acid (12 %). Oxalates, flavonoids (isoquercetin and quercetin glycosides), and carotinoids (flower pigments lutein and zeaxanthin) are also present.
  - *Pharmacological properties:* Benzyl isothiocyanate has bacteriostatic, virustatic, and antimycotic effects in vitro. Isothiocyanates mainly accumulate in and are eliminated via the respiratory air and urine. Nasturium induces local hyperemia when applied externally.
➤ **Indications**
  - Urinary tract infections
  - Coughs, acute or chronic bronchitis
  - Diseases of the kidney and ureter
  - Urethritis and urethral syndrome
  - Cystitis
  - Menstrual complaints.
➤ **Contraindications:** Nasturium should not be used by infants and small children or patients with gastrointestinal ulcers or renal diseases.
➤ **Dosage and duration of use**
  - *Tea infusion:* 30 g herb per liter of water.
    - *Dosage:* One cup, 2 to 3 times a day.
  - *Expressed juice:* Daily dose: 30 g.
➤ **Adverse effects:** Higher doses in fresh plant or essential oil preparations can lead to gastrointestinal irritation. Prolonged intensive contact with the fresh plant can cause skin irritation, as it has a slight potential for sensitization.
➤ **Herb–drug interactions:** None known.
➤ **Summary assessment:** Accurate information on the safety and effectiveness of nasturium is not yet available.
✿ **Literature**
  - Monographs: Commission E
  - Scientific publications: see p. 478; Fanutti C, Gidley MJ, Reid JS: Tropaeolum majus and contact dermatitis. Br J Dermatol, 200 (1996) 221–228; Franz G: Kapuzinerkresse (Tropaeolum majus L.) Portrait einer Arzneipflanze. Z Phytother 17 (1996), 255–622; Pintao AM, Pais MS, Coley H, Kelland LR, Judson IR: In vitro and in vivo antitumor activity of benzyl isothiocyanate: a natural product from Tropaeolum majus. Planta Med, 61 (1995) 233–236, Jun.

Nettle: Stinging Nettle (*Urtica dioica* L.), Small Nettle (*Urtica urens*)

➤ **Synonyms:** Common nettle; Brennesselkraut (Ger.)
➤ **General comments:** The fresh or dried aerial and subterranean parts of *Urtica* spp., collected at the time of flowering, are used in medicine.

Nettle Leaf/Herb (Urticae folium/herba)

➤ **Pharmacology**
  – *Herb:* Nettle leaf/herb (Urticae folium/herba). The herb consists of the fresh or dried aerial parts of *Urtica dioica* L., *Urtica urens* L. and/or their hybrids collected at the time of flowering, and preparations of the same.
  – *Important constituents:* Histamine, serotonin, leukotriene, acetylcholine, formic acid, 0.7 – 1.8 % flavonoids (rutin, 0.1 – 0.6 %, isoquercetin, 0.2 %), and silicic acid (1 – 5 %).
  – *Pharmacological properties:* Nettle leaf/herb is an aquaretic that also promotes the excretion of uric acid. It can eliminate edemas when taken with an ample volume of fluids. Local anesthetic and analgesic effects have been observed in animals by external use of the tincture. The drug inhibits leukotriene and prostaglandin synthesis in vitro. Significant antirheumatic and antiarthritic effects have been observed in studies with large numbers of patients.

➤ **Indications**
  – Rheumatic complaints
  – Urinary tract infections
  – Renal or urinary calculi
  – External use for rheumatic pain (nettle spirit).

➤ **Contraindications:** The drug is not recommended in patients with cardiac or renal edema.

➤ **Dosage and duration of use**
  – *Internal use:* Daily dose: 4 – 6 g drug. An adequate intake of fluids (at least 2 liters per day) is essential for aquaresis.
  – *Tea:* Place 1.5 g (2 teaspoons) of the finely chopped herb in cold water, bring to a boil and steep for 10 minutes (1 teaspoon = ca. 0.8 g drug).
    • *Dosage*: One cup, several times a day.
  – *External use:* Tincture/spirit (1 : 10).

➤ **Adverse effects:** None known.

➤ **Herb–drug interactions:** None known

➤ **Common misconceptions:** In folk medicine, nettle herb is used for treatment of diabetes mellitus, but the efficacy of the herb in this indication has never been scientifically validated.

➤ **Summary assessment:** The anti-inflammatory effect of the drug has been evaluated in an increasing number of uncontrolled clinical studies.

✿ **Literature**
  – Monographs: BHP 96; DAB 1998; DAB 86; ESCOP; Commission E, Mar 31
  – Scientific publications: see p. 478; Anon: Vet Hum Toxicol 24 (1982), 247; Chaurasia N, Wichtl M: Planta Med 53 (1987), 432; Hughes RE et al: J Sci Food Agric 31 (1980), 1279; Kern W, List PH, Hörhammer L (Ed): Hagers Handbuch der Pharmazeutischen Praxis. 4. Aufl., Bde. 1 – 8, Springer Verlag Berlin, Heidelberg, New York 1969; Lewin L: Gifte und Vergiftungen.

6. Aufl., Nachdruck, Haug Verlag, Heidelberg, New York 1992; Schiebel-Schlosser G: Die Brennessel. PTA 8 (1994), 53; Schilcher H: Urtica-Arten – Die Brennessel. Z Phytother 9 (1988), 160; Schomakers J, Bollbach FD, Hagels H: Brennesselkraut – Phytochemische und anatomische Unterscheidung der Herba-Drogen von Urtica dioica und U. urens. Deutsche Apotheker Ztg 35 (1995), 578–584.

Nettle Root (Urticae radix et rhizoma)

➤ General comments: See page 97.
➤ **Pharmacology**
  – *Herb:* Nettle root and rhizome (Urticae radix et rhizoma). The drug consists of the dried roots and rhizomes of *Urtica dioica* L. (common nettle), *Urtica urens* L. (small nettle), hybrids of these species, and/or other wild species in North America.
  – *Important constituents:* Sterols (0.03–0.6 % β-sitosterol), 0.1 % lectins (Urtica dioica agglutinin) and polysaccharides (glucans, glucogalacturonans, acid arabinogalactans).
  – *Pharmacological properties:* Immunomodulation (due to lectin content); inhibits the transformation of testosterone to estradiol in the prostate; increases the flow of urine and decreases irritation and discomfort in stages I to II of benign prostatic hyperplasia.
➤ **Indications**
  – Prostate problems
  – Irritable bladder
➤ **Contraindications:** The herb is not recommended in patients with cardiac or renal edema.
➤ **Dosage and duration of use**
  – *Tea:* Place 1.5 g (1 heaped teaspoon) coarsely powdered drug in a vessel containing at least 200 mL of cold water, boil for 1 minute, then cover and steep for 10 minutes.
  – *Dry extract:* Manufactured with 8.3–12.5 parts herb to 1 part ethanol 60 %. Dosage: 120 mg, two times a day in capsule or tablet form.
  – *Daily dose:* 4–6 g herb.
➤ **Adverse effects:** Mild gastrointestinal symptoms can occur as an occasional side effect.
➤ **Herb–drug interactions:** None known.
➤ **Summary assessment:** Clinical studies on the efficacy of nettle root in benign prostatic hyperplasia are highly suggestive of efficacy, but not conclusive.
✿ **Literature**
  – Monographs: DAB 1998; ESCOP; Commission E
  – Scientific publications: see p. 478; Ganßer D, Spiteller G: Aromatase inhibitors from Urtica dioica. Planta Med 61 (1995), 138–140; Sonnenschein R: Untersuchung der Wirksamkeit eines prostatotropen Phytotherapeutikums (Urtica plus) bei benigner Prostatahyperplasie und Prostatitis – eine prospektive multizentrische Studie. Urologe [B] 27 (1987), 232–237; Wagner H et al: Studies on the binding of Urtica dioica agglutinin (UDA) and other lectins in an in vitro epidermal growth factor receptor test. Phytomedicine 1 (1994), 287–290; Wagner H, Willer F, Samtleben R, Boos G: Search for the antiprostatic principle of stinging nettle (Urtica dioica) roots. Phytomedicine 1 (1994), 213–224.

Oak (*Quercus robur* L.) _____

➤ **General comments:** The common or pedunculate oak (*Quercus robur*) is distinct from the sessile or durmast oak (*Quercus petraea*). There are no significant differences in the concentrations of active substances in the bark of the two species. The tree is common in Europe, Asia Minor, and the Caucasus. Bark from a number of oak species is collected in North America, especially *Quercus alba*, white oak.

➤ **Pharmacology**
  – *Herb:* Oak bark (Quercus cortex), consists of the dried bark from young branches and twigs of *Quercus robur* L. and/or *Quercus petraea* (M.) L. collected in the spring and preparations of the same.
    • *Important constituents:* Tannins (12–16 %), including catechins, oligomeric proanthocyanidins, and gallotannins.
    • *Pharmacological properties:* The tannins have astringent, anti-inflammatory, antiviral, and anthelmintic effects.

➤ **Indications**:
  – External use for: inflammatory skin complaints of various causes and
  – Topical treatment of mild inflammations of the mouth and throat or genital and anal region
  – Internal use for unspecific acute diarrhea.
  ◉ *Warning:* A physician should be consulted if diarrhea persists for more than 3 to 4 days.

➤ **Contraindications:** External use: extensive skin damage.

➤ **Dosage and duration of use**
  – *Internal use*: Tea: Add 1 g finely chopped or coarsely powdered dried bark to cold water, bring to a boil and steep (1 teaspoon = ca. 3 g drug).
  – *Daily dose*: 3 g dried bark.
  – *External use*
    • *Gargles and compresses:* Bring 2 tablespoons of the finely cut dried bark to a boil in 3 cups of water. For inflammations of the mouth and throat, gargle with the solution several times a day.
    • *For hydrotherapy:* Boil 5 g of the dried bark in 1 liter of water. Use the infusion to prepare a full or partial bath. The patient should bathe for 20 minutes at 32–37 °C once a week initially, then 2 to 3 times a week thereafter.

➤ **Adverse effects:** No known health hazards. When used internally, the secreto-inhibitory effects of the drug can cause indigestion. Tannins can cause bowel irritation in some individuals when the strong tea is taken on an empty stomach.

➤ **Herb–drug interactions:** Oak bark interferes with the absorption of alkaloids and other alkaline drugs.

➤ **Summary assessment:** Oak bark has an empirically proven efficacy for the specified indications.

✿ **Literature**
  – Monographs: Commission E
  – Scientific publications: see p. 478; König M et al: Ellegitannins and complex tannins from Quercus petraea bark. J Nat Prod 57 (1994), 1411–1415; Pallenbach E, Scholz E, König M, Rimpler H: Proanthocyanidins from Quercus petraea bark. Planta Med 59 (1993), 264.

Oregon Grape (*Mahonia aquifolium* [Pursh.] Nutt.)

➤ **Synonyms:** *Berberis aquifolia*, holly-leaved barberry; Mahonie (Ger.)

➤ **General comments:** Oregon grape is a shrub native to the Pacific region of the United States. In Europe, it is grown as an ornamental plant and can sometimes be found growing wild.

➤ **Pharmacology**
  – *Herb:* Oregon grape bark (Mahoniae cortex). The herb consists of the bark of the branches and twigs as well as the branch tips of *Mahonia aquifolium* (Pursh.) Nutt.
  – *Important constituents:* Isoquinoline alkaloids (root bark 7–16 %, trunk bark 2–4.5 %), berberine, berbamine, oxyacanthine, and isocorydine.
  – *Pharmacological properties:* Oregon grape bark contains bitters that are useful for treating lack of appetite. The herb also may have antipsoriatic effects when applied externally.

➤ **Indications**
  – Dyspeptic complaints
  – Eczema, boils, and acne
  – Psoriasis

➤ **Contraindications:** None known.

➤ **Dosage and duration of use**
  – *Decoction or powder:* One dose equals: 1–2 g of the herb.
  – *Fluid extract:* Maximum dose: 1–2 mL, 3 times a day.

➤ **Adverse effects:** There are no known health hazards or side effects in conjunction with proper administration of the designated therapeutic doses of the herb.

➤ **Herb–drug interactions:** None known.

➤ **Summary assessment:** Oregon grape bark can be tried in mild to moderate psoriasis.

✿ **Literature**
  – Monographs: HAB 1
  – Scientific publications: see p. 478; Augustin M: Mahonia aquifolium bei Psoriasis. Z Phytother 17 (1996), 44; Misik V et al: Lipoxygenase inhibition and antioxidant properties of protoberberine and aporphine alkaloids isolated from Mahonia aquifolium. Planta Med 61 (1995), 372–373.

Oxlip (*Primula elatior*)

➤ **See Primula**

Parsley (*Petroselinum crispum* Mill. Nymph.)

➤ **General comments:** Parsley herb and root are widely used in cooking and herbal medicine.
➤ **Pharmacology**
  – *Herb*
    • *Parsley herb* (Petroselini herba). The herb consists of the fresh or dried aerial parts of *Petroselinum crispum* (M.) N. et A. W. H. and preparations of the same.
    • *Parsley root* (Petroselini radix). The herb consists of the dried subterranean parts of Petroselinum crispum (M.) N. et A. W. H. and preparations of the same.
  – *Important constituents*
    • *Parsley herb:* Essential oil (0.02–0.3 % in fresh parsley, ca. 1.2 % in dried parsley) and up to 90 % apiol and myristicin, depending on the variety. Other constituents include furanocoumarins, flavonoids (1.9–5.6 %), and vitamins, especially vitamin C (up to 165 mg per 100 g fresh herb).
    • *Parsley root:* 0.05–0.12 % essential oil (apiol, myristicin), furanocoumarins, and 0.2–1.3 % flavonoids (apiin).
  – *Pharmacological properties:* The efficacy of parsley in humans has not been clearly demonstrated. Stimulation of the renal parenchyma due to the essential oils is assumed to occur.
➤ **Indications**
  – Urinary tract infections
  – Renal or urinary calculi
➤ **Contraindications:** Known allergy to parsley or apiol; nephritis; pregnancy. Irrigation therapy is contraindicated in cardiac or renal edema.
➤ **Dosage and duration of use**
  – *Tea:* Infuse 2 g in a cup of boiled water for 20 minutes, 2–3 times a day.
  – *Daily dose:* 6 g herb.
  ◉ *Important:* An adequate intake of fluids (at least 2 liters per day) is essential during irrigation therapy.
➤ *Adverse effects:* There are no known health hazards or side effects in conjunction with proper administration of the designated therapeutic doses of the herb. Contact allergy is a rare side effect.
➤ **Herb–drug interactions:** None known.
➤ **Summary assessment:** Parsley herb and root should be combined with other herbal preparations with aquaretic and urinary antiseptic effects.
✿ **Literature**
  – Monographs: Commission E

Passion Flower (*Passiflora incarnata* L.)

➤ **General comments:** Several species of passion flowers, of which some are known to be toxic, are native to North and South America, Mexico, and West Indies. The plant supplies a tasty fruit. The herb is used in medicine.
➤ **Pharmacology**
  – *Herb:* Passion flower herb (Passiflorae herba). The herb consists of the fresh or dried aerial parts of *Passiflora incarnata* L. and preparations of the same.
  – *Important constituents:* Up to 2.5 % flavonoids (mainly C-glycosylflavone), and cyanogenetic glycosides (up to 1 % gynocardin).

– *Pharmacological properties:* Cyanogenetic glycosides were found to reduce the blood pressure and stimulate the respiratory center in animals. There is still no unequivocal proof of the herb's sedative or spasmolytic effects.
➤ **Indications:** States of nervous unrest.
➤ **Contraindications:** None known.
➤ **Dosage and duration of use**
– *Tea:* Steep 1 teaspoon (2 g) of the herb in 150 mL of hot water for 10 minutes.
• *Dosage:* One cup, 2 to 3 times a day and 30 minutes before retiring.
– *Daily dose:* 4–8 g.
➤ **Adverse effects:** There are no known health hazards or side effects in conjunction with proper administration of the designated therapeutic doses of the herb.
➤ **Herb–drug interactions:** None known.
➤ **Summary assessment:** Hardly any scientific research on the herb has been performed. Passion flower should be used in combination with other sleep-promoting herbal preparations.
✿ **Literature**
– Monographs: DAB 1998; ESCOP; Commission E
– Scientific publications: see p. 478; Anon: Phytotherapeutika: Nachgewiesene Wirkung, aber wirksame Stoffe meist nicht bekannt. Deutsche Apotheker Ztg 137 (1997), 1221–1222.

Peppermint (*Mentha piperita* L.):

➤ **General comments:** Peppermint is widely distributed throughout Europe and North America. The leaves and the oil extracted from them are used in medicine.

Peppermint Leaf (Menthae piperitae folium)

➤ **General comments:** See Peppermint Oil, p. 478.
➤ **Pharmacology**
– *Herb:* Peppermint leaf (Menthae piperitae folium). The herb consists of the dried leaves of *Mentha piperita* L. and preparations of the same.
– *Important constituents:* Essential oil (0.5–4.0 %) consisting mainly of menthol (35–45 %), menthone (15–20 %), menthyl acetate (3–5 %), and 1,8-cineole (6–8 %). Flavonoids are also present.
– *Pharmacological properties:* Antiviral, antimicrobial, aquaretic, choleretic, and mildly sedative.
➤ **Indications**
– Dyspeptic complaints
– Liver and gallbladder complaints
➤ **Contraindications:** None known.
➤ **Dosage and duration of use**
– *Tea:* Steep 1 tablespoon (3–6 g) of the herb in 150 mL of boiled water for 10 minutes. Sip slowly while hot.
• *Dosage:* One cup, between meals, 3 to 4 times a day.
➤ **Adverse effects:** Owing to its cholagogic action, the herb can induce acute abdominal pain in patients with gallstones.
➤ **Herb–drug interactions:** None known.
➤ **Summary assessment:** Peppermint leaf combines well with other herbal preparations that induce spasmolysis and improve digestive function.

✿ **Literature**
- Monographs: ESCOP; HAB 34; Commission E
- Scientific publications see p. 478; Nöller HG: Elektronische Messungen an der Nasenschleimhaut unter Mentholwirkung. In: Menthol and menthol-containing external remedies. Thieme, Stuttgart 1967, S 146–153, 179.

Peppermint Oil (Menthae piperitae aetheroleum)

➤ **Pharmacology**
- *Herb:* Peppermint oil (Menthae piperitae aetheroleum). The herb consists of the essential oil distilled from the fresh, flowering branch tips of *Mentha piperita* L. and preparations of the same.
- *Important constituents:* Menthol (35–45%), menthone (15–20%), menthyl acetate (3–5%), neomenthol (2.5–3.5%), isomenthone (2–3%), mentho-furan (2–7%), and 1,8-cineole (6–8%).
- *Pharmacological properties:* Peppermint oil has antimicrobial, insecticidal, choleretic, and carminative effects. It induces smooth-muscle spasmolysis and produces a cooling sensation when applied to the skin.

➤ **Indications**
- Dyspeptic complaints
- Colds and fever, runny nose
- Coughs and bronchitis
- Decreased resistance to infections
- Liver and gallbladder complaints
- Inflammations of the mouth and throat

➤ **Contraindications**
- *Internal use:* Individuals with biliary tract obstruction, inflammation of the gallbladder or severe liver damage should not use peppermint oil. Owing to its cholagogic action, the herb can induce acute abdominal pain in patients with gallstones.
- *External use:* Peppermint oil preparations should not be applied to the face, especially the nose or the eyes, of infants and small children due to the risk of respiratory side effects such as respiratory arrest.

➤ **Dosage and duration of use**
- *Daily dose:* 6 to 12 drops. Daily dose for irritable colon: 0.6 mL; individual dose in enteric coated preparations: 0.2 mL.
- *Inhalation:* Add 3 to 4 drops to hot water and inhale the vapors.
- *External use:* Apply several drops of peppermint liniment to the affected area of the skin 2 to 4 times a day. Analgesic effects after application on the temples in tension headache could be proven in clinical studies.
- *Pediatric use:* Apply 5 to 15 drops to the chest and back.

➤ **Adverse effects:** Peppermint oil can upset the stomach of sensitive individuals. Persons who tend to develop gastroesophageal reflux should avoid peppermint oil. Menthol-containing essential oils can increase the spasms of bronchial asthma. Because of its menthol content, peppermint oil has a weak potential for sensitization.

➤ **Herb–drug interactions:** None known.

◉ *Warning:* See Contraindications.

➤ **Summary assessment:** Peppermint oil is an extremely popular herbal remedy with a relatively wide therapeutic range.

✿ **Literature**
- Monographs: ESCOP; Commission E
- Scientific publications: see p. 478; Gräfe AK: Besonderheiten der Arznei-mitteltherapie im Säuglings- und Kindesalter. PZ 140 (1995), 2659–2667.

Pine (*Pinus* spp. L.):
Pine Needle Oil (Pini aetheroleum)

➤ **Pharmacology**
- *Herb:* Pine needle oil (Pini aetheroleum). The preparation consists of the essential oil derived from the fresh needles and branch tips collected in the springtime of *Pinus sylvestris* L., *Pinus mugo* spp. *pumilio* (H.) F., *Pinus nigra* Arnold, or *Pinus pinaster* S. or preparations of the same.
- *Important constituents*
  - *P. sylvestris* L.: α-pinenes (10–50%), δ-3-carene (20%), camphene (12%), β-pinene (10–25%), limonene (10%), myrcene, terpinolene, and bornyl acetate
  - *P. mugo* Turra: δ-3-carene (35%), α- and β-pinenes (20%), and β-phellandrene (15%)
  - *P. nigra* Arnold: α-pinene (48–65%), β-pinene (32%), and germacrene-D (19%)
  - *P. pallustris* Mill.: α- and β-pinenes (95%).
- *Pharmacological properties:* The essential oil has antimicrobial and expectorant effects and induces local hyperemia.

➤ **Indications**
- Coughs and acute bronchitis
- Decreased resistance to infections
- Inflammations of the mouth and throat
- Rheumatism and acute rheumatic fever
- Acute infections of the upper or lower respiratory tract
- Acute (obstructive) laryngitis, pharyngitis, or tracheitis
- Acute rhinopharyngitis or tonsillitis
- Arthropathies
- Neuralgia, neuritis, radiculopathy

➤ **Contraindications:** Bronchial asthma, whooping cough. Individuals with extensive wounds, acute skin diseases, febrile and infectious diseases, heart failure and/or hypertension should not use pine oils as a bath additive.

➤ **Dosage and duration of use**
- *Inhalation:* Add 2 g (9 to 10 drops) of pine oil to 2 cups of hot water and inhale the vapors. Repeat several times a day.
- *Bath additive:* Add one drop of the oil per liter of water. Bathe for 10 to 20 minutes at a water temperature of 35–38°C.
- *Externally:* Apply a few drops of the oil to the affected areas of the skin and rub in thoroughly.
- *Ointment:* Apply a 10–50% ointment several times a day.

➤ **Adverse effects:** Can irritate the skin and mucous membranes or worsen bronchospasms.

➤ **Herb–drug interactions:** None known.

➤ **Summary assessment:** Pine oil is a well-known herbal medicament with established effectiveness.

✿ **Literature**
  – Monographs: DAB 1998; Commission E, Mar 31
  – Scientific publications: see p. 478; Glasl H et al: Gaschromatographische Untersuchung von Arzneibuchdrogen 7. Mitt.: GC-Untersuchung von Pinaceen-Ölen des Handels und Versuche zu ihrer Standardisierung. Deutsche Apotheker Ztg 120 (1980), 64–67; 455; Leung Ay: Encyclopedia of Common Natural Ingredients Used in Food Drugs and Cosmetics. John Wiley & Sons Inc. New York 1980.

Pine Sprouts (Pini turiones)

➤ **Pharmacology**
  – *Herb:* Pine sprouts (Pini turiones). The herb consists of the fresh or dried sprouts (3–5 cm in length) of *Pinus sylvestris* L., collected in the spring, and preparations of the same.
  – *Important constituents:* Essential oil (0.2–0.5%) consisting mainly of bornyl acetate, cadinene, δ-3-carene, limonene, phellandrene, and α-pinene. Resins, bitter principles, pinicrin, and ascorbic acid (vitamin C) are also present.
  – *Pharmacological properties:* The essential oil has bronchosecretolytic and weakly antiseptic effects. It induces local hyperemia when applied to the skin.
➤ **Indications and contraindications:** See Pine needle oil.
➤ **Dosage and duration of use**
  – *Bath additive:* Add 100 g alcohol extract to a full tub of bath water.
  – *Semisolid forms:* Apply the ointment (20–50%) to the affected areas of the skin several times a day.
➤ **Adverse effects:** There are no known health hazards or side effects in conjunction with proper administration of the designated therapeutic doses of the herb.
➤ **Herb–drug interactions:** None known.
➤ **Summary assessment:** Pine sprouts is a well-known herb in Europe with proven effectiveness in clinical experience.
✿ **Literature**
  – Monographs: Commission E
  – Scientific publications: See Pine needle oil.

Primula (*Primula veris* L.)

➤ **Synonyms/related species:** Cowslip (*Primula veris*), oxlip (*Primula elatior* L. (Hill)); Schlüsselblume (Ger.)
➤ **General comments:** *Primula veris* and *Primula elatior*, the species native to Europe, are used in medicine. The parts used are the roots and flowers.
➤ **Pharmacology**
  – *Herb*
    • *Primula flower* (Primulae flos cum calycibus). The herb consists of the dried, entire flowers (with calyx) of *Primula veris* L. and/or *Primula elatior* (L.) H. and preparations of the same.
    • *Primula root* (Primulae radix). The herb consists of the dried rhizomes (with roots) of *Primula veris* L. and/or *Primula elatior* (L.) H. and preparations of the same.
  – *Important constituents*
    • *Primula flower:* Up to 2% triterpene saponins (primula acid A), flavonoids (ca. 3%), phenol glycosides (primverin and primulaverin).

- *Primula root:* 5–10% triterpene saponins (primula acid A), phenol glycosides (0.2–2.3%), with the highest concentrations in the spring (primulaverin).
  - *Pharmacological properties*
    - *Primula flower:* The flavonoids and saponins in primula flower have bronchosecretolytic and expectorant action. In animal studies, the herb was found to increase the volume of bronchial secretions. The herb also contains saponins with antimycotic effects.
    - *Primula root:* The herb contains saponins with bronchosecretolytic and expectorant effects. The herb takes effect by stimulating the gastric mucosa. This triggers the increased production of bronchial secretions due to a CNS reflex possibly transmitted by the vagal nucleus.
- ➤ **Indications:** Acute and chronic coughs and bronchitis.
- ➤ **Contraindications:** Known allergy to primula.
- ➤ **Dosage and duration of use**
  - *Primula flower tea:* Steep 1.3 g (1 teaspoon) of the herb in boiled water for 10 minutes.
    - *Dosage:* One cup, several times a day, especially in the morning and before retiring at night.
    - *Daily dose:* 3 g herb.
    - May be sweetened with honey when used as a bronchial tea.
  - *Primula root tea:* Add 0.2–0.5 g of the finely cut or pulverized herb (1 teaspoon = ca. 3.5 g herb) to cold water and bring to a boil. Steep for 5 minutes, then strain. Sweeten with honey.
    - *Dosage:* One cup every 2 to 3 hours.
    - *Daily dose:* 1 g herb.
- ➤ **Adverse effects:** There are no known health hazards or side effects in conjunction with proper administration of the designated therapeutic doses of the herb. It can upset the stomach or cause nausea if overdosed.
- ➤ **Herb–drug interactions:** None known.
- ➤ **Summary assessment:** Primula flower and, especially, primula root can be recommended for treatment of persistent productive coughs.
- ✿ **Literature**
  - Monographs: Commission E; ESCOP (Primulae radix)
  - Scientific publications: see p. 478; Büchi S: Antivirale Saponine, pharmakologische und klinische Untersuchungen. Deutsche Apotheker Ztg 136 (1996), 89–98.

Psyllium (*Plantago ovata* L. [psyllium])

- ➤ **General comments:** Psyllium and Indian plantain (*Plantago ovata* Forssk.) are related species.
- ➤ **Pharmacology**
  - *Herb:* Psyllium (Psyllii semen). The herb consists of the dried mature seeds of *Plantago psyllium* L., and other species, and preparations of the same. The swelling index of the preparations used in medicine should be no less than 10.
  - *Important constituents:* 10–12% mucilage (arabinoxylans) in the seed coat and iridoid glycosides (ca. 0.14% aucubin).
  - *Pharmacological properties:* Regulates the bowels owing to the swelling capacity of its mucilages. The stool volume increases, the transit time

decreases (a desirable effect in constipation), and intestinal peristalsis is stimulated. When used to treat diarrhea, the herb leads to fluid binding, thereby normalizing the transit time.

▶ **Indications**
  – *For all psyllium species:* Irritable colon, chronic constipation
  – *Additional indications for Indian psyllium*
    • Diarrhea of various origin
    • Intestinal diseases in which stool softening is desired to facilitate defecation

▶ **Contraindications:** Gastrointestinal tract stenosis, inflammation of the gastrointestinal tract (risk of irritation and spasm), imminent or existent bowel obstruction, difficult to manage diabetes mellitus.

▶ **Dosage and duration of use**
  – *Daily dose:* 12–40 g seeds. Allow whole or coarsely crushed seeds to swell in water, then take with plenty of water (150 mL for each 5 g of the drug). Psyllium is best taken on an empty stomach in the morning.
  – Onset of effect after a single dose occurs within 12 to 24 hours. The maximum effect can be observed within 2 to 3 days. A physician should be consulted in any case when diarrhea lasts for more than 3 to 4 days.

▶ **Adverse effects:** Hypersensitivity reactions (rhinitis, conjunctivitis, asthma, urticaria) have been reported in isolated cases. Blockage of the esophagus or intestine and choking attacks can occur if the patient, especially when elderly, does not take an ample supply of water. Drinking two 8-ounce glasses of water is recommended to prevent this effect.

▶ **Herb–drug interactions:** The herb can delay the absorption of other drugs if used concomitantly. Psyllium polysaccharides can increase the effects of insulin or oral antidiabetic drugs.

▶ **Summary assessment:** Psyllium is an herb with proven effects. It is well tolerated, even by children. Clinical studies on the efficacy of psyllium are available.

✿ **Literature**
  – Monographs: DAB 10; ESCOP; Commission E
  – Scientific publications: see p. 478; Anon: Pharmaceutical Care: „Den Mißbrauch von Laxanzien vermeiden helfen". Deutsche Apotheker Ztg 135 (1995), 1867–1868.

Purple Butterbur (*Petasites hybridus* L. Gaertn., Mey. et Scherb.) ___

▶ **General comments:** Purple butterbur has the largest leaves of all the German native plants. The rhizome is used in herbal medicine.

▶ **Pharmacology**
  – *Herb:* Butterbur rhizome (Petasitidis rhizoma). The herb consists of the dried subterranean parts of *Petasites hybridus* L. P. G. M. et S. and preparations of the same.
  – *Important constituents:* Petasins (petasin, neopetasin, isopetasin), sesquiterpenes, furanopetasin, 9-hydroxyfuranoeremophilane, and pyrrolizidine alkaloids (0.0001–0.5 %).
  – *Pharmacological properties:* Petasins inhibit leukotriene synthesis and have spasmolytic, analgesic, and cytoprotective effects in animals. In humans, they have analgesic effects in headaches caused by nervous tension and are effective in treating psychasthenic neuroses.

> ◉ *Warning:* When pyrrolizidine alkaloid-containing herbs are adminis-
tered at high doses or chronically, they can induce hepatotoxic, mutagenic, teratogenic, and carcinogenic effects.

➤ **Indications**
   – Renal or urinary calculi
   – Headaches

➤ **Contraindications:** Pregnancy and breast feeding.

➤ **Dosage and duration of use:** We do not recommend the use of purple butterbur teas. Only industrially manufactured butterbur extracts should be used. In
that case, they should be used according to the instructions supplied by the
manufacturers.

➤ **Adverse effects:** Purple butterbur tea and native extract contain pyrrolizidine
alkaloids with hepatotoxic and carcinogenic effects. Industrial manufacturers
are able to prepare extracts that are (virtually) pyrrolizidine alkaloid-free.

➤ **Herb–drug interactions:** None known.

➤ **Summary assessment:** Interest in purple butterbur has grown in recent years
because of its efficacy in preventing headaches, especially migraine which
could be demonstrated in clinical trials. We advise against using the tea or
native extracts.

✿ **Literature**
   – Monographs: Commission E
   – Scientific publications: see p. 478

Pumpkin (*Cucurbita pepo* L.)

➤ **General comments:** Pumpkin is native to the Americas, where it is used to
make a variety of dishes. The seeds are a foodstuff, but are also used as an herbal remedy for prostate and irritable bladder complaints.

➤ **Pharmacology**
   – *Herb:* Pumpkin seed (Cucurbitae peponis semen). The herb consists of the
ripe, dried seeds of *Cucurbita pepo* L. and other varieties cultivated from it.
   – *Important constituents:* Steroids (1%), especially 24-alkylsterols, δ-5-ster-
ols, and δ-7-sterols (ca. 0.5%), clerosterol, isofucosterol, β-sitosterol, fatty
oils (35–53%) including oleic and linoleic acids (35–68%), and amino acids
(cucurbitin, 0.2–0.7%).
   – *Pharmacological properties:* The conformation of δ-7-sterols is very similar
to that of dihydrotestosterone. δ-7-sterols have antiphlogistic, antioxidant,
and diuretic effects. The experimental data are hardly sufficient to document the clinical efficacy of the herb. There is empirical evidence of the efficacy of the herb in treating prostatic hyperplasia but clinical studies are
still not sufficient.

➤ **Indications**
   – Prostate complaints associated with stage I–II prostatic adenoma
   – Benign prostatic hyperplasia (BPH)
   – Irritable bladder

➤ **Contraindications:** None known.

➤ **Dosage and duration of use**
   – *Daily dose:* 10 g of the coarsely ground seeds.
   – *Dosage:* 1 to 2 heaped teaspoons in the morning and at night. The dose
should be chewed and swallowed with fluid or mixed with food.

➤ **Adverse effects:** There are no known health hazards or side effects in conjunction with proper administration of the designated therapeutic doses of the herb.
➤ **Herb–drug interactions:** None known.
➤ **Summary assessment:** Pumpkin seed is safe for unrestricted over-the-counter use. The use of commercial preparations is recommended.
✿ **Literature**
  – Monographs: DAB 1998; Commission E
  – Scientific publications: see p. 478; Koch E: Pharmakologie und Wirkmechanismen von Extrakten aus Sabal fructus, Urticae radix und Cucurbitae peponis semen bei der Behandlung der benignen Prostatahyperplasie. Loew D (Ed): Phytopharm. in Forsch. und klin. Anwend. Darmstadt, 1995.

Rauwolfia (*Rauwolfia serpentina* L. Benth.) _____

➤ **General comments:** Rauwolfia is native to Southeast Asia, where the root is used to treat insect bites, snake bites and diarrhea and as a sedative.
➤ **Pharmacology**
  – *Herb:* Rauwolfia root (Rauwolfiae radix). The herb consists of the dried roots of *Rauwolfia serpentina* (L.) Benth. ex Kurz and preparations of the same.
  – *Important constituents:* Indole alkaloids (1–2.5 %) including reserpine, serpentinine, raubasine, and ajmaline.
  – *Pharmacological properties:* Reserpine and other rauwolfia root alkaloids induce sympathicolytic effects by depleting the stores of norepinephrine and inhibiting its reabsorption at the nerve endings, thus inducing blood pressure reduction. Ajmaline has membrane-stabilizing and antiarrhythmic effects. A central sedative effect was observed in animals.
➤ **Indications**
  – Hypertension
  – Nervousness and insomnia
➤ **Contraindications:** Depression, ulcers, pheochromocytoma, pregnancy, breast feeding.
➤ **Dosage and duration of use:** Daily dose of 600 mg herb, equivalent to a total alkaloid content of 6 mg. Rauwolfia can be taken for several years.
➤ **Adverse effects:** Stuffy nose, depressive mood, tiredness, reduced potency. Rauwolfia can impair the responsiveness to external stimuli, thus impairing one's ability to drive a motor vehicle or operate machinery.
➤ **Herb–drug interactions**
  – The responsiveness to external stimuli slows down considerably when rauwolfia is used in combination with alcohol.
  – Combination with neuroleptics and barbiturates leads to a mutual increase in potency.
  – Combining rauwolfia with digitalis glycosides results in severe bradycardia.
  – Rauwolfia decreases the potency of levodopa while causing an undesirable increase in extrapyramidal and motor symptoms.
  – When combined with sympathicomimetics (contained in cold and flu remedies, for example), it can cause a large initial increase in blood pressure.
➤ **Summary assessment:** Rauwolfia is hardly ever used owing to its numerous side effects. Reserpine, one of its alkaloids, is used in multidrug antihypertensive medications.
✿ **Literature**
  – Monographs: DAB 1998; Commission E
  – Scientific publications: see p. 478; Lounasmaa M et al: On the structure of the indole alkaloid ajmalicidine. Planta Med 60 (1994), 480.

Red Squill (*Urginea maritima* L. Bak.) _____

➤ **General comments:** Red squill is distributed through the entire Mediterranean region and is sometimes cultivated in Germany. The cardiotonic effects of the plant have been known since ancient times.
➤ **Pharmacology**
  – *Herb:* Squill (Scillae bulbus). The herb consists of the dried, fleshy, central bulb sections of the white onion species *Urginea maritima* (L.) B., collected

after the time of flowering and cut in to transverse or longitudinal strips, and preparations of the same.

– *Important constituents:* Steroid cardiac glycosides (bufadienolide, 1–3 %), glucoscillaren A, proscillaridin A, and scillaren A.

– *Pharmacological properties:* Squill has potent diuretic, positive inotropic and negative chronotropic effects. It also lowers left ventricular end diastolic pressure.

➤ **Indications**
– Heart failure (NYHA classes I and II)
– Cardiac arrhythmias
– Nervous heart disorders

➤ **Contraindications:** Individuals with AV block classes II or III, hypercalcemia, hypokalemia, hypertrophic cardiomyopathy, carotid sinus syndrome, ventricular tachycardia, aneurysm of the thoracic aorta, or Wolff–Parkinson–White (WPW) syndrome should not use squill or glycosides isolated from it.

➤ **Dosage and duration of use**
– One dose equals 60–200 mg herb.
– *Daily dose:* 180–200 mg herb.
– *Standardized powder:* 0.1–0.5 g.
– *Extractum Scillae:* 1.0 g.
– *Fluid extract:* 0.03–2.0 mL.
– *Tincture:* 0.3–2.0 mL.
◉ *Important:* Because squill is so difficult to standardize, the isolated glycosides (e. g., proscillaridin A) should preferentially be used.

➤ **Adverse effects:** Because steroid cardiac glycosides have a narrow therapeutic range, therapeutic doses of these drugs can induce side effects in some individuals. These include increased muscle tone in the gastrointestinal region, lack of appetite, nausea, diarrhea, headaches, and irregular pulse.

◉ *Warning:* Symptoms of overdose
– Cardiac symptoms can range from cardiac arrhythmia to life-threatening tachycardia and/or atrial tachycardia with AV block.
– CNS symptoms are stupor, impaired vision, depression, confusion, hallucination, and psychoses.
– In lethal poisoning, the cause of death is cardiac arrest or asphyxia.

➤ **Herb–drug interactions:** The concomitant administration of arrhythmogenic substances such as sympathomimetics, methylxanthines, phosphodiesterase inhibitors, and quinidine increases the risk of cardiac arrhythmia.

➤ **Summary assessment:** Red squill is a cardiac glycoside-containing herb that can effectively replace synthetic glycosides, especially in cases of mild kidney dysfunction. It should be used only under medical supervision.

✿ **Literature**
– Monographs: DAB 1998; Commission E
– Scientific publications: see p. 478; Eichstädt H, Hansen G, Danne O et al: Die positiv inotrope Wirkung eines Scilla-Extraktes nach Einmal-Applikation. Z Phytother 12 (1991), 46; Majinda RRT et al: Bufadienolides and other constituents of Urginea sanguinea. Planta Med 63 (1997), 188–190.

Rhatany (*Krameria lappacea* Ruiz et Par.)

➤ **Synonyms:** Krameria, Peruvian rhatany; Rhatania (Ger.)
➤ **General comments:** Rhatany is a shrub that grows wild in the Central Andes, especially in Peru. The dried root is used in medicine.
➤ **Pharmacology**
  - *Herb:* Rhatany root (Rhataniae radix). The herb consists of the dried roots of *Krameria trianda* R. et P. and preparations of the same.
  - *Important constituents:* Tannins, 10–15 % (oligomeric proanthocyanidins), tanner's red compounds (phlobaphenes, polymers, insoluble products of tannin oxidation), and neolignans (0.3 % rhatany phenols I–III).
  - *Pharmacological properties:* Rhatany root has antimicrobial and fungitoxic effects in vitro. It also has astringent effects due to its content of tannins and lignans.
➤ **Indications:** Applied topically for gum inflammations and inflammations of the mouth and throat.
➤ **Contraindications:** None known.
➤ **Dosage and duration of use**
  - *Tea:* Steep 1.5–2 g (1 teaspoon) of the coarsely powdered herb in 1 cup of boiled water for 10 to 15 minutes. Rinse the mouth or gargle with the freshly prepared infusion 2 to 3 times a day. Use as long as the symptoms persist.
➤ **Adverse effects:** There are no known health hazards or side effects in conjunction with proper administration of the designated therapeutic doses of the herb. Allergic skin reactions have been observed as a rare side effect.
➤ **Herb–drug interactions:** None known.
➤ **Summary assessment:** Rhatany root is well-tolerated when used externally.
✿ **Literature**
  - Monographs: DAB 1998; Commission E

Rosemary (*Rosmarinus officinalis* L.)

➤ **General comments:** Rosemary has been used as a medicinal herb since ancient times. Its leaves are used in herbal medicine.
➤ **Pharmacology**
  - *Herb:* Rosemary leaf (Rosmarini folium). The leaves consist of the fresh or dried foliage leaves of *Rosmarinus officinalis* L. collected during the time of flowering, and preparations of the same.
  - *Important constituents:* Essential oil (1.0–2.5 %) consisting mainly of 1,8-cineole (20–50 %), α-pinene (15–25 %), and camphor (10–25 %). Diterpenes (bitter-tasting substances), caffeic acid derivatives (rosmarinic acid), flavonoids, and triterpenes are also present.
  - *Pharmacological properties:* Rosemary leaf has weakly antimicrobial and antiviral action, presumably due to its diterpene content. In animals, the herb was found to have spasmolytic (biliary tract, small intestine), choleretic, and hepatoprotective effects. In humans, rosemary oil irritates the skin and increases the circulation when applied topically.
➤ **Indications**
  - Dyspeptic complaints
  - Supportive treatment of rheumatic diseases
  - Circulatory complaints
➤ **Contraindications:** Pregnancy.

➤ **Dosage and duration of use**
  – *Tea:* Steep 2 g (ca. 1 teaspoon) of the finely chopped herb in boiled water for 25 minutes and strain.
    • *Dosage:* One cup, several times a day.
    • *Daily dose:* 4 – 6 g herb.
  – *Internal use:* Because they contain higher concentrations of the essential oil, alcohol extracts are more effective for treating circulatory complaints than the tea.
  – *External use*
    • Semisolid and liquid analgesic preparations containing 6 – 10 % essential oil: Apply 2 to 3 times daily.
    • *Bath additive:* Infuse 50 g of the herb in 1 liter of water. Add to bath water or use to make a sitz bath.
➤ **Adverse effects**
  – Contact allergies have been observed as an occasional side effect. Pregnant women should avoid rosemary.
  – Very large quantities of rosemary leaves are said to cause deep coma, convulsions, vomiting, gastroenteritis, uterine bleeding, kidney irritation and, are severe cases, pulmonary edema and death in humans. However, no concrete cases of this have been reported.
➤ **Herb–drug interactions:** Can accelerate the metabolism of some pharmaceutical medications when taken concomitantly.
➤ **Summary assessment:** Rosemary is a popular herbal medicament, but there are hardly any clinical data to support its uses.
✿ **Literature**
  – Monographs: DAB 1998; ESCOP; Commission E
  – Scientific publications: see p. 478; Czygan I; Czygan FC: Rosmarin – Rosmarinus officinalis L. ZPZ 18 (1997), 182 – 186.

Sage (*Salvia officinalis* L.)

➤ **General comments:** In folk medicine, sage is used to treat a variety of diseases. The leaves of the plant are used in herbal medicine.

➤ **Pharmacology**
   – *Herb:* Sage leaf (Salviae folium). The herb consists of the fresh or dried foliage leaves of *Salvia officinalis* L. and preparations of the same.
   – *Important constituents:* Essential oil (1.5–3.5%) consisting mainly of α- and β-thujone (20–60%), 1,8-cineole (6–16%), and camphor (14–37%). Caffeic acid derivatives (3–6%) consisting mainly of rosmarinic acid and chlorogenic acid. Diterpenes (carnosolic acid, 0.2–0.4%), flavonoids (apigenin- and luteolin-7-*O*-glucosides), and triterpenes (ursolic acid, 5%) are also present.
   – *Pharmacological properties:* The thujone-rich essential oil and the diterpenoid substance carnosol have antimicrobial, antimycotic, and antiviral effects. Flavonoids are spasmolytic and choleretic. In animals, carnosolic acid and carnosol act in the central nervous system. The tannins (rosmarinic acid) have anti-inflammatory, astringent, and antihydrotic effects.

➤ **Indications**
   – Lack of appetite
   – Excessive perspiration
   – Inflammations of the mouth and throat

➤ **Contraindications:** Pure sage oil should be avoided during pregnancy. High-dose or prolonged internal use of sage is not recommended.

➤ **Dosage and duration of use**
   – *Internal use:* Steep 1–2 g of the herb in 150 mL of hot water for 15 minutes. Sweeten with honey or sugar.
      • *Dosage:* One cup, several times a day.
      • For gastrointestinal complaints, drink 1 cup of the warm tea 30 minutes before meals.
      • For excessive perspiration, allow the tea to cool before drinking.
   – *External use:* For mouthwash or gargle, steep 2.5 g of the herb in 100 mL of hot water for 15 minutes. Use several times a day.

➤ **Adverse effects:** There are no known health hazards or side effects in conjunction with proper administration of the designated therapeutic doses of the herb.

➤ **Herb–drug interactions:** None known.

◉ *Warning:* Heat sensations, tachycardia, vertigo, and epileptiform convulsions can occur after prolonged use (of ethanolic sage extracts or sage oil) or overdose (>15 g sage leaf).

➤ **Summary assessment:** Sage is a well-known herbal medicament that is generally regarded as safe for short-term use.

✿ **Literature**
   – Monographs: DAB 1998; ESCOP; Commission E
   – Scientific publications: see p. 478; Paris A, Strukelj B, Renko M et al: Inhibitory effects of carnosolic acid on HIV-1 protease in cell free assays. J Nat Prod 56 (1993), 1426–1430; Tada M et al: Antiviral diterpenes from Salvia officinalis. Phytochemistry 35 (1994), 539.

Saint John's Wort (*Hypericum perforatum* L.)

➤ **General comments:** In earlier times, Saint John's wort was used to treat a variety of ailments. It has only recently become known as a remedy for psychological disorders. *Dioscorides* recommended the herb for easing pain of sciatica.

➤ **Pharmacological properties**
  – *Herb:* Saint John's wort (Hyperici herba). The herb consists of the fresh plant material or dried aerial parts of *Hypericum perforatum* L., collected during the time of flowering, and preparations of the same.
  – *Important constituents:* Anthracene derivatives, 0.1–0.15 % (hypericin, pseudohypericin), flavonoids, 2–4 % (hyperoside, 0.7 %, quercetin, rutin), acylphloroglucinols, 2–4 % (hyperforin), essential oil (0.1–1 %), oligomeric procyanidins, and other catechinic tannins (6.5–15 %).
  – *Note:* Plants with the highest hypericin content generally have the highest content of all other constituents.
  – *Pharmacological properties*
    • Oral hypericum preparations have mild sedative, antidepressant, and anxiolytic effects (probably due to synergistic effects of the constituents).
    • Oily topical hypericum preparations have mainly antiphlogistic effects due to their high content of flavonoids; they also exhibit antibacterial, antiviral, and immunomodulatory action.

➤ **Indications**
  – *Internal use:* Depressive mood, anxiety
  – *External use* (oily preparations): Contusions, wounds, burns

➤ **Contraindications:** None known.

➤ **Dosage and duration of use**
  – *Tincture:* Extract 20 g of the herb in 100 g of 70 % ethanol and filter. Store away from light. Take 3–4 mL three times a day. The mean daily dose should be 0.2–1 mg total hypericin in any dosage form.
  – *For depressive mood:* The herb preparations should be taken for a period of at least 4 to 6 weeks to assess benefit. Solid and liquid hypericum preparations should be given at doses corresponding to 300 mg native extract (standardized to 0.3 % hypericin, and/or 2–3 % hyperforin), 2 to 3 times a day.

➤ **Adverse effects**
  – Photosensitization (hypericism) has been observed in animals that consume large quantities of the herb, but this is unlikely to occur in humans following administration of the designated therapeutic doses. Nonetheless, fair-skinned individuals should take due precaution when using Hypericum.

➤ **Herb–drug interactions:** Recently reduction of plasma concentrations of digoxin and cyclosporin and some antiretroviral drugs has been described. Further intense research is going on in this field.

➤ **Summary assessment:** Hypericum is an effective herb for treatment of mild to moderate depression and in the other specified indications. The effectiveness of the drug has been investigated quite thoroughly in a large number of human studies. Some controlled studies show equivalent antidepressive effects to tricyclic and SSRI antidepressants with less than half the side effects.

✿ **Literature**
  – Monographs: ESCOP; Commission E
  – Scientific publications: see p. 478; Saint John's wort for depression: a meta-analysis of well-defined clinical trials. Kim HL, Streltzer J, Goebert D. J Nerv Ment Dis 187(9) (1999), 532–538; Hänsgen KD: Vesper, J.: Antidepressive Wirksamkeit eines hochdosierten Hypericum-Extraktes. Münch Med Wschr 138 (1996), 29–33; Rammert K: Phytopharmaka: Johanniskraut als Antidepressivum. Deutsche Apotheker Ztg 136 (1996), 4131–4132; Teuscher E, Lindequist U: Biogene Gifte – Biologie, Chemie, Pharmakologie 2. Aufl., Fischer Verlag Stuttgart 1994.

Saw Palmetto (*Serenoa repens* Bartram Small)

➤ **General comments:** Saw palmetto grows wild in the southeastern region of the United States. Its berries were first introduced to contemporary herbal medicine towards the beginning of the twentieth century.

➤ **Pharmacology**
  – *Herb:* Saw palmetto fruit (Sabal fructus, Serenoae repentis fructus). The herb consists of the ripe, dried fruit of *Serenoa repens* (B.) S. (syn. *Sabal serrulata* [M] N. et S.) and preparations of the same.
  – *Important constituents:* Steroids (β-sitosterol and its glucosides), flavonoids, water-soluble polysaccharides, and a fatty oil consisting of 80 % lauric, myristic, and oleic acids, two-thirds of which are present as free fatty acids.
  – *Pharmacological properties:* In animals, lipophilic saw palmetto fruit extracts inhibited testosterone production at the cytosol receptors, thus causing significant inhibition of prostatic growth. Owing to its β-sitosterol content, it increases the uterine weight of female mice after injection. Saw palmetto extracts have antiandrogenic and antiestrogenic effects. Lipophilic extracts of the herb induce spasmolysis of the smooth muscles of organs. The extract was found to have antiexudative and decongestive effects in animals and also promotes the degradation of prostaglandins and leukotrienes. Saw palmetto improves the urinary flow rate and reduces the residual urine volume in patients with grades I and II of prostatic hyperplasia (Alken).

➤ **Indications**
  – Urinary tract infections
  – Benign prostatic hyperplasia grades I and II

➤ **Contraindications:** None known.

➤ **Dosage and duration of use**
  – *Daily dose:* 1–2 g herb or 320 mg lipophilic extract (standardized preparations made with supercritical carbon dioxide or hexane extraction techniques). (Supercritical carbon dioxide extracts are made with carbon dioxide at a temperature and pressure at which it is in a state between liquid and gas [the "supercritical state"], which preserves delicate fatty acids, and leaves no residues in the finished product as with hexane-extracted fruits. Supercritical extracts are preferred in North America.

➤ **Adverse effects:** There are no known health hazards or side effects in conjunction with proper administration of the designated therapeutic doses of the herb. Stomach complaints have been observed as a rare side effect.

➤ **Herb–drug interactions:** None known.

◎ *Warning:* Malignant disease or retention of urine should be ruled out before taking saw palmetto.

▶ **Summary assessment:** Saw palmetto fruit extracts are effective in treating problems associated with prostatic hyperplasia and irritable bladder, but do not affect the size of the prostate.

▶ **Literature**
  - Monographs: ESCOP; Commission E
  - Scientific publications: see p. 478; Bach D, Ebeling, L: Long-term drug treatment of benign prostatic hyperplasia – Results of a prospective 3-year multicenter study using Sabal extract IDS 89. Phytomedicine 3 (1996), 105–111; Engelmann U: Phytopharmaka und Synthetika bei der Behandlung der benignen Prostatahypertrophie. Z Phytother 18 (1997), 13–19; Plosker GL, Brogden RN: Serenoa repens (Permixon): A review of its pharmacological and therapeutic efficacy in benign prostatic hyperplasia. Drugs & Aging 9 (1996), 379–395; Ravenna L et al: Effects of the lipidosterolic extract of Serenoa repens (Permixon) on human prostatic cell lines. Prostate 29 (1996), 219–230; Shimada H et al: Biological active acylglycerides from the berries of saw-palmetto (Serenoa repens). J Nat Prod 60 (1997), 417–418.

Silverweed (*Potentilla anserina* L.)

▶ **Synonyms:** Goosewort, wild agrimony; Gänsefingerkraut (Ger.)
▶ **Pharmacology**
  - *Herb:* Silverweed (Potentillae anserinae herba). The herb consists of the fresh or dried leaves and flowers of *Potentilla anserina* L. collected shortly before or during the time of flowering, and preparations of the same.
  - *Important constituents:* 5–10 % tannins (ellagitannins).
  - *Pharmacological properties:* Tannins have astringent action.
▶ **Indications**
  - Unspecific diarrhea
  - Inflammations of the mouth and throat
  - Symptoms of dysmenorrhea (traditional use)
▶ **Contraindications:** None known.
▶ **Dosage and duration of use**
  - *Tea:* Steep 2 g of the finely chopped herb in 1 cup of boiled water for 10 minutes (1 teaspoon = ca. 0.7 g drug).
    • *Dosage:* One cup of the freshly prepared tea between meals, 3 times a day.
  - *Daily dose:* 4–6 g herb.
  - *Topical use:* Rinse the mouth with an infusion of the herb several times a day. The infusion is made by steeping 4 g of the herb in ¹/₂ liter of hot water for 15 minutes.
▶ **Adverse effects:** None known.
▶ **Herb–drug interactions:** None known.
▶ **Summary assessment:** This drug is safe for unrestricted over-the-counter use.
✿ **Literature**
  - Monographs: Commission E
  - Scientific publications: see p. 478; Kombal R, Glasl H: Flavan-3-ols and flavonoids from Potentilla anserina. Planta Med 61 (1995), 484–485; Schimmer O, Lindenbaum M: Tannins with antimutagenic properties in the herb of Alchemilla species and Potentilla anserina. Planta Med 61 (1995), 141–145.

Sundew (*Drosera rotundifolia* L.)

- ➤ **Synonyms:** Round-leaved sundew; Sonnentau (Ger.)
- ➤ **General comments:** Sundew is distributed through the entire Northern Hemisphere and is typically found on moist or marshy soils. Various sundew species are used in medicine.
- ➤ **Pharmacology**
  - *Herb:* Sundew herb (Droserae herba). The herb consists of the dried aerial and subterranean parts of *Drosera rotundifolia* L.
  - *Important constituents:* Flavonoids, anthocyans, and naphthalene derivatives (naphthoquinones, 0.5 %, such as plumbagin).
  - *Pharmacological properties:* The herb was found to exert antimicrobial, secretolytic, bronchospasmolytic, and antitussive effects in animals. Plumbagin inhibits the synthesis of prostaglandins in vitro. An immunomodulatory effect has also been proposed.
- ➤ **Indications:** Coughs and bronchitis.
- ➤ **Contraindications:** None known.
- ➤ **Dosage and duration of use**
  - *Tea:* Steep 1–2 g of the herb in boiled water for 10 minutes.
    - *Dosage:* One cup, 3 to 4 times a day.
    - *Mean daily dose:* 3 g herb.
  - *Tincture (1 : 5):* 1–3 mL, 2 or 3 times a day.
- ➤ **Adverse effects:** Plumbagin can induce allergic side effects.
- ➤ **Herb–drug interactions:** None known.
- ➤ **Summary assessment:** Sundew tinctures and extracts are used in many industrial pharmaceutical preparations. The herb is seldom used for tea preparation. No controlled clinical studies on the herb are available.
- ➤ **Literature**
  - Monographs: Commission E
  - Scientific publications: see p. 478; Wunderer H: Zentral und peripher wirksame Antitussiva: eine kritische Übersicht. PZ 142 (1997), 847–852.

Thuja (*Thuja occidentalis* L.)

▶ **Synonyms:** Arbor vitae, tree of life, Northern white cedar; Lebensbaum (Ger.)
▶ **Pharmacology**
  – *Herb:* Thuja herb (Thujae herba). The herb consists of the branch tips and young shoots of *Thuja occidentalis* (Thujae occidentalis stipites).
  – *Important constituents:* Polysaccharides (immunostimulants), glycoproteins (immunostimulants), essential oil (1.4–4%), (–)-thujone (α-thujone, 49–59%), (+)-isothujone (β-thujone, 7–10%), fenchone (10–15%), flavonoids (quercetin, mearusitrin and the biflavonoids hinokiflavone, amentoflavone, and bilobetin), proanthocyanidins, lignans, and tannins.
  – *Pharmacological properties:* The antiviral effect of thujone has been demonstrated in various trials. Topical application of the herb is therefore recommended for viral warts. The polysaccharides in the herb promote T cell proliferation (especially of CD4+ T-helper and inducer cells) and increase the production of interleukin-2. The essential oil is spasmogenic and, when administered in high doses, can induce clonic-tonic convulsions, damage to the renal parenchyma, and cause severe metabolic disorders due to fatty degeneration of the liver. Various *Thuja* species were among the most frequently used medicinal agents, both externally and internally, for treating infections, in native American medicine and in other cultures.
▶ **Indications**
  – Colds and fever
  – Decreased resistance to infections
  – Psoriasis
  – Warts
▶ **Contraindications:** None known.
▶ **Dosage and duration of use**
  – *Extract:* 1–2 mL, 3 times a day.
  – *Tincture (undiluted):* No more than 0.5 g, to be painted onto the affected site.
▶ **Adverse effects:** Arbor vitae is toxic. Symptoms of poisoning, especially after abuse of the herb as an abortifacient, include nausea, vomiting, painful diarrhea, and mucosal bleeding. Fatalities have been reported.
◉ *Warning*
  – **Poisoning:** All cases of poisoning reported since 1980 were attributable to consumption of the leaves and young shoots of the fresh thuja plant. The toxic effect of the herb is attributable to its high content of thujone. The toxic threshold for safe oral administration of thujone is reported to be 1.25 mg/kg body weight. When herbal remedies are administered at the designated therapeutic doses, the thujone concentration remains far below the toxic threshold. A tea is the safest form of administration because thujone is not easily soluble in water.
▶ **Herb–drug interactions:** None known.
▶ **Summary assessment:** Use of thuja should be restricted to commercial preparations and tea infusions.
▶ **Literature**
  – Monographs: BHP 83; EB 6, Mar 31
  – Scientific publications: see p. 478; Anon: Behandlung mit pflanzlichen Immunmodulatoren. Symbiose 5 (1993), 9; Baba T, Nakano H, Tamai K, Sawamura D, Hanada K, Hashimoto I, Arima Y: Inhibitory effect of beta-

thujaplicin on ultraviolet B-induced apoptosis in mouse keratinocytes. Invest Dermatol, 110 (1998) 24–8; Baumann J: Vergleichende pharmako gnostisch-phytochemische Untersuchungen an Drogen der Familie de Cupressaceae. Diplomarbeit Göttingen 1987; Gohla SH: Dissertation Uni versität Hamburg 1988; Gross G: Papillomvirus-Infektionen der Haut. Me Welt 36 (1985), 437–440.

Thyme (*Thymus vulgaris* L.)

➤ **General comments:** Thyme has been revered as a remedy for pulmonary anc bronchial diseases since the Middle Ages. Its use as a culinary herb also date back to the Middle Ages.

➤ **Pharmacology**
 – *Herb:* Thyme (Thymi herba). The herb consists of the stripped and dried fo liage leaves and flowers of *Thymus vulgaris* L and/or *Thymus zygis* L. anc preparations of the same.
 – *Important constituents:* Essential oil (1.0–2.5%) consisting mainly of thy mol (20–55%), *p*-cymene (14–45%), and carvacrol (1–10%). Caffeic aci derivatives (rosmarinic acid, 0.15–1.35%) and flavonoids (luteolin, apigen in) are also present.
 – *Pharmacological properties:* Thyme has primarily expectorant effects base on the herb's underlying bronchospasmolytic and secretomotor action. Ir addition, thymol and carvacrol have antimicrobial, antimycotic, and anti viral effects. The herb has spasmolytic effects (due to its flavone fraction and expectorant effects in animals due to the action of terpenes on ciliar activity. Thyme has excellent antioxidant effects. Controlled clinical studie are not available.

➤ **Indications**
 – Internal use for coughs and bronchitis.
 – External use for supportive treatment of acute and chronic respiratory trac diseases
 – External use for dermatosis-related pruritus

➤ **Contraindications:** Long-term or high-dose administration of thymol and car vacrol, and thyme preparations such as alcoholic tinctures and distilled oil that contain them, can be toxic.
 ◉ *Important:* Use by patients with severe liver damage or impaired thyroic function can aggravate these conditions. These individuals should there fore use thyme preparations with due caution.

➤ **Dosage and duration of use**
 – *Internal use*
  • *Tea:* Steep 1.5–2 g (1 to 1 $^1/_2$ teaspoons) of the herb in 1 cup of boile water for 10 minutes. Dosage: One cup, several times a day.
  • *Daily dose:* 10 g herb with a 0.3% phenol content, calculated as thymol
 – *External use*
  • *Compresses:* Prepare using 5% infusion.
  • *Baths:* Steep 500 g of the herb in 4 liters of boiled water for 10 minutes then add to bath water.

➤ **Adverse effects:** Health hazards in conjunction with proper administration c the designated therapeutic doses of the herb are not known. Thyme has a sligh potential for sensitization.

➤ **Herb–drug interactions:** None known.

➤ **Summary assessment:** Thyme fluid extracts, tinctures, and teas are commonly added to preparations involving multiple herbal constituents. Thyme is an herbal medicament with demonstrated effects.

➤ **Literature**
  – Monographs: DAB 1998; ESCOP; Commission E
  – Scientific publications: see p. 478; Haraguchi H et al: Antiperoxidative components in Thymus vulgaris. Planta Med 62 (1996), 217–221.

Tormentil (*Potentilla erecta* L. Raeuschel)

➤ **General comments:** Tormentil is a plant native to the entire European continent. It has long been revered for its astringent effects. The rhizome is used in medicine.

➤ **Pharmacology**
  – *Herb:* Tormentil rhizome (Tormentillae rhizoma). The herb consists of the rootless dried rhizomes of *Potentilla erecta* (L.) R. (syn. *Potentilla tormentilla* N.) and preparations of the same.
  – *Important constituents:* Tannins (17–22%), tannins of the catechin type (15–20%), gallotannins (ca. 3.5%), flavonoids, and triterpenes (tormentoside, tormentillic acid glucoside).
  – *Pharmacological properties:* The tannins in tormentil have astringent, antibacterial, and hemostyptic effects. Clinical studies are not yet available.

➤ **Indications**
  – Diarrhea
  – Inflammations of the mouth and throat

➤ **Contraindications:** None known.

➤ **Dosage and duration of use**
  – *Tea:* Steep 3–4 g herb in 150 mL of hot water. For diarrhea: One cup, between meals, 2 to 3 times a day.
  – *Daily dose:* 4–6 g herb.

➤ **Adverse effects:** Tormentil can cause nausea or vomiting in sensitive individuals, especially on an empty stomach.

➤ **Herb–drug interactions:** None known.

➤ **Summary assessment:** Tormentil is a useful tannin-bearing herb that is suitable for unrestricted over-the-counter use.

✿ **Literature**
  – Monographs: DAB 1998; Commission E
  – Scientific publications: see p. 478; Geiger C et al: Ellagitannins from Alchemilla xanthochlora and Potentilla erecta. Planta Med 60 (1994), 384.

Turmeric (*Curcuma longa, C. xanthorriza* Valeton)

➤ **General comments:** Turmeric was originally native to India but has now become naturalized in tropical regions of Southeast Asia. The rhizome is used as both a culinary and medicinal herb. *Curcuma longa* and *Curcuma xanthorriza* are used in herbal medicine.

➤ **Pharmacology**
  – *Herb:* Turmeric rhizome (Curcumae rhizoma). The herb consists of the fingerlike or cylindrical rhizomes of *Curcuma longa* L. (syn. *Curcuma domestica* V.) or *Curcuma xanthorriza* Val., which are scalded and dried after harvesting.

- *Important constituents:* Essential oil (3–4%) containing *ar*-turmerone, α- and β-turmerones, zingiberene, α- and γ-atlantones, curlone, and curcumol. Curcuminoids (3–5%) such as curcumin and desmethoxycurcumin are also present. *Curcuma longa* contains di-*p*-coumaroylmethane, a chemical that reduces the effects of the other curcuminoids.
- *Pharmacological properties:* Curcumin counteracts hepatotoxic effects and has antilipemic, anti-inflammatory (in chronic inflammation), antioxidant antimicrobial, choleretic, and cholekinetic action. Curcumin is poorly absorbed from the gut.

➤ **Indications**
  - Lack of appetite
  - Dyspeptic complaints

➤ **Contraindications:** Individuals with biliary tract obstruction or gallstones should not use turmeric, or should consult a physician if in doubt.

➤ **Dosage and duration of use**
  - *Tea:* Pour 1 cup of boiled water onto 0.5–1 g (1 teaspoon) of the herb, then cover and steep for 5 to 10 minutes. Drink between meals.
  - *Daily dose:* 2 g of the herb.

➤ **Adverse effects:** Prolonged use or overdose can cause stomach disorders.

➤ **Herb–drug interactions:** None known.

➤ **Summary assessment:** *Curcuma xanthorriza* is superior to *Curcuma longa* in the treatment of dyspeptic complaints according to empirical reports.

✿ **Literature**
  - Monographs: Commission E; ESCOP (Curcumae longae rhizoma)
  - Scientific publications: see p. 478; Babu PS, Srinivasan K: Hypolipidemic action of curcumin the active principle of turmeric (Curcuma longa) in streptozotocin induced diabetic rats. Mol Cell Biochem, 30 (1997), 169–75; Bonte F, Noel-Hudson MS, Wepierre J, Meybeck A: Protective effect of curcuminoids on epidermal skin cells under free oxygen radical stress Planta Med, 8 (1997), 265–6; Hanif R, Qiao L, Shiff SJ, Rigas B: Curcumin a natural plant phenolic food additive inhibits cell proliferation and induces cell cycle changes in colon adenocarcinoma cell lines by a prostaglandin-independent pathway. J Lab Clin Med, 42 (1997), 576–84; Sikora E, Bielak-Zmijewska A, Piwocka K, Skierski J, Radziszewska E: Inhibition of proliferation and apoptosis of human and rat T lymphocytes by curcumin, a curry pigment. Biochem Pharmacol, 54 (1997), 899–907; Verma SP, Salamone E Goldin B: Curcumin and genistein plant natural products show synergistic inhibitory effects on the growth of human breast cancer MCF-7 cells induced by estrogenic pesticides. Biochem Biophys Res Commun, 233 (1997), 692–6.

Uva-ursi (*Arctostaphylos uva-ursi* L. Sprengel) _____

➤ **Synonyms:** Bearberry, Bärentraube (Ger.)
➤ **General comments:** The dried leaves (bearberry leaf) and preparations made from the fresh leaves are used in medicine. In Europe, bearberry is a protected species and cannot be collected in the wild, but is not considered threatened in North America.
➤ **Pharmacology**
  – *Herb:* Bearberry leaf (Uvae ursi folium). The herb consists of the fresh or dried young foliage leaves of *Arctostaphylos uva-ursi* (L.) Sprengel and preparations of the same. The chopped or powdered drug and dry extracts are used to prepare infusions, macerations, and other dosage forms intended for internal use.
  – *Important constituents:* Hydroquinone glycosides including arbutin, arbutoside, hydroquinone-*O*-β-D-glucoside (5 – 16 %) and methylarbutin, *O*-galloylhydroquinone-*O*-β-D-glucoside (*p*-galloyloxyphenyl-*O*-β-D-glucoside), 2´-*O*-galloylarbutin, 6´-*O*-galloylarbutin, free hydroquinone (0.3 %) and flavonoids consisting mainly of flavonol glycosides such as hyperoside (0.8 – 1.5 %), quercetin, and isoquercetin. Phenolcarbonic acids (free gallic acid: 180 mg/100 g), *p*-coumaric acid (18.0 mg/100 g), syringic acid (16.8 mg/100 g), salicylic acid (12.0 mg/100 g), *p*-hydroxybenzoic acid (9.6 mg/100 g), and 7 – 18 % tannins (gallotannins, proanthocyanidins) are also present.
  – *Pharmacological properties:* Phenol glycosides have antibacterial effects, and tannins have astringent action. Hydroquinone conjugates of glucuronic acid and sulfuric acid have bacteriostatic and urinary antiseptic effects.
➤ **Indications**
  – Urinary tract infections
  – Cystitis
➤ **Contraindications:** Pregnant or nursing mothers and children under 12 years of age should not use uva-ursi. The duration of treatment should be restricted to no more than one week at a time or five times a year.
➤ **Dosage and duration of use**
  – *Tea with bearberry content of up to 30 %:* Steep 2 g of the finely chopped or coarsely powdered drug in 150 mL of boiled water for 15 minutes. Teas with a higher bearberry content must be prepared as macerations (macerated in cold water for 6 to 12 hours). This prevents the extraction of excess quantities of tannin to ensure better tolerability.
  – *Daily dose:* 10 g finely chopped or powdered drug (equivalent to 400 – 840 mg arbutin).
➤ **Adverse effects:** Preparations with high tannin contents can induce nausea and vomiting. Prolonged use may result in liver damage.
➤ **Herb–drug interactions:** Drugs that produce acidic urine weaken the effects of bearberry. A plant-rich diet enhances its effect by alkalinizing the urine.
➤ **Summary assessment:** Definitive clinical studies are not currently available.
✿ **Literature**
  – Monographs: ESCOP; Commission E
  – Scientific publications: see p. 478; Matsuo K, Kobayashi M, Takuno Y, Kuwajima H, Ito H, Yoshida T: Anti-tyrosinase activity constituents of Arctostaphylos uva-ursi. Yakugaku Zasshi, 117 (1997), 1028 – 32; Ng TB et al:

Examination of coumarins, flavonoids and polysaccharopeptides for anti
bacterial activity. General Pharmacology 27 (1996), 1237–1240; Ritch-Kr
EM, Thomas S, Turner NJ, Towers GH: Carrier herbal medicine: traditiona
and contemporary plant use. J Ethnopharmacol, 117 (1996), 85–94
Stammwitz U: Pflanzliche Harnwegsdesinfizienzien – heute noch aktuell
Z Phytother 19 (1998), 90–95.

Uzara (*Xysmalobium undulatum* L. R. Br.) _____

➤ **General comments:** The native inhabitants of South Africa have long used the
root of the uzara plant to treat digestive complaints. In Europe, it was first in
troduced as an antidiarrheal herb in the early 1900s, and is also commonly
recommended for digestive cramps and irritable bowel syndromes today
because of its spasmolytic effect. To date, this herb has not found common
usage in North America.

➤ **Pharmacology**
  – *Herb:* Uzara root (Uzarae radix). The herb consists of the dried, subterrane
    an parts of two- to three-year-old *Xysmalobium undulatum* (L.) R. B. plant
    and preparations of the same.
  – *Important constituents:* Steroid glycosides (cardenolides, their mixture i
    also called uzarone or xysmalobin), uzarin (5.5 %), xysmalorin (1.5 %), and
    pregnane derivatives.
  – *Pharmacological properties:* Cardenolide glycosides (uzarin and xysma
    lorin) inhibit motility in the small intestine and urogenital tract. Because o
    its glycoside content, higher doses of the herb have digitalis-like effects o
    the heart. Clinical studies are not available.

➤ **Indications:** Acute, unspecific diarrhea.

➤ **Contraindications:** Use of cardiac glycosides, such as digoxin.

➤ **Dosage and duration of use**
  – *Daily dose:* 45–90 mg total glycosides, calculated as uzarin.
  – Use of uzara root should be limited to industrially produced tablets or tinc
    tures (to date only available in Europe), to be taken as instructed by the
    manufacturer.

➤ **Adverse effects:** There are no known health hazards or side effects in conjunc
tion with proper administration of the designated therapeutic doses of th
herb. Poisoning is unlikely when the herb is taken by the oral route because the
glycosides in the herb are poorly absorbed and their cardiac action is ver
weak.

➤ **Herb–drug interactions:** Digitalis preparations and other cardiac glycosides

➤ **Summary assessment:** Uzara is an effective herbal antidiarrheal agent, eve
in cases of diarrhea with vomiting. Because of its excellent tolerability, it ca
be safely administered to infants and young children.

✿ **Literature**
  – Monographs: Commission E
  – Scientific publications: see p. 478; Schmidt M: Uzarawurzel. PTA 8 (1994
    498.

Valerian (*Valeriana officinalis* L.)

▶ **Synonyms:** Garden heliotrope; Baldrian (Ger.)

▶ **General comments:** The subterranean root parts of *Valeriana officinalis* L., dried at temperatures below 40 °C, are used in medicine. The drug consists of the rhizomes, roots, and stolons of the plant and preparations of the same.

▶ **Pharmacology**

  – *Drug:* Valerian root (Valerianae radix).

  – *Important constituents:* Iridoids (valepotriate, 0.5–2.0%); essential oil, 0.2–1.0% (bornyl-isovalerianate, isovalerianic acid; sometimes also valerenal and valeranone), and sesquiterpenes (valerenic acid, 0.1–0.9%).

  – *Pharmacological properties:* Valerian has central depressant, sedative, anxiolytic, spasmolytic, and muscle relaxant effects in animals and has a benzodiazepine-like effect on the GABA system. Valepotriates have a sedative effect on the autonomic nervous system. The essential oil has sedative and spasmolytic effects on the central nervous system. The efficacy of valerian preparations depends largely on the quality and freshness of the starting material, the extraction process, and the freshness of the extract. In humans it reduces the sleep induction time and has sedative action during the daytime.

  ◉ *Warning:* Although Valerian tea and tincture do not contain any valepotriates (because they are unstable), they do contain degradation products with similar action. The long-term safety of these products has not been determined.

▶ **Indications**

  – Difficulty in falling asleep due to nervous tension

  – Restlessness, anxiety, nervous agitation

  – Lack of concentration, decreased mental performance

▶ **Contraindications:** None known.

▶ **Dosage and duration of use:** Used internally and externally (hydrotherapy).

  – *Tea:* Steep 1 teaspoonful (3–5 g) of the chopped roots and rhizomes in 150 mL of hot water for 10 to 15 minutes.

    • *Dosage:* 2 to 3 cups a day, plus 1 cup before retiring.

    • *Daily dose:* 15 g herb.

  – *1 : 5 tincture:* 15–20 drops several times a day.

  – *Extract:* 2–3 g herb, one to several times a day.

▶ **Adverse effects:** No known health hazards. Gastrointestinal symptoms are rare side effects and contact allergies are very rare. Headaches, anxiety, insomnia, mydriasis and disturbance of heart action occasionally occur during prolonged use of high doses.

▶ **Herb–drug interactions:** None known

◉ *Warning:* Valepotriate-free preparations are currently recommended for pediatric use since the potential risk of mutagenic and/or genotoxic effects has not yet been satisfactorily defined.

▶ **Summary assessment:** Valerian tea, tincture, and other valepotriate-free preparations promote the induction of sleep. Preparations containing valepotriates are effective in the treatment of daytime mental and motor agitation and lack of concentration; they have a calming effect when taken prior to stress situations. The ability to drive a motor vehicle or operate machinery is not impaired.

▶ **Literature**

  – Monographs: DAB 1998; ESCOP; Commission E

– Scientific publications: see p. 478; Amon: Phytotherapeutika: Nachgewiesene Wirkung, aber wirksame Stoffe meist nicht bekannt. Deutsche Apotheker Ztg 137 (1997), 1221–1222; Bodesheim U, Hölzl J: Isolation and receptor binding properties of alkaloids and lignans from Valeriana officinalis L. PA 52 (1997), 386–391; Hiller K-O, Zetler G: Neuropharmacological Studies on Ethanol Extracts of Valeriana officinalis: Behavioural, Anticonvulsant Properties. Phytotherapy Res 10 (1996), 145–151; Hölzl J: Baldrian ein Mittel gegen Schlafstörungen. Deutsche Apotheker Ztg 136 (1996) 751–759; Jansen W: Doppelblindstudie mit Baldrisedon. Therapiewoche 27 (1977), 2779–2786.

White Deadnettle (*Lamium album* L.)

➤ **General comments:** White deadnettle is widely distributed throughout Europe and Central Asia. It has been used as a remedy for inflammations since ancient times.

➤ **Pharmacology**
  – *Herb:* White deadnettle flower (Lamii albi flos). The herb consists of the dried petals and stamens of *Lamium album* L. and preparations of the same.
  – *Important constituents:* Iridoids, triterpene saponins, caffeic acid derivatives (rosmarinic acid, chlorogenic acid), and mucilage.
  – *Pharmacological properties:* The mucilage and saponins have expectorant effects; the tannins have astringent effects. Clinical studies are not available.

➤ **Indications**
  – Skin inflammations
  – Coughs and bronchitis
  – Inflammations of the mouth and throat

➤ **Contraindications:** None known.

➤ **Dosage and duration of use**
  – *Tea:* Steep 1 g of the herb in 150 mL of hot water for 5 minutes. Sip slowly.
  – *Mean daily dose:* 3 g.
  – *Sitz baths:* Add 5 g of the herb to 1 liter of hot water; add more water as needed.
  – *Compresses:* Soak in infusion made by steeping 50 g of the finely chopped herb in 500 mL of hot water.

➤ **Adverse effects:** There are no known health hazards or side effects in conjunction with proper administration of the designated therapeutic doses of the herb.

➤ **Summary assessment:** White deadnettle is a well-tolerated though weakly affective herbal remedy that combines well with other herbal remedies with soothing and expectorant effects.

✿ **Literature**
  – Monographs: Commission E
  – Scientific publications: see p. 478

White Mustard (*Sinapis alba* L.)

➤ **General comments:** White mustard is an ancient garden and medicinal plant. Its seeds are used externally and internally. Black mustard (*Brassica nigra* L.) has the same uses as white mustard.

➤ **Pharmacology**
  – *Herb:* White mustard seed (Sinapis albae semen). The herb consists of the ripe, dried seeds of *Sinapis alba* L. and preparations of the same.
  – *Important constituents:* Glucosinolates such as sinalbin (2.5 %), which yields hydroxybenzyl mustard oil when the seeds are ground and stirred to a paste with warm water or chewed. Phenylpropane derivatives such as sinapine, a choline ester of sinapic acid (1.5 %), are also present.
  – *Pharmacological properties:* p-hydroxybenzyl mustard oil induces bacteriostatic, skin irritant, and hyperemic effects in the acral regions.

➤ **Indications**
  – Coughs and bronchitis
  – Rheumatic complaints
  – Head colds

➤ **Contraindications:** Gastric and intestinal ulcers, inflammatory nerve diseases. Should not be used by children under 12 years of age.
➤ **Dosage and duration of use**
  – *External use*
    • *Poultices:* Mix 4 tablespoons of the powdered herb with water immediately prior to use (see p. 298 for standard treatment instructions). The poultice is applied to the skin for 10 to 15 minutes in adults, and for 5 to 10 minutes in children. Patients with sensitive skin should reduce the application time.
    • *Baths:* Tie 150 g of mustard flour in a bag and add to bath water (35–45 °C).
    • *Footbaths:* Add 20–30 g of mustard flour per liter of water.
    • Maximum duration of treatment: 2 weeks. Rinse with water after application.
  – *Daily dose:* 60–240 g herb.
➤ **Adverse effects:** Long-term topical use of mustard can damage the skin. The herb has a slight potential for sensitization (and is a potential cause of food allergies). Caution: supervision is always necessary because of the possibility of falling asleep with the plaster in place, which can cause severe burns.
➤ **Herb–drug interactions:** None known.
➤ **Summary assessment:** Mustard is a very effective inducer of hyperemia.
➤ **Literature**
  – Monographs: Commission E

Witch Hazel (*Hamamelis virginiana* L.)

➤ **General comments:** The bark and leaves of the witch hazel bush are used in medicine.
➤ **Pharmacology**
  – *Herb*
    • Witch hazel bark (Hamamelidis cortex) consists of the dried bark of the branches and twigs of *Hamamelis virginiana* L. and preparations of the same.
    • Witch hazel leaf (Hamamelidis folium) consists of the dried foliage leaves of *Hamamelis virginiana* L. and preparations of the same.
  – *Important constituents*
    • *Bark:* 12% tannins (hamamelitannin, catechins, oligomeric procyanidins)
    • *Leaves:* 5% tannins (hamamelitannin, catechins, oligomeric procyanidins)
  – *Pharmacological properties:* Tannins have astringent, anti-inflammatory, venotonic, and local hemostyptic effects.
➤ **Indications**
  – Hemorrhoids
  – Skin inflammations
  – Varicose veins
  – Wounds and burns
➤ **Contraindications:** None known.
➤ **Dosage and duration of use**
  – *External use*

- *Rinses and compresses:* Use a decoction containing 5 – 10 g of the herb and 250 mL water.
- *Gargle:* Mix 2 – 3 g of the herb with 150 mL water and use several times a day.
  - *Internal use:* One suppository 3 times a day; each suppository should contain 0.1 – 1 g herb.

➤ **Adverse effects:** Health hazards in conjunction with proper administration of the designated therapeutic doses of the drug are not known. High tannin contents in preparations of the drug can cause indigestion.

➤ **Herb–drug interactions:** None known.

➤ **Summary assessment:** Witch hazel is a tried and tested herb that has been subjected to intense scientific study in recent years. Only few clinical trials of any significance have been performed.

✿ **Literature**
  - Monographs: ESCOP; Commission E
  - Scientific publications: see p. 478; Erdelmeier CAJ et al: Antiviral and antiphlogistic activites of Hamamelis virginiana bark. Planta Med 62 (1996), 241 – 245; Hartisch C et al: Dual inhibitory activities of tannins from Hamamelis virginiana and related polyphenols on 5-lipoxygenase and Lyso-PAF: Acetyl-CoA-Acetyltransferase. Planta Med 63 (1997), 106 – 110; Mennet-von Eiff M, Meier B: Phytotherapie in der Dermatologie. Z Phytother 16 (1995), 2001 – 2010.

Wormwood (*Artemisia absinthium* L.)

➤ **Pharmacology**
  - *Herb:* Wormwood (Absinthii herba). The herb consists of the dried top parts (shoot tips and foliage leaves) and/or the dried basal foliage leaves of *Artemisia absinthium* L., collected at the time of flowering.
  - *Important constituents:* Essential oil (0.2 – 1.5 %) containing (+)-thujone, α-bisabolol, and *trans*-sabinyl acetate or chrysanthenyl acetate (content of each over 40 %). Sesquiterpene lactones, including absinthin, artabsin, and matricin, are also present.
  - *Pharmacological properties:* The essential oils and bitter substances in wormwood have cholagogue and digestant effects. They also stimulate the appetite and promote wound healing. Sesquiterpene lactones stimulate the bitter receptors at the base of the tongue, thus triggering a reflex to increase the secretion of gastric juices with higher acid concentrations. In patients with liver diseases, 20 mg of wormwood extract administered through a gastric tube increased the levels of α-amylase, lipase, bilirubin, and total cholesterol in the duodenal fluid. The essential oil has antimicrobial effects in vitro.

➤ **Indications**
  - Lack of appetite
  - Dyspeptic complaints
  - Biliary dyskinesia

➤ **Contraindications:** Pregnancy, liver disease.

➤ **Dosage and duration of use**
  - *Tea:* One cup, 30 minutes before meals, 3 times a day.

– *Tincture:* 10 to 30 drops in 150 mL of water, 3 times a day (not for long-term use).
– *Daily dose:* 2 – 3 g herb.

➤ **Adverse effects:** The concentration of thujone may be high enough to cause vomiting, stomach cramps, enterospasms, headaches, dizziness, and central nervous disorders if high doses of the alcoholic extract are used internally. Tea preparations contain much less thujone.

◉ *Warning:* Prolonged use (more than 2 weeks) is not recommended; also contraindicated for pregnancy, lactation, and liver disease.

➤ **Herb–drug interactions:** None known.

➤ **Summary assessment:** Wormwood combines well with other bitter herbs.

➤ **Literature**
– Monographs: DAB 1998; ESCOP; Commission E
– Scientific publications: see p. 478; Roth L, Daunderer M, Kormann K: Gift-pflanzen, Pflanzengifte. 4. Aufl., Ecomed Fachverlag, Landsberg/Lech.

Yarrow (*Achillea millefolium* L.)

> **General comments:** Yarrow has long been revered for its wound-healing properties. It is now used to relieve gastrointestinal complaints. There are numerous subspecies of yarrow such as Achillea asiatica which is used medicinally in Asia.

> **Pharmacology**
>   – *Herb:* Yarrow herb (Millefolii herba). The herb consists of the fresh or dried aerial parts of *Achillea millefolium* L., collected at the time of flowering, and preparations of the same.
>   – *Important constituents:* Essential oil (0.2–1.0 %) containing chamazulene (6–40 % max.), camphor (20 %), β-pinene (23 %), and 1,8-cineole (up to 10 %). Sesquiterpene lactones (mainly guaianolides) and flavonoids (apigenin-7-O-glucoside and rutin) are also present. Azulenes tend to occur in the tetraploid subspecies growing in meadows, rather than hexaploid subspecies growing in forests.
>   – *Pharmacological properties:* The bitter principles (guaianolides) have cholagogic effects, whereas the flavonoids are spasmolytic. The interaction of different compounds (chamazulene and flavonoids) renders the herb anti-edematous, anti-inflammatory, and antibacterial.
>   – *Achillea asiatica*: Has antiulcerogenic activity in rats, and anti-inflammatory effects; contains high levels of chamazulene. Only a few varieties of *A. millefolium* contain chamazulenes. The German Pharmacopeia specifies that yarrow flowers for tea should contain not less than 0.2 %, the Austrian and French Pharmacopeias specify at least 0.3 % essential oil, with 0.02 % proazulenes, calculated as chamazulene.

> **Indications**
>   – *Internal use:* Lack of appetite, dyspeptic complaints, liver and gallbladder complaints.
>   – *External use:* For treatment of spasmodic pain in the minor pelvis.

> **Contraindications:** Allergy to yarrow or other composite plants.

> **Dosage and duration of use**
>   – *Tea:* Pour boiling water onto 2–5 g of the finely chopped herb, cover and steep for 10 to 15 minutes.
>   • *Dosage:* One cup, between meals, 3 to 4 times a day.
>   – *External use:* Steep 100 g yarrow herb in 1 to 2 liters of water for 20 minutes, then add to bathwater.

> **Adverse effects:** There are no known health hazards or side effects in conjunction with proper administration of the designated therapeutic doses of the herb. The herb has a weak to moderate potential for sensitization.

> **Herb–drug interactions:** None known.

> **Summary assessment:** Yarrow is a well-known and well-tolerated herbal remedy. Some species, including most varieties of *A. millefolium*, have little or no chamazulenes, reducing their anti-inflammatory effects. Products from cultivated varieties in Europe, but not North America are required to contain not less than 0.2 % proazulenes.

✿ **Literature**
  – Monographs: DAB 1998; Commission E
  – Scientific publications: see p. 478; Kastner U, Glasl S, Jurenitsch J: Achillea millefolium – ein Gallentherapeutikum. Z Phytother 16 (1995), 34–36, Müller-Jakic B et al: In vitro inhibition of cyclooxygenase and 5-lipoxygenase by alkamides from Echinacea and Achillea species. Planta Med 60 (1994), 37.

Clinical Considerations _____

➤ **General comments**
  – In heart failure, the heart is unable to maintain adequate circulation owing to a decrease in heart muscle function (cardiac output) resulting from cardiac myocyte death. The main causes are hypertension (see p. 138) with increased venous pressures or cardiac volumes, valvular defects, and ischemia due to sclerotic coronary artery disease (see p. 134).
  – The body attempts to compensate for the circulatory deficiency by stimulating mechanisms such as the sympathetic nervous system and by narrowing the blood vessels, resulting in a higher workload on the heart. Additional compensatory mechanisms lead to a further decrease in cardiac performance.
  – Effective treatment measures should be initiated as early as possible to prevent the progression of heart failure.
➤ **Prognosis:** The overall prognosis for heart failure remains poor although the conventional treatments (diuretics, ACE inhibitors, beta blockers, AT_1-blockers, digitalis) are effective.
➤ **Classification:** According to the system of the New York Heart Association (NYHA), heart failure is divided into four clinical stages:
  – NYHA I: Symptoms do not occur during normal physical exercise.
  – NYHA II: Symptoms occur during more strenuous exercise.
  – NYHA III: Symptoms occur during light exercise.
  – NYHA IV: Symptoms occur even at rest.
➤ **Clinical value of herbal medicine:** Hawthorn and digitaloid herbs are used in NYHA I and II heart failure. The current knowledge does not support treatment of NYHA III and IV heart failure by herbal remedies.

Recommended Herbal Remedies _____

Flavonoid-containing Herbs

➤ **Hawthorn leaf and flower** (Crataegie folium cum flore; see p. 74).
  – *Action*: Procyanidins enhance the influx of calcium into cardiac muscle fibers while only moderately increasing the oxygen demand. These compounds widen the coronary arteries and other cardiac vessels, thereby extending the refractory time. This results in an antiarrhythmic effect.
  – *Advantages of hawthorn*
    • Effective and well-tolerated in the early stages of heart failure, especially in patients with age-related degenerative changes in the heart muscle.
    • With a high rate of acceptance by patients, hawthorn leaf and flower have only few side effects.
    • Since flavonoids do not reduce the afterload, hawthorn can also be used by patients with low blood pressure.
    • Hawthorn can be recommended for long-term use, and it combines well with cardiac glycosides, but may have a synergistic effect. This potential interaction should be watched. It may allow a reduction in medications like digoxin while maintaining the same overall therapeutic effect.
  – *Dosage and administration*: One oral dose, 2 to 3 times daily. Relatively large doses over time are needed for sufficient effects. A daily dose of ca. 900 mg hawthorn total extract is generally recommended. The herbal remedy takes around 4 weeks to become fully effective.

◉ *Note:* Tea infusion is not the best way to extract water-soluble compounds from hawthorn. Hawthorn tea therefore has only weak effects and can be recommended, at best, only for a health-promoting effect in the very early stages of cardiac insufficiency, or as a long-term preventative measure.

Digitaloid Herbs

➤ **Adonis** (Adonidis herba; see p. 33), **lily-of-the-valley** (Convallariae herba; see p. 86), and **squill root** (Scillae bulbus; see p. 110).

  – *Action*: The effects are comparable to those of the isolated substances digoxin and digitoxin, but the herbal preparations have secondary effects such as increased urinary excretion (squill) or frequency (lily-of-the-valley).

  – *Advantages*: The herbal preparations have a somewhat wider therapeutic range than the isolated substances, but their concentrations can extend into the toxic range.

  – *Disadvantages*: The absorption of the active compounds in the herbal preparations is generally poor and variable. Hence, their bioavailabilities and potencies are usually low.

  – *Dosage and administration*: One oral dose, 2 to 3 times daily. Individualized dose setting is required.

  ◉ *Warning:* All digitaloid preparations can be toxic (similar to the glycosides digoxin and digitoxin), producing symptoms such as nausea, vomiting, stomach complaints, diarrhea, and cardiac arrhythmias.

Combinations of Flavonoid and Digitaloid Herbs

  – *Advantages*: The tolerance is said to be better than that of preparations containing digitaloid herbs alone.

  – *Disadvantages*: Their therapeutic range is smaller than that of pure hawthorn preparations, and their toxic effects are similar to those of digitaloid drugs.

4.2 Coronary Artery Disease

Clinical Considerations

➤ **General comments**
- The prevalence of coronary artery disease (CAD) is increasing in industrialized countries. This is certainly attributable to a general lack of physical exercise, increased consumption of fatty foods, and cigarette smoking, but is also due to the fact that people now live longer.
- Despite intensive research, some risk factors of CAD are still unknown or untreatable.

➤ **Herbal treatment measures**
- In Germany, topical heart ointments containing aromatic herbs that increase local blood flow of cutivisceral reflex regions are thought to be beneficial in acute functional coronary artery spasms.
- Flavonoids in hawthorn extract reduce wall tension in normal and sclerotic blood vessels. These chemicals are also presumed to stimulate beta-2 receptors and, thus, to widen coronary arteries and blood vessels in skeletal muscle. The usefulness of hawthorn in CAD is therefore arguable, but has not yet been confirmed in clinical studies.

➤ **Clinical value of herbal medicine**
- The recommendations in this section are solely based on empirical experience. Clinical study data or controlled studies on most of these indications are not yet available.
- Once CAD has become manifest, herbal measures should be restricted to adjunctive treatment only.

➤ **Herbal measures to help counteract risk factors**
- Antilipemic herbs: Garlic (see p. 70), artichoke (see p. 36).
- Antithrombotic herbs: Garlic (see p. 70).
- Antihypertensive herbs: Garlic (see p. 70).

➤ **Clinical value of herbal medicine for risk factors of CAD**
- The herbal treatments outlined here are purely prophylactic and adjunctive measures that can be recommended as home remedies. Clinical studies are available.

Recommended Herbal Remedies (Overview)

External Remedies

➤ Aromatic plant medicaments such as **camphor** (Cinnamomic camphorae aetheroleum), **rosemary leaf** (Rosmarini folium; see p. 112), **pine needles** (Pini aetheroleum), **eucalyptus leaf** (Eucalypti folium; see p. 61), and **menthol** (Menthae aetheroleum).
- *Action*: Stimulate cutivisceral reflexes, blood flow and spasmolysis, thereby reducing CAD-related pain.
- *Dosage and administration*: The preparations are applied to the left precordial region of the chest and rubbed into the skin as often as needed.
- ◉ *Warning:* Ointments containing camphor can cause skin irritation and inflammation and should not be applied to damaged skin.

Internal Remedies

➤ **Hawthorn** (see p. 74).

Range of Applications _____

Acute Angina Pectoris

➤ **Hawthorn leaf** and **flower** (see p. 74).
   – *Dosage and administration*: Dose is diluted oil or other balm applied several times daily or as needed for mild pain of angina. Apply twice daily to the left precordial region, or as needed when chest pain occurs.
   – *Clinical value*: Clinical studies have not been conducted. Large inter-individual differences in the effects of these remedies can be observed.

Prevention and Treatment of Early-stage CAD

➤ **Hawthorn leaf** and **flower** (see p. 74).
   – Steep 2 teaspoons of the herb in 150 mL of boiling water for 20 minutes. Sweeten lightly. This mild infusion should be used only for health-promoting benefits.
   – **Hawthorn tincture** (see p. 74): 2–4 mL several times a day.
   – **Extract** standardized to flavonoids and/or proanthocyanins: 1 to 2 capsules or tablets.
   – *Dosage and administration*: One dose, 2 to 3 times daily.
   – *Clinical value*: For low-potency treatment, hawthorn extracts that are not standardized have a smaller therapeutic range than the corresponding standardized commercial products.

Early-stage CAD with Mild Hypertension

➤ **Tea *Rx***: Crataegi flos; Crataegi folium; Visci albi, aa ad 100.0.
   – *Dosage and administration*: 1 to 2 teaspoons per cup, 2 times daily.
   – *Clinical value*: For low-potency treatment. The extract is not standardized and has a smaller therapeutic range than commercial products.

CAD with Gastrocardiac Symptom Complex (Roemheld's Syndrome)

➤ **Tincture *Rx***: Ol. Carvi 5.0; Tinct. Convallariae, Tinct. Crataegi, Tinct. Carminativa, Spirit. Aetheris Nitrosi, ad 10.0.
   – *Dosage and administration*: 20 drops, 3 times a day.
   – *Clinical value*: This has proved to be a very useful remedy in elderly patients, who often develop Roemheld's syndrome.

Long-term Treatment of CAD

➤ **Hawthorn preparations** (see p. 74), garlic (see p. 70).

4.3 Functional Heart Disorders

Clinical Considerations

➤ **General comments**
  – The diagnosis of functional heart disorder is a diagnosis of exclusion. The typical patient complains of heart palpitations.
  – The most common symptoms are "loud" heartbeat, cardiac arrhythmias, subjective feeling of unrest, diffuse left precordial, non-load-dependent pressure sensation, sudden shortness of breath, nervousness, anxiety, rapid fatigability, insomnia, lack of concentration, tendency to sweat heavily, symptoms of heart "agitation."
  – The cardiac work-up usually does not reveal any abnormalities. If any changes are found, they are usually harmless extrasystoles or functional coronary spasms.
➤ **Clinical value of herbal medicine:** Herbal preparations can be helpful because no specific synthetic drugs or chemical remedies for functional heart disorders exist. Beta blockers are, in many cases, either contraindicated or not accepted by the patients.

Recommended Herbal Remedies (Overview)

External Remedies: See Coronary Artery Disease, p. 134.

Internal Remedies (nonglycoside drugs)

➤ **Hawthorn leaf** and **flower** (Crataegi folium cum floribus; see p. 74), **motherwort herb** (Leonuri cardiacae herba).
  – *Action:*
    • *Hawthorn*, see p. 74 ff.
    • *Motherwort* has mild negative chronotropic, antihypertensive, and calming effects. Its use is recommended only as an additive to other cardiac remedies or sedatives.

Internal Remedies (glycoside drugs)

➤ **Adonis** (Adonidis herba, see p. 33) and **lily-of-the-valley** (Convallariae herba, see p. 86).
  ◉ *Note:* Larger doses of any preparation containing cardiac glycosides are toxic.
  – For further information, see Heart Failure, section 4.1.

Range of Applications

Functional Heart Disorders

➤ **Tincture *Rx*:** Extract. Adonidis Fluid., Tinct. Convallariae, Tinct. Valerianae, aa 10.0.
  – *Dosage and administration:* 30 drops, 3 times a day.
  – *Clinical value:* Mild cardiac sedative, useful in nervous palpitations.
➤ **Tea *Rx*:** Leonuri cardiacae herba, Convallariae herba, Melissae folium, aa 100.0.
  – *Dosage and administration:* Steep 2 teaspoons in 1 cup of boiling water. Take 1 cup, twice daily, for several weeks.
  – *Clinical value:* Somewhat less potent than the first formulation.

➤ **Leonuri cardiacae herba** (motherwort)
- *Dosage and administration:* Steep 2 teaspoons in 1 cup of boiling water, or add 1–2 mL of the 1 : 5 tincture to a cup of water. Take 1 cup, 3 times daily.
- *Clinical value:* This prescription is very mild and can be recommended for long-term use.

➤ **Tea *Rx*:** Crataegi flos, Crataegi folium, Visci albi, aa ad 100.0.
- *Dosage and administration:* Steep 1 to 2 teaspoons of the herbs in 1 cup of boiled water, or add 1–2 mL Tinct. Crataegi tincture and 1 mL Tinct. Visci to 1 cup of boiled water. Take 1 cup, 2 times a day.
- *Clinical value:* For mild antihypertensive action.

Functional Heart Disorders with Gastrocardiac Symptoms Complex (Roemheld's Syndrome): see p. 178.

Functional Heart Disorders with Severe Anxiety

➤ **Tincture *Rx*:** Tinct. Convallariae 5.0, Tinct. Crataegi 10.0, Tinct. Valerianae ad 30.0.
- *Dosage and administration:* 15 drops, 3 times a day.
- *Clinical value:* The valerian component provides an additional sedative effect

4.4 Hypertension

Clinical Considerations

➤ **General considerations and classification**
- Hypertension is defined by the World Health Organization (WHO) as systolic blood pressure >139 mmHg and/or diastolic pressure >90 mmHg.
- *Classification according to severity*
  - First degree: 140–159/90–99 mmHg
  - Second degree: 160–179/100–109 mmHg
  - Third degree: ≥180/≥110 mmHg
  - Isolated systolic hypertension: ≥140/<90 mmHg
- Arterial hypertension can be found in 25–30% of the population. The incidence increases with age.

➤ **General treatment measures:** Lifestyle changes should be carried out before initiation of therapy (e. g., endurance sports, dietary measures such as reduced refined fat and sugar intake, weight and stress reduction).

➤ **Clinical value of herbal medicine**
- Although a number of very safe and effective synthetic drugs are available, the patient compliance rates with these drugs are rather low.
- Although few study data are available on herbal antihypertensives, and although they tend to be low-potency medications, many European patients request them.
- We feel that medically supervised attempts to manage hypertension using herbal preparations are justifiable in the initial stages of the disease. Moreover, herbal preparations make it easier for relatively young and older patients to accept the lifelong need for treatment.

Recommended Herbal Remedies (Overview)

Sympatholytics

➤ **Rauwolfia** (Rauwolfia serpentina, see p. 110).
- *Action:* Rauwolfia total extract has antihypertensive and sympatholytic effects due to various constituents, especially reserpine and raubasine.
  - Immediate blood pressure reduction cannot be expected.
- *Contraindications*: Depression, peptic ulcer, pheochromocytoma, pregnancy and lactation.
- *Dosage and administration*: To ensure consistency of potency and for safety, use should be restricted to commercial oral rauwolfia products.
- *Side effects*: Sedation, dryness of the mouth, nasal congestion, reduced sex drive, depression. These effects can be reduced or avoided by reducing the dose.
- *Interactions*: Digitalis or other cardiac glycosides, neuroleptics, barbiturates, levodopa.

Vasodilators

➤ **Garlic cloves** (Allii sativi bulbus, see p. 70).
- *Action*
  - The constituents allicin and ajoene cause hyperpolarization of vascular smooth-muscle cells, resulting in vasodilatation. This is presumably due to a non-potassium channel-related reduction in the intracellular calcium concentration.

- Thanks to their wide therapeutic range (e. g., antioxidant, slightly anti-lipemic, fibrinolytic, and inhibitory of platelet aggregation), garlic extracts are useful for adjunctive treatment of all forms of arteriosclerosis (cf. p. 70).
- The antihypertensive effect of garlic takes a while to become noticeable. The maximum effect develops after around 6 months of treatment. Dry garlic powder extracts have the largest therapeutic effect.
  - *Contraindications*: Hemophilia A and other coagulation disorders.
  - *Dosage and administration*: 600–900 mg per day, equivalent to 1.8–2.7 g of fresh garlic.
  - *Side effects*: Gastrointestinal irritation and allergic reactions are rare side effects. Typical smelling.
  - ◉ *Warning:* Although garlic preparations are unlikely to affect blood coagulation enough to contraindicate it before or after surgery, it is safest to discontinue use before or after major surgery.

Drugs with Unclear Effects

➤ **Mistletoe** (Visci albi herba, see p. 93).
  - *Action*: The antihypertensive constituents in aqueous mistletoe extracts have not yet been identified. They are said to reduce occasional symptoms such as headaches, dizziness, restlessness, nervousness, and reduced exercise tolerance.
  - *Dosage and administration*
    - *Tea:* Pour 1 cup of cold water onto 2.5 g (1 teaspoon) of the finely chopped herb, allow to stand at room temperature for 12 hours, then strain.
    - *Dosage:* One to two cups per day. Tincture (1 : 1) 20 to 30 drops, several times daily.

4.5 Hypotension

Clinical Considerations

➤ **General comments**
  - Hypotension is defined as a chronic reduction in the systolic blood pressure to < 100 mmHg.
  - *Primary hypotension* is common, but clinically significant only if the symptoms are severe. The causes of hypotension are unknown. Fatiguability and orthostasis are typical symptoms.
  - *Secondary hypotension* is rare. It can occur secondary to cardiac or adrenal insufficiency, or as the result of liver disease or cancer. When possible, the causes of the disease should be treated. No clinical data on herbal treatment of hypotension are currently available.

➤ **Clinical value of herbal medicine**
  - Primary hypotension can usually be managed by nonpharmaceutical measures, such as exercise and physical therapy. It does not appear wise to prescribe medications unless the patient is recovering from illness of surgery or is under great physical and mental stress.
  - Herbal remedies for primary hypotension are low-side-effect alternatives to synthetic drugs and chemical remedies, which often fail to provide satisfactory results, especially in long-term treatment. The herbal remedies are safe to use for self-treatment. Clinical studies are not available.

Recommended Herbal Remedies (Overview)

External Remedies

➤ **Rosemary leaf** (Rosmarini folium, see p. 112).
  - *Action*: The essential oil in rosemary leaves stimulates the blood flow and has central analeptic effects attributed to the constituents camphor and cineol. A circulatory tonic effect of the herbal remedy has been empirically demonstrated.
  - *Contraindications:* Heart failure (see p. 132). (See Herbal Hydrotherapy, p. 282).
  - *Dosage and administration*: Steep 50 g of rosemary leaf in 1 liter of boiled water for 30 minutes, then strain and add to full bath or hip bath. Bathe for 10 minutes at 34–36 °C after getting up in the morning and rest for 1 hour afterward.
    - 🔍 *Note:* Rosemary baths are stimulating, they should not be taken before retiring at night.

Internal Remedies

➤ **Rosemary leaf** (Rosmarini folium, see p. 112).
  - *Action*: See above.
  - *Dosage and administration*: Take 5 drops of rosemary tincture (1 : 5) in a little warm water, 15 minutes before meals, 3 times a day.

Clinical Considerations _____

➤ **General comments**
  – The incidence of peripheral and/or cerebral circulatory disturbances is growing since the average age of the population is increasing in many states.
  – Peripheral vascular disease (PVD) is characterized by the development of arteriosclerotic vessel changes, especially in the extremities. Low-density lipoprotein (LDL), elevated cholesterol levels, the coagulatory system, and platelet function play a decisive role in these changes. Their interactions are responsible for the deposition of arteriosclerotic plaques on blood vessel walls. This ultimately leads to narrowing and occlusion of the blood vessels. Since this is related to an oxygen deficiency, larger quantities of free radicals develop and damage the vessel walls by way of oxidized LDL.

➤ **General treatment measures**
  – It is essential to eliminate the risk factors (e. g., smoking and lack of exercise) and to ensure optimal management of diabetes, elevated serum lipid levels, and arterial hypertension.
  – Regular physical therapy and physical exercise are achieved in only one-third of all patients with peripheral vascular disease because of concomitant cardiological or orthopedic diseases and/or lack of motivation.

➤ **Clinical value of herbal medicine:** *Ginkgo biloba* extracts are useful alternatives to the corresponding synthetic drugs and chemical remedies.

Recommended Herbal Remedies (Overview) _____

Symptomatic Treatment

➤ **Ginkgo leaf** (Ginkgo bilobae folium, see p. 71).
  – *Action*: The acetone-based dry ginkgo biloba leaf extract (35:1 to 67:1) received a positive monograph rating. The therapeutic effects of ginkgo biloba extract (GBE) are largely determined by its flavone glycoside and sesquiterpene lactone components.
    • Positive rheological effect (reduction of erythrocyte and platelet aggregation)
    • Inhibits free radical production
    • Increases prostacyclin synthesis
    • Antagonizes platelet-activating factor (PAF)
    • Neuroprotective
    • Improves cellular energy metabolism
  – *Dosage and administration*: Daily dose of 120–160 mg, taken orally in 2 or 3 divided doses, for a period of at least 6 weeks.
  – *Side effects*: Although very rare, mild gastrointestinal complaints, headaches, and allergic reactions can occur.

Prophylactic Treatment

➤ **Garlic** (Allii sativi bulbus, see p. 70).
  – *Action, formulations, and dosage:* See p. 70.

Clinical Considerations _____

➤ **General comments**
  – *Systemic vertigo*: Usually occurs as a result of microcirculatory and macrocirculatory disturbances in the inner ear and is often associated with tinnitus and other hearing problems.
  – *Nonsystemic vertigo*: This form of vertigo is much more common and usually occurs as a result of hypertension, hypotension, cardiac arrhythmias, or decreased mental performance.
  – *Tinnitus*: The subjective perception of sounds (whistling, rustling, or ringing noises) in one or both ears, often due to microcirculatory disturbances.
➤ **Clinical value of herbal medicine:** Combinations of physical therapy and herbal remedies that modify the cerebral metabolism have proved to be effective. The effectiveness of *Ginkgo biloba* on aural vertigo has been demonstrated in clinical studies. Benefit should be assessed after three months of application.
◉ *Note:* Sudden hearing loss is characterized by a unilateral loss of hearing of rapid onset with or without tinnitus. The patient should receive immediate medical attention, because complete restoration of health is possible only if treatment is initiated within the first 24 hours. Herbal remedies are not recommended for causative treatment.

Recommended Herbal Remedies (Overview) _____

Symptomatic Treatment

➤ **Ginkgo leaf** (Ginkgo bilobae folium, see p. 71).
  – *Action, dosage, and administration:* See p. 72.

Clinical Considerations

➤ **General comments**
- *Mental functional disorders* present with unspecific symptoms such as headaches, vertigo, insomnia, lack of concentration, and depression. The later reduction of cognitive and perceptive abilities as well as a loss of intellectual abilities, an impaired sense of time and space, and changes in personality develop as the disease progresses. In the final stages, these patients exhibit affective disorders, lack of motivation, impaired social behavior, and mental confusion.
- *Primary dementia*
  - In around 80% of cases, the death of nerve cells (usually cholinergic neurons in the basal forebrain) or the destruction of synaptic junctions (Alzheimer's dementia) is the underlying cause of primary dementia. Multi-infarct dementia (10%) and mixed types of dementia (10%) are less common causes.
  - Increased oxidative stress due to increased generation of oxygen radicals during ATP production from glucose is a possible cause of nerve cell loss. The radicals lead to lipid peroxidation and sodium-potassium-ATPase inhibition. This, in turn, causes pathological changes in the cell's electrolyte distribution and, ultimately, cell death. In Alzheimer's dementia, β-amyloid is deposited in nerve cells, the role of which is still discussed. At least 30% of persons over 80 years are affected.
  - Multi-infarct dementia is characterized by the increasing recurrence of lacunar infarcts and damage to the cerebral medulla near the lateral ventricle. The high level of platelet-activating factor (PAF) activity is of pathogenetic importance. The increased activity results in increased platelet aggregation, microcirculatory impairment, increased vessel permeability and, ultimately, edema formation.
- *Secondary dementia* occurs as a result of cardiovascular diseases, hormone changes, infections, and poisoning (e.g., drug poisoning).

➤ **Clinical value of herbal medicine**
- Acetylcholinesterase inhibitors have recently been adopted in the treatment of dementia. These herbal remedies should always be administered under the watchful eye of a physician. The effectiveness of so-called nootropic drugs such as piracetam is debated.
- The efficacy of ginkgo extract for symptomatic treatment of all types of primary dementia has been demonstrated in various clinical studies.
- Treatment of primary dementia must be started in the early stages in order to slow down the progression of the disease. A psychometric test should be conducted after 3 months of therapy to assess treatment success.
- In secondary dementia, eliminating the underlying cause is the primary goal of treatment.

Recommended Herbal Remedies (Overview)

Symptomatic Treatment

➤ **Ginkgo leaf** (Ginkgo bilobae folium, see p. 71).
- *Action, dosage, commercial products:* See p. 72.

4.9 Atherosclerosis

Clinical Considerations

➤ **General comments**
  – Half of all mortality in Germany is attributed to atherosclerosis, a disease in which the walls of the arteries degenerate progressively over the course of several decades. Free radicals of oxidized lipoproteins have been implicated as cofactors in the etiology of atherosclerosis.
  – Individuals with high serum cholesterol levels and LDL : HDL ratios of more than 4.0 have a particularly high risk of developing atherosclerosis. This constellation is most prevalent in men of all ages and in postmenopausal women.

➤ **General treatment measures:** Dietary measures are the first and foremost treatment measures. The patient should be placed on a reduced fat diet and use dietary fats high in polyunsaturated or monosaturated fatty acids (e. g., olive oil, flaxseed oil), as well as fatty fish with DHA and EPA (salmon, halibut). Foods with both added refined sugar and saturated fatty acids should be strictly avoided. Therapy should be combined with regular aerobic exercise for best results, according to recent research.

➤ **Clinical value of herbal medicine**
  – Herbal medicinal preparations play an especially important role in prevention. Their therapeutic action is directed against important mechanisms involved in the development of atherosclerosis.
  – Synthetic antilipemic drugs clearly reduce cardiovascular mortality, but are expensive and sometimes highly prone to side effects. Moreover, they are not covered by most health care insurers when used primarily for prophylactic purposes.
  – The herbal alternatives have a very low incidence of side effects and can be recommended for medically supervised self-treatment.

Recommended Herbal Remedies (Overview)

Antilipemic Herbs

➤ **Artichoke leaf** (Cynarae folium, see p. 36).
  – *Action*: Standardized artichoke leaf extract inhibits cholesterol biosynthesis on various levels and increases the biliary elimination of cholesterol, resulting in an overall antilipemic effect. Antioxidant effects have also been observed in pharmacological experiments.
  – *Contraindications*: Hypersensitivity to artichoke or other composite plants; biliary tract obstruction; cholelithiasis.
  – *Dosage and administration*: 320–640 mg extract, 3 times a day, equivalent to 960–1920 mg per day.

Antiatherosclerotic Herbs

➤ **Garlic bulb** (Allii sativi bulbus, see p. 70).
  – For further details, see p. 70.

Clinical Considerations

➤ **General comments**

– In a recent survey on the German population, 70 % of all females and 50 % of all males over 30 years of age were found to have some type of venous disease. Up to 86 % of the US population will have venous disease at some time in their lives.

– Lack of physical exercise, prolonged sitting or standing on the job, and obesity contribute to the development of venous insufficiency (varicose veins). The disease occurs when the supporting and stabilizing connective tissue structures around the veins weaken due to congenital factors, fat deposition, or hormonal changes, resulting in damage to the venous walls and incompetence of the valves.

➤ **Symptoms:** Venous insufficiency develops gradually, with the first signs being tired and heavy legs and swelling of the ankles (edema) in the evening. Increased venous pressure and oxygen free radicals render the venous walls increasingly permeable, allowing fluids, leukocytes, and proteins to escape into the adjacent tissues. This results in edema formation and a reduced supply of nutrients and oxygen to the surrounding tissues. In severe cases, necrotic leg ulceration can also develop.

➤ **General treatment measures**

– It is important to start treatment early, that is, as soon as the first symptoms develop, to delay the progression of the disease.

– Physical treatment measures can be very helpful: for example, regular leg elevation, leg exercises, short exercise breaks to interrupt prolonged sitting activity, treading cold water, losing weight, and endurance sports.

– Elastic stockings should be used regularly, but most patients refuse to wear them.

– In certain rare cases, short-term treatment with diuretics may be necessary. Loop diuretics are not suitable for this indication.

➤ **Clinical value of herbal medicine**

– The efficacy of "vein ointments" has not been conclusively demonstrated. Use of these preparations should be limited to adjuvant therapy of varicose veins parallel to physical therapy and treatment with oral preparations.

– Treatment with herbal medicinal compounds should be initiated in the early stages of chronic venous insufficiency to maintain the decongestant effects of treatment. The herbal measures combine well with physical treatment measures.

Recommended Herbal Remedies (Overview)

External Remedies

➤ **Witch hazel bark** (Hamamelidis cortex, see p. 128), **horse chestnut seed** (Hippocastani semen, see p. 77), **red** or **white grape leaf** (Vitis viniferae folium).

– *Action*: These herbs reduce leakage from the capillaries and have astringent, antiphlogistic, and antiedematous effects.

– *Dosage and administration*: These preparations are gently applied to the affected area, several times a day. Gels are suitable for long-term use with elastic bandages and stockings. Ointments penetrate into the deeper tissues and are therefore more suitable for inflammatory processes.

◉ *Warning:* Inflamed areas of the skin should not be massaged, to avoid the potential detachment of blood clots. Topical remedies should never be applied to mucous membranes or broken skin.
– *Side effects*: Although rare, allergic skin reactions may occur.

Internal Remedies

➤ **Horse chestnut seed** (Hippocastani semen, see p. 77).
– *Action:* The therapeutic action of horse chestnut seed can mainly be attributed to β-aescin, a complex saponin with antiexudative, membrane-stabilizing, antiphlogistic, diuretic, and venotonic effects. Preparations containing aescin stabilize the lysosomal membrane. The therapeutic effects should develop within around 3 to 5 days of oral administration.
– *Contraindications:* Pregnant or nursing mothers should not use preparations containing alcohol. High-dose horse-chestnut formulations should not be used in the last two trimesters of pregnancy or when nursing a baby unless absolutely necessary.
– *Dosage and administration:* One oral 50 mg dose, twice daily.
– *Side effects:* Horse chestnut seed can irritate the stomach and should therefore be administered as an enteric-coated, slow-release dosage form.
➤ **Melilot** (Meliloti herba): The herb is derived from *Melilotus alba* or *M. officinalis* (sweet clover).
– *Action:* Melilot contains antiedemic flavonoids and coumarins with antioxidant, antiphlogistic, antiedematous, antispasmodic, and lymphokinetic effects. The herb does not affect coagulation of the blood.
– *Dosage and administration:* Up to 30 mg coumarin per day (oral).
– *Side effects:* Headache is a rare side effect. Preparations with a high coumarin content can also cause hepatitis.
➤ **Butcher's broom** (Rusci aculeati rhizoma, see p. 43).
– *Action:* Contains steroid saponins with antiexudative, antiphlogistic, and venotonic effects.
– *Contraindications:* None known.
– *Dosage and administration:* Oral commercial preparations should be used as directed on the product label. Daily dose: 7–11 mg total ruscogenins.
– *Side effects:* Although rare, gastrointestinal complaints and skin rashes may occur.
➤ **Grape leaf** (Vitis viniferae folium)
– *Action:* The herbal remedy contains caffeic acid derivatives, tannins, organic acids, and flavonoids such as quercetin-3-glucuronide and isoquercetin and has antiedemic and antiphlogistic effects.
– *Dosage and administration:* Oral commercial preparations should be used as directed on the product label.

Clinical Considerations

➤ **General comments**
  – *Acute catarrhal rhinitis (head cold)*
    • Head colds are most commonly caused by viruses, especially rhinoviruses.
    • The preliminary stage is marked by nasal dryness, often with sneezing or severe itching.
    • This is followed by a catarrhal stage with profuse discharge of watery mucus. Yellowish-green mucus is indicative of a secondary bacterial infection.
    • After a few days, the viscosity of the nasal mucus increases, and the nasal membranes become inflamed, swollen, and congested. Drainage of mucus is impaired, and the local immune defenses are weakened. Sinusitis can develop if marked swelling of the paranasal sinuses occurs.
    • The symptoms of a harmless head cold normally subside within a week.
  – *Acute sinusitis*
    • Acute sinusitis is characterized by congestion of the entire nasal sinus system. Individuals with congenitally narrow sinuses or narrowing of the sinuses due to chronic allergy-related inflammation are especially prone to sinusitis.
    • Sinusitis often occurs secondary to rhinitis.
    • The lack of sufficient drainage of mucus leads to an oxygen deficiency and inadequate mucous membrane function. The membranes start to produce a very thick discharge (dyscrinism) that is an ideal breeding ground for bacteria. The mucociliary clearance mechanisms responsible for transporting the discharge out of the mucous membranes become inactivated.
    • Acute sinusitis is marked by a clear feeling of malaise, usually with fever and unpleasant sensations in the cheeks, eyes, or temples ranging from pressure sensations to severe pain. Earaches can also occur. The condition can become chronic if acute episodes do not fully subside before the next bout. Chronic sinusitis can lead to massive changes in the mucous membranes.

➤ **Herbal and general treatment measures**
  – All patients with respiratory tract infections should drink plenty of fluids.
  – Nasal douches with isotonic saline solution are helpful, especially in the first two stages of acute rhinitis.
  – The sooner herbal remedies are administered, the better the chance of successful treatment.
  – Different herbal remedies have different effects. Some stimulate the immune system, whereas others counteract inflammation. Combinations of remedies can therefore be very useful.

➤ **Clinical value of herbal medicine:** Herbal remedies for acute rhinitis (head colds) are cheap and safe. They do not damage the mucous membranes of the nose, even when used for long periods of time, if administered at low doses. In the case of sinusitis, a qualified physician should determine whether antibiotic treatment is necessary. Herbal treatments are always useful adjunctive measures.

Recommended Herbal Remedies (Overview) ▬▬▬▬▬▬▬▬▬

Antiphlogistics

➤ **Chamomile flower** (Matricariae flos, see p. 47).
  - *Indications*: Acute rhinitis.
  - *Contraindications*: Known allergy to plants from the Asteraceae (aster or daisy family).
  - *Action:* The essential oil in chamomile is not irritating to the mucous membranes. Two of its constituents, β-bisabolol and chamazulene, counteract inflammation.
  - *Dosage and administration*: Inhalation: Add 2 to 3 tablespoons dried chamomile flower, 1 teaspoon chamomile extract, or 5 drops of the essential oil to boiling water and inhale, several times daily (see p. 18). If this is not possible, administer chamomile nose drops or chamomile cream to each nostril, 3 to 4 times a day.
  - *Side effects*: None known.

Cold Receptor Stimulators

➤ **Peppermint oil** (from the leaves of *Mentha* piperita L. (see p. 103)); *Mentha arvensis* var. *piperascens* (mint oil; sometimes mislabeled as peppermint oil) **menthol**; **camphor tree** (see p. 45).
  - *Action*: These preparations stimulate cold receptors in the nose, making it easier to breathe. They also have secretolytic, antimicrobial, and antiviral effects, but do not reduce swelling of the mucous membranes. The remedies are generally safe, except in the specified contraindications.
  - *Indications*: Acute rhinitis.
  - *Contraindications*: Exanthematous skin and childhood diseases, bronchial asthma. Infants and small children should not inhale peppermint oil or use nasal ointments containing menthol. Camphor should not be used during pregnancy or lactation. Individuals with hypertension or heart failure should use it with caution.
  - ◉ *Warning*
    • When administered to infants and small children, peppermint oil and preparations containing menthol and camphor can trigger respiratory problems ranging from shortness of breath and choking to laryngeal spasms or cardiovascular problems. These herbal remedies should never be applied to the face or to large areas of the chest or back of infants and small children.
    • Do not apply peppermint oil, mentholated nasal ointments or camphor to the eyes or to broken skin. Camphor should not be allowed to come in contact with the mucous membranes.
  - *Dosage and administration*: Peppermint oil: Add 2 to 4 drops of peppermint oil to boiling water and inhale, several times a day, or apply 1 drop of the oil directly below the nostrils (school-aged children and adults only). Camphor: Apply the ointment directly to the chest, several times a day, to inhale the vapors. Nasal ointment: Apply a pea-sized amount to the nostrils, 3 to 4 times daily.
  - *Side effects*: Allergic skin reactions and unpleasant local sensations can occur in isolated cases (in conjunction with mentholated nasal ointments). Rare incidences of contact eczema (camphor) have also been reported.

Immunostimulants

➤ **Purple echinacea herb** (Echinaceae purpureae herba, see p. 56);
Paleflowered echinacea root (Echinaceae pallidae radix, see p. 56).
- *Action*: Increases the ability of granulocytes and macrophages to ward off disease. The immunostimulatory effect of echinacea develops over a few days of oral administration. No comparable synthetic preparations exist. See pp. 150, 153 for other therapeutic actions.
- *Indications*: Chronic sinusitis.
- *Contraindications*: Chronic-progressive systemic diseases (e. g., tuberculosis), leukoses, inflammatory rheumatic diseases, multiple sclerosis, HIV infection, known hypersensitivity to composite plants, autoimmune diseases.

  ◉ *Warning:* In severely ill patients, the patient's immune status should be checked before starting immunostimulatory therapy. The expected benefits of treatment must clearly outweigh the potential risks.
- *Dosage and administration*: Liquid tinctures are widely available that include either or both of *E. purpurea* and *E. angustifolia*. The roots, leaves, seeds, or flowers are included in many products, and are sometimes blended.
  • Flavored liquid products that include glycerin instead of alcohol are popular, especially for children.
- *Side effects*: Rarely, allergic skin reactions, which disappear after use is discontinued.
- None of the available data confirms the efficacy of oral echinacea preparations for sinus infections.

Compound Remedies for Acute Sinusitis

➤ We do not recommend single-component commercial preparations for this indication.
- *Action*: See those of the individual herbs contained in compound remedies. Herbal remedies are highly recommended for adjunctive treatment of acute sinusitis.
- *Indications*: Acute sinusitis; adjunctive treatment of chronic sinusitis.
- *Contraindications*: See cautions noted on labels of commercial products.

  ◉ *Warning:* The patient should consult a physician if the symptoms persist for more than 7 to 14 days or re-occur periodically. Pregnant women should not use **echinacea** unless directed by a qualified health care practitioner.
- *Dosage and administration*: Oral preparations should be used as directed on the product label.
- *Side effects*: Occasionally allergic reactions in the skin, respiratory tract, and gastrointestinal tract. Although rare, stomach complaints, nausea, vomiting, and diarrhea can occur.
- *Interactions:* See cautions noted on labels of commercial products.

5.2 Colds and Flu

Clinical Considerations

➤ **General comments**
- Colds and flu are the most common reasons for the loss of working hours.
- Around 90 % of all catarrhal disorders are caused by viruses, especially rhinoviruses. Secondary bacterial infection can also develop. Viral and secondary bacterial infections are especially common in individuals with temporary or permanent asthenia of the unspecific (congenital) or specific (acquired) immune system.
- Drafts, cold weather, excessive indoor heating, stress, and loss of sleep are factors that promote the development of colds. When the body (especially lower body) is subjected to hypothermia or ischemia, it responds by reducing the blood flow to the mucous membranes in the upper respiratory passages. This and the drying of the mucous membranes due to excessive room heating promote the growth of pathogens.

➤ **Herbal and general treatment measures**
- Once a cold has fully developed, treatment focuses on alleviating typical symptoms, such as a runny nose, sore throat, and hoarseness with or without fever. Nasal douches, throat wraps, inhalation, sweat-inducing agents (diaphoretics), and baths with aromatic herbs have proved to be effective. Cold remedies usually contain secretolytic and expectorant herbs with essential oils, mucilage, and saponins.
- Hot baths for colds and flu are prepared with aromatic oils, such as spruce oil, pine needle oil, eucalyptus oil, thyme oil, camphor and/or menthol. See p. 283 for details.
- The administration of a *diaphoretic tea* after a hot bath can enhance the febrifuge effects of the treatment.

➤ **Clinical value of herbal medicine:** All measures that improve the natural function of the mucous membranes of the upper respiratory tract, alleviate cold symptoms, and strengthen the immune system, can be recommended for symptomatic treatment of all virally induced catarrhal disorders. There are no comparable synthetic drug preparations. Self-treatment measures should be coordinated with the help of a physician.

Recommended Herbal Remedies (Overview)

Immunostimulants

➤ **Purple echinacea herb** (Echinaceae purpureae herba, see p. 150); **paleflowered echinacea root** (Echinacea pallidae radix, see p. 150); **wild indigo** (Baptisiae tinctoriae radix); and **arbor vitae tips** (Thujae occidentalis stipites, see p. 119).

  ◉ *Note:* The efficacy of other plant parts of the two *Echinacea* species has not been convincingly demonstrated, although the roots of *E. purpurea*, and especially *E. angustifolia* are frequently thought to be more potent in North America.

- *Action*
  - *Echinacea:* Certain compounds in echinacea (arabinogalactans, arabinogalactan proteins) enhance the body's nonspecific immune defenses by activating the granulocytes and macrophages, thereby improving the body's capacity to phagocytose viruses and bacteria. Activated macrophages secrete interleukin-1, interleukin-6, and tumor necrosis factor-α,

substances that stimulate the specific immune system and protect the cells from viral attacks. These mechanisms are activated when the pathogen comes in contact with the oral mucous membranes.

- Caffeic acid derivatives such as chicoric acid and alkylamides are responsible for the antiviral effect of purple echinacea juice.
- Echinacea juice inhibits hyaluronidase, thereby reducing the permeability of the blood vessels and inhibiting the spread of local infection.
- Clinical and postmarketing surveillance studies indicate that echinacea juice and alcoholic extracts of *Echinacea pallida* root increase the time until the occurrence of a new infection. In those who already have a cold, the course of the infection is less severe and the symptoms subside more quickly. Since many antibiotics can suppress the immune system, these herbal remedies should be helpful in patients with bacterial infections.
- *Wild indigo* promotes the release of interleukin 1 and stimulates the production of interferons.
- *Arbor vitae* stimulates the T cells, increases interleukin-2 secretion, and has a direct antiviral effect.

- *Indications*: Viral and bacterial infections of the upper respiratory passages.
- *Contraindications:* See cautions noted on labels of commercial products. See p. 149.
- *Dosage and administration:* Oral echinacea preparations are available. See p. 57 for dosage instructions. Based on the current data, combinations of *Echinacea* root (*E. purpurea, E. pallida*), wild indigo (*Baptisia tinctoria*), and arbor vitae tips (*Thuja occidentalis*) appear to be superior to preparations with *Echinacea* alone. Further in-depth studies are needed for final clarification.
  - Flavored liquid products containing coneflower preparations that include glycerine instead of alcohol are popular for children.
- *Side effects:* None known for oral administration.

Diaphoretics (Sweat Inducers)

➤ **Elder flower** (Sambuci flos, see p. 62); **yarrow flower** and **leaf** (Millefolii herba, see p. 131); and **linden flower** (Tiliae flos, see p. 87).
- *Action*: Elder, yarrow, and linden flowers have febrifuge and anti-inflammatory effects due to the inhibition of prostaglandins by their flavonoid constituents. Prostaglandins play a role in fever development. Linden flower tea also induces nonspecific activation of the immune system. Yarrow has anti-inflammatory properties.
- *Indications*: Viral and bacterial infections of the upper respiratory passages.
- *Contraindications*: None known.
- *Dosage and administration*: Elder flower: see p. 62.
- *Side effects*: None known.

➤ **Vitamin C Supplements**
- **Black currant** (Ribes nigrae fructus); **rose hip peel** (Rosae pseudofructus).
- *Action*: Increases the stores of vitamin C, yielding unspecific enhancement of the immune system.
- *Indications*: For prevention and treatment of upper respiratory tract infections.
- *Contraindications*: None known.
- *Dosage and administration*:

- *Black currant juice:* Dilute with hot water. Drink 1 glass with meals at noon and in the evening. Can be used by patients in all age groups.
- *Rose hip tea:* Steep 2–5 g of the herb in 1 cup of boiled water for 15 to 30 minutes. Take one cup, several times a day.
- Cold rose hips tea is an effective thirst quencher for patients with fever.
- ◉ *Note:* These preparations have relatively low concentrations of vitamin C, and their beneficial action depends also on their flavonoid or anthocyanin content. Their effectiveness is not proven with clinical trials; they fall more into the realm of pleasant-tasting home remedies.
- – *Side effects:* None known.

Remedies to Apply at the First Signs of a Cold

Circulatory Stimulants

➤ Powdered **black mustard seed** (Sinapis nigrae semen) or **white mustard seed** (Sinapis albae semen, see p. 127).
- – *Action*: Mustard stimulates the blood flow in the mucous membranes of the mouth and nose by reflex mechanisms. It can prevent the outbreak of a cold if treatment by footbath is started early enough.
- – *Contraindications*: Powdered mustard seed should not be used by patients with kidney diseases or by children under 6 years of age due to transdermal absorption of mustard oil.
- – *Dosage and administration*: Powdered mustard seed should not be applied to mucous membranes. When used for footbaths, add enough warm water to cover the feet and ankles (see p. 312 for standard treatment instructions).
- ◉ *Warning:* After treatment, all mustard particles should be removed by rinsing the skin with warm water. Prolonged exposure can cause skin irritation and blistering, especially in patients with sensitive skin.
- – *Side effects:* Prolonged use (>2 weeks) of strongly heated preparations externally can lead to skin burns and nerve damage.

Diaphoretics (Sweat Inducers)

➤ See Recommended Herbal Remedies (Overview) on p. 151.
- – *Contraindications:* None known.
- – *Dosage and administration:* The tea should be taken as hot as tolerable during the early afternoon.
- – *Linden flower tea:* 2 teaspoons per cup (see p. 87).
- – *Diaphoretic tea **Rx***: Sambuci flos 35.0, Tiliae flos 25.0, Liquiritiae radix 10.0, Rosae pseudofructus 30.0. Use 1 teaspoon per cup of boiled water.
- ◉ *Warning:* Diaphoretic teas should not be taken on a full stomach.

Nonspecific Immunostimulants

➤ **Vitamin C supplements:** see p. 151.
➤ **Immunomodulators:** see p. 150.
- – *Dosage and administration:* Oral dosage forms are used. Treatment should be continued for at least 5 to 6 days.
  - *Liquids:* 20 to 40 drops (up to 2–4 mL [2 to 4 droppersful]), 3 to 4 times a day.
  - *Solids:* 1 to 2 lozenges, tablets or capsules, 3 times a day, as directed on the product label.

◉ *Note:* Echinacea should be taken at the first signs of a cold. The efficacy of the herbal remedy is questionable when treatment is started at the climax of the disease. The preventive effect of echinacea is still under investigation.

Chronic Infections of the Upper Respiratory Tract _____

➤ Purple echinacea leaf juice, liquid extracts of the root of *E. purpurea* or *E. angustifolia*, or a combination of various parts of the two species can be very helpful in chronic upper respiratory tract infections and recurrent colds. Products manufactured from the fresh, or recently-dried plants are preferred by most herbalists.

➤ The usefulness of echinacea preparations past 2 weeks or so is still controversial and requires further clinical studies. Oral administration of alcoholic extracts and homeopathic tinctures (mother tinctures to D2 tinctures) is reported to be more effective than other preparations. The current data suggest that preparations combining echinacea with other herbs are more effective than echinacea alone.

➤ Siberian ginseng (*Eleutherococcus senticosus*) may also be useful (see notes on the immune system on p. 226).

◉ *Warning:* The immune status of severely ill patients should be checked before starting immunostimulatory therapy. Supposed risks must be carefully weighed against the expected but unproven benefits of treatment.

Patients with Low Resistance to Infection

➤ **Echinacea** (see pp. 56, 149).
  – *Dosage and administration*: Oral dosage forms are used. In the early phases of manifest disease, administer for a period of no less than 6 days and no more than 14 days.
    • *Liquids:* 30 to 40 drops, 3 to 4 times a day.
    • *Solids:* 1 to 2 lozenges, tablets of capsules, 3 times a day, as directed on the label.

Chronic Recurrent Respiratory Tract Infections

➤ **Echinacea** (see pp. 149 and 56).
  – *Dosage and administration*: Liquid oral preparations: See p. 56.
  – *Side effects*: See p. 149.

5.3 Bronchitis

Clinical Considerations

➤ **General comments**

– *Acute bronchitis*

- Usually caused by an ascending viral infection. Irritant bronchitis is due to the inhalation of toxic or allergic substances.
- The disease is marked by abnormal mucus production and impaired ejection of mucus from the bronchi. The bronchial passages become obstructed owing to the thick mucous secretions and inflammation. Coughing and phlegm production, the hallmark symptoms of bronchitis, ultimately occur.
- The initial symptoms are dry cough accompanied by a burning sensation in the chest. The cough gradually becomes productive and increasingly troublesome. The viscosity of the mucus starts to decrease over the course of time (2 to 3 weeks).
- Yellowish-green mucus is indicative of secondary bacterial infection.
- ◉ *Note:* If there is severe coughing (especially with a presumed lung involvement), frequent relapsing, or persistent coughing with expectoration, the patient should consult a physician to assess the need for antibiotic treatment.
- *Complications:* The primary complication is chronic bronchitis, which can cause irreversible damage to the mucous membranes. The damaged membranes provide a foundation for further complications, such as pulmonary emphysema, bronchiectasis, and bronchopneumonia.

– *Chronic bronchitis*

- Smoking is usually responsible for the persistence of bronchitis. Chronic adenovirus infection may be another cause.
- Increased quantities of CD8+ T lymphocytes can be found in the larger airways (beneath the basal membrane). The bronchial glands are swollen, and large quantities of neutrophil granulocytes and macrophages are present, even in the alveolar fluid.

➤ **Herbal and general treatment measures**

– Increasing the fluid intake is essential. In mild cases, the patient should drink large quantities of tea made from herbs selected according to the type of cough.

– Herbal preparations with soothing effects are to be applied first. Expectorants, preferably those with antispasmodic or immunostimulatory effects, can be prescribed later if necessary.

➤ **Clinical value of herbal medicine**

– The objective of herbal treatment is to prevent complications. Treatment should therefore be initiated in the early stages of disease.

– Herbal medicinal products containing single or multiple ingredients can decrease the viscosity of mucus, counteract inflammation, ease bronchospasms, and stimulate the immune system.

– In chronic bronchitis, herbal remedies are used for adjunctive treatment.

Recommended Herbal Remedies (Overview)

Demulcents

➤ **Marshmallow root** (Althaeae radix, see p. 91); **mallow leaf** and **flower** (Malvae folium cum flores, see p. 89); **ribwort plantain** (Plantaginis herba, see

p. 60); **Iceland moss** (Lichen islandicus, see p. 79); **mullein** (Verbasci flos, see p. 94).
- *Action:* Antitussive; see p. 158.
- *Contraindications:* None known.
- *Dosage and administration:* Oral dosage forms should be used. For dosage recommendations, see the application in question.
- *Side effects:* None known.

Secretolytics and Expectorants

➤ **Aromatic herbs and pure essential oils: Aniseed** (Anisi fructus, see p. 34); **fennel seed** (Foeniculi fructus, see p. 65); **thyme** (Thymi herba, see p. 120); **eucalyptus oil** (cineol); **camphor tree** Cinnamomum camphorae aetheroleum, see p. 45); **peppermint oil** (menthol, see p. 103); **pine needle oil** (Pini aetheroleum, see p. 104).

➤ **Saponin-containing herbs:** Primula root (Primulae radix, see p. 105); mullein flower (Verbasci flos, see p. 94); licorice (Liquiritiae radix, see p. 85).
- *Action*: Mucolytic and expectorant.
- *Contraindications*: Peppermint oil and preparations containing menthol and camphor (see p. 45) as well as eucalyptus, pine, and spruce needle oils should never be applied to the face, especially the nose, of infants.
- *Dosage and administration*: See instructions for the specific application in question.
- *Side effects*
  • *Eucalyptus oil:* Internal administration of large quantities of eucalyptus oil can lead to the passage of gallstones or kidney stones or to stomach irritation, cramps, tachycardia, and cyanosis. Eating large amounts of eucalyptus candy can induce nausea and vomiting in children.
  • *Licorice:* Aldosterone-like side effects such as edema and hypokalemia, when larger quantities are consumed.
  • *Saponin-containing herbs:* The consumption of large quantities can irritate the stomach.
  • *Cineol* activates the hepatic enzyme system that metabolizes foreign substances, possibly weakening and/or shortening the therapeutic action of other active principles.
  • Although rare, contact eczema may occur.

Bronchospasmolytics

➤ **Thyme** (Thymi herba); **ivy leaf** (Hederae helicis folium, see p. 58); **primula root** (Primulae radix, see p. 105); **licorice root** (Liquiritiae radix, see p. 85).
- *Action:* Relieve bronchial muscle spasms.
- *Contraindications:* None known.
- *Dosage and administration:* See instructions for the specific disease in question.
- *Side effects*
  • *Licorice* (see p. 86).
  • *Ivy leaf and primula root:* Large quantities of saponin-bearing herbs can irritate the stomach.

5.3 Bronchitis

Antiphlogistics

➤ **Ivy leaf** (Hederae helicis folium, see p. 58); **primula root** (Primulae radix, see p. 105); **ribwort plantain** (Plantaginis herba, see p. 60); **licorice** (Liquiritiae radix, see p. 85); **Iceland moss** (Lichen islandicus, see p. 79).
  – *Action:* Anti-inflammatory.
  – *Contraindications:* None known.
  – *Dosage and administration:* See instructions for the specific application in question.
  – *Side effects:* Described above.

Antibiotics and Immunomodulators

➤ **Thyme** (Thymi herba, see p. 120); **ivy leaf** (Hederae helicis folium, p. 58); **nasturium** (Tropaeoli herba, see p. 96); **horseradish root** (Amoraciae radix).
  – *Action*: Reduces the likelihood of a secondary bacterial infection.
  – *Contraindications*: Horseradish should not be used by individuals with peptic ulcers or nephritis, and should not be administered to children under 4 years of age.
  – *Dosage and administration*: See instructions for the specific disease in question.
  – *Side effects*: Those of ivy leaf are described above. Horseradish root can cause isolated allergic side effects; higher doses of the herbal remedy can cause gastrointestinal upsets.

Antitussives

➤ **Sundew herb** (Droserae herba, see p. 118).
  – *Action:* Relieves dry cough by reducing the cough reflex.
  – *Contraindications:* None known.
  – *Dosage and administration:* See instructions for the specific disease in question.
  – *Side effects:* None known.

Range of Applications in Acute Bronchitis

Internal Remedies

➤ See overview on p. 154.
➤ **Chest tea, *Rx*:** Standard license: Anisi fructus (chopped) 15.0, Liquiritiae radix 25.0, Althaeae radix 35.0, Malvae folium 25.0.
➤ **Cough and bronchial tea *Rx*:** Anisi fructus 10 g, Plantaginis herba 30 g, Liquiritiae radix 30 g, Thymi herba 30 g.
  – *Dosage and administration*: One teaspoon of either tea mixture per cup, 3 to 4 times a day. Commercial preparations should be used as directed on the product label.
  – *Clinical value*: When treatment is initiated early, the combined administration of oral herbal remedies with topical remedies and inhalants (see p. 157) can be sufficient treatment in many cases.

External Remedies

➤ **Thyme**; **eucalyptus oil**; **dwarf pine oil**; **peppermint oil**; **spruce needle oil**; **camphor** (see p. 45).

– *Dosage and administration*: Apply to the skin or use for inhalation several times a day. Should be used as directed on the product label.
– *Clinical value*: See internal remedies.

Range of Applications in Chronic Bronchitis

Immunostimulants

➤ **Purple echinacea herb** (Echinaceae purpureae herba) and **paleflowered echinacea root** (E. pallida radix); see p. 56.

– *Dosage and administration*: Liquid tinctures, 1:4, 2–4 mL are added to a little water and taken orally, 4 to 5 times daily.
– *Clinical value*: No comparable synthetic drug preparations exist. Echinacea's immunostimulatory action takes effect within 24 hours. These products are safe to use, even by patients on concomitant antibiotic treatment.

Symptomatic Treatment

➤ The purpose of *symptomatic treatment* is to promote the ejection of mucus in subacute or chronic bronchitis and to counteract inflammation.

➤ **Thyme herb**; **primula root**; **ribwort plantain herb**; **ivy leaf** (use commercial products only); **cineol**. See overview on p. 155.

– **Tea *Rx*:** Primulae radix, Thymi herba, Plantaginis herba, aa ad 100 g.
– *Dosage and administration*: 1 teaspoon per cup, 3 to 4 times a day. Commercial preparations should be used as directed on the product label.
– *Clinical value*: The specified herbal remedies are generally well tolerated and useful for adjunctive treatment.

5.4 Symptomatic Cough

Clinical Considerations _____

➤ **General comments**
  – Coughing clears foreign particles and accumulated mucus from the respiratory passages.
  – Coughing is a response to foreign particles caused by stimulation of neuroreceptors located on the larynx and esophageal bifurcation at the opening of the stem bronchi. The stimulus is usually mechanical, but sometimes also chemical or thermal in nature. The cough reflex travels through the afferent nerve fibers to the cough center of the medulla oblongata. Additional cough receptors are located in the bronchi, alveoli, and throat. A smaller number of receptors can be found in the nose and paranasal sinuses. Connected to the cough center are receptors in the auditory canal, esophagus, and stomach. Coughing is induced when these receptors are stimulated.
  – Coughing for reasons other than to eject mucous secretions and foreign particles places unnecessary strain on the respiratory tract and should therefore be treated. Expectoration should be boosted through appropriate measures.
  – If the cough becomes chronic, a thorough work-up should be performed to determine the cause and to initiate the proper treatment measures. Apart from lung and heart disease, other common causes include medications, such as ACE inhibitors, and environmental factors, such as irritant gases, cigarette smoke, and solvents.

➤ **Herbal and general treatment measures**
  – Herbal remedies that quiet coughing (antitussives) or promote the ejection of mucus (expectorants) are delivered either by inhalation or orally.
  – *Herbal antitussives with central effects:* The essential oil in eucalyptus leaves (cineol) and licorice root may have central effects.
  – *Herbal antitussives with peripheral effects* reduce the sensitivity of cough receptors in the mucous membranes of the mouth and throat as well as in the esophagus and stomach.
  – *Anticoughing teas* can help to liquefy thick mucous secretions. The secretolytic and expectorant actions of certain essential oils develops more effectively when the preparations are inhaled or taken in extract form. Saponin-containing herbs, on the other hand, should be administered by mouth since they work by stimulating the sensitive fibers of the gastric mucosa. The reflex stimulus is then passed on to the bronchial mucosa.
  – Some herbal remedies have an additional anti-inflammatory effect (e. g., licorice root and sundew herb) or bronchospasmolytic effect (e. g., sundew herb, peppermint oil, and licorice root).

➤ **Clinical value of herbal medicine**
  – Herbal remedies that liquefy the mucus have antitussive efficacy.
  – All the specified herbal preparations are used for symptomatic treatment of coughs.

Recommended Herbal Remedies (Overview) _____

Demulcents

➤ See p. 154.
  – *Action*: Reduction of coughing. The active constituents in some herbal demulcents (e. g., marshmallow root, ribwort plantain herb, Iceland moss) are

transported by the mucus to the receptors in the mucous membranes of the mouth and throat. Those of others (e. g., naphthoquinone derivatives in sundew herb) take effect in the bronchial mucosa. Iceland moss contains bitter principles that additionally stimulate the production of saliva and digestive juices, thereby triggering a swallowing reflex that decreases the cough reflex.

Antitussives

➤ See p. 156.

Secretolytics and expectorants

➤ See p. 155.

Antispasmodics

➤ See p. 155.

Antiphlogistics

➤ See p. 156.

Range of Applications in Unspecific Dry Cough _____

➤ **General comments**
  – Symptomatic treatment is justifiable if the cause of coughing cannot be identified or if the environmental factors causing the coughing cannot be eliminated. Herbal remedies with primarily antitussive and anti-inflammatory effects should be used.
  – Aromatic oils such as anise oil, eucalyptus oils, fennel oil, menthol, peppermint oil, and thyme oil are useful. When allowed to dissolve in the mouth, they not only have a pleasant taste but also stimulate the swallowing reflex, which can be further enhanced by adding sugar or other sweeteners.

Demulcents

➤ See p. 154.

Antitussives

➤ See p. 156.

Antiphlogistics

➤ See p. 156.
➤ **Tea *Rx*:** Althaeae radix 25.0, Foeniculi fructus 10.0, Lichen islandicus 10.0, Plantaginis lanceolatae herba 15.0, Liquiritiae radix 10.0, Thymi herba 30.0. Steep 1 tablespoon in 1 cup of boiled water. Sweeten and drink the fresh tea slowly and as hot as tolerable. Take 1 cup, several times a day.
➤ *Dosage and administration:* Commercial preparations (e. g., capsules, cough drops, lozenges, cough syrup) should be taken several times a day, as directed on the product label.
➤ *Clinical value:* For adjunctive treatment.
➤ *Differential diagnosis:* Chronic bronchitis, see p. 154.

5.4 Symptomatic Cough

Range of Applications in Bronchial Asthma —————————

➤ **Preliminary remarks**
  - The chronic inflammatory process associated with bronchial asthma is controlled by T-helper cells and effector cells involved in the inflammatory response. Eosinophil granulocytes and other cells are typically found in inflamed bronchial tissues and bronchoalveolar fluids.
  - The main goals of therapy are to reduce inflammation and eliminate bronchospasms.

➤ **Recommended herbal preparations: Eucalyptus oil in various forms**
  - Eucalyptus oil is often used in steam inhalers, or as a rub. Small amounts can be found in cough lozenges or cough syrups.
  - Eucalyptus oil is is only rarely availaible in capsule or tablet form in the United States and is little used in these forms.
  - *Clinical value:* For adjunctive treatment. A cortisone-reducing effect has also been reported.
  - ◉ *Warning:* Asthma patients are often allergic to essential oils.

Clinical Considerations

➤ **General comments:** Mouth and throat diseases can be caused by bacteria, (e. g., *Streptococcus* or *Staphylococcus* species), viruses, mycoses (e. g., *Candida albicans*), allergies, pseudoallergies, and autoimmune diseases.

➤ **Herbal and general treatment measures:** Mouth washes and gargles are mechanical measures for cleansing the mouth and increasing the blood flow in the oral mucous membranes. Depending on which secondary herbal substances they contain, they can also relieve pain and speed up the healing process.

➤ **Clinical value of herbal medicine**
  – Herbal preparations are effective in counteracting bacterial, viral or non-specific mouth and throat diseases. They can be used alone or for adjunctive treatment parallel to established synthetic drugs.
  – There are no known herbal remedies for fungal diseases of the mouth and throat.
  – Astringents help to clear up drug-related oral eruptions, and bitters are used to counteract dryness of the mouth.

Recommended Herbal Remedies (Overview)

Demulcents

➤ **Marshmallow root** (Althaeae radix, see p. 91); **mallow leaf** (Malvae folium, see p. 89); **ribwort plantain** (Plantaginis lanceolatae folium, see p. 60); **sage leaf** (Salviae folium, see p. 114).
  – *Action*: Antitussive.
  – *Contraindications:* None known.
  – *Side effects*: None known.

Astringents

➤ **Myrrh** (Myrrhae); **dried bilberries** (Myrtilli fructus); **silverweed** (Potentillae anserinae herba, see p. 117); **rhatany root** (Rhataniae radix, see p. 111); **sage leaf** (Salviae officinalis folium, see p. 114); tormentil root (Tormentillae rhizoma, see p. 121).
  – *Action*: Anti-inflammatory, antimicrobial, promotes wound healing.
  – *Side effects*: None known.

Aromatic Herbs

➤ **Clove oil** (Caryophylli aetheroleum, see p. 49); **chamomile flower** (Matricariae flos, see p. 47) **myrrh**; **lemon balm leaf** (Melissae folium, see p. 84).
  – *Action*: Bacteriostatic, bactericidal, virustatic. Some are antiphlogistic.
  – *Contraindications*: Chamomile: Known allergy to chamomile.
  – *Side effects*: None known.

Bitters

➤ **Centaury herb** (Centaurii herba, see p. 84); **bogbean leaf** (Menyanthidis folium); **gentian root** (Gentianae radix).
  – *Action*: Increases the flow of saliva by stimulating bitter receptors on the tongue.
  – *Contraindications*: Individuals with gastric or duodenal ulcers should not use gentian root.
  – *Side effects*: Although rare, headaches may occur.

6.1 Diseases of the Mouth and Throat

Range of Applications in Acute Mouth and Throat Diseases _____

Acute Stomatitis (with less severe pain)

➤ **Mallow leaf**, **marshmallow root**, and **sage leaf**, either alone or using equal parts of each, as an infusion.
  – *Dosage and administration*: Use as a mouthwash or gargle, 3 to 6 times a day.
  – *Clinical value*: Herbal treatment alone is usually sufficient in mild cases. Otherwise, the herbal remedies can be applied for adjunctive treatment.

Acute Stomatitis (painful)

➤ **Chamomile flower** and **sage leaf** (1 : 1) for infusions.
  – *Alternative:* **Clove oil** 5 % in water base.
  – *Suggested combination:* Commercial slippery elm bark (*Ulmus rubra*) preparations.
  – *Dosage and administration*: Place herbs in water, bring to a boil, then cover and steep for 14 minutes. Rinse mouth or gargle with 1 tablespoon infusion in a cup of warm milk, 3 to 10 times a day as needed.
  – *Clinical value*: Can be used alone to treat mild or moderate disorders. Also combines well with synthetic drugs and chemical remedies (e. g., lidocaine or tetracaine).

Isolated Mouth and Throat Ulcers (Aphthae)

➤ **Myrrh tincture**; **sage leaf**.
  – *Dosage and administration*
    • Apply a few drops of myrrh tincture 1 : 5 to the affected sites, 2 to 3 times a day.
    • *Gargle:* Briefly boil sage leaves in water (1:1) and steep for 14 minutes.
  – *Clinical value*: The effects of these herbs are comparable to those of their active constituents' synthetic counterparts.

Pharyngitis with Dry Cough and Problems in Swallowing

➤ **Mallow leaf**; **sage leaf**; **marshmallow root**.
  – *Dosage and administration*: Prepare an infusion using one or more of these herbs. Gargle with the infusion several times a day.
  – *Clinical value*: The effects of these herbs are comparable to those of their active constituents' synthetic counterparts. Clinical studies to confirm this are, however, not available.

Acute Glossitis and Aphthous Stomatitis

➤ **Dried bilberry**.
  – *Dosage and administration*: Steep 1 to 3 tablespoons of dried bilberries in 1 liter of water for around 15 minutes. Gargle with the infusion several times a day.
  – *Clinical value*: Studies comparing bilberry to its active constituents' synthetic counterparts are not available.

Angina Tonsillaris

➤ **Chamomile tea** (see p. 47) and **extract**.
➤ **Chamomile–sage tincture** *Rx:* Extract. Salviae Fluidum, Extract. Chamomillae Fluidum, aa 20.0.
  - *Dosage and administration*
    • Freshly made chamomile infusion from good-quality dried flowers should always be used. Gargle or rinse the mouth at hourly intervals.
    • *Chamomile extract:* Add 10 drops to a glass of water, or apply directly to the affected sites, 2 to 3 times a day. Also rinse the mouth with an astringent.
    • Chamomile–sage tincture: Add 20 to 30 drops to a glass of water and gargle.
    • *Arnica tincture (1:10):* Add 1 teaspoon to a glass of water as hot as tolerable, gargle or rinse the mouth at hourly intervals, but *do not swallow the preparation.*
    ◉ *Important:* Arnica flower should not be used by persons allergic to the plant. When selecting the remedy, the individual preferences of the patients should be taken into consideration.
  - *Clinical value*: Studies comparing these herbal remedies to their active constituents' synthetic counterparts are not available.

Peritonsillar Abscess

➤ **Arnica** (see above) and **chamomile** (see Angina Tonsillaris).
  - *Dosage and administration*: Use arnica and chamomile preparations alternately. Gargle intensively, every half hour, with the infusion as hot as tolerable.
  - *Clinical value*: For adjunctive treatment.

Range of Applications in Chronic Mouth and Throat Diseases _____

Chronic Stomatitis, Chronic Pharyngitis, Smoker's Catarrh

➤ We recommend the alternating use of **demulcents** (see p. 161), **astringents** (see p. 161), and **bitters** (see p. 161).
  - Mucilaginous coverage on the free nerve endings responsible for pain development is best produced by alternately using astringents and demulcents. The above conditions are characterized by permanent atrophy of most mucous glands. Bitters stimulate the remaining intact mucous glands.
  - *Dosage and administration*: The patient should intensively rinse the mouth with infusions made from the recommended preparations, alternating between the different types.
    • *Astringents:* 1 to 3 tablespoons of dried bilberry fruit (or 1 tablespoon of bayberry root and dried bilberry fruit 1:1) per liter of water.
    Tincture *Rx* 1: Tinct. Myricae 15.0. Take 1 teaspoon diluted in a glass of water.
    Tincture *Rx* 2: Tinct. Myricae, Tinct. Salviae, aa 10.0. Take 1 teaspoon diluted in a glass of water.
    Tincture *Rx* 3, for patients with severe inflammation: Tinct. Myricae, Tinct. Arnicae, aa 20.0. Take 1 teaspoon diluted in a glass of water.
    • *Demulcents:* Mallow leaves, slippery elm bark, marshmallow root. Prepare an infusion using one or more of these herbal remedies.

- *Bitters:* Century herb, bogbean, and gentian root. Prepare an infusion using one or more of these herbs. Add 1 to 2 teaspoons of the tea mixture to 1 liter of water.
  - *Clinical value*: Comparable treatment regimens with synthetic drugs do not exist. The elimination of harmful factors (e. g., cigarette smoking) can greatly improve the symptoms.

Chronic Gingivitis and Periodontal Disease

➤ **Undiluted rhatany** (*Krameria* spp.) **tincture**.
  - **Tincture *Rx*:** Tinct. Krameriae, Tinct. Arnicae, aa 20.0.
  - *Dosage and administration*: Dilute 1 teaspoon in 1 glass of water and rinse or apply undiluted tincture to gums, 2 to 3 times a day.
  - *Clinical value*: Useful alternative to synthetic drugs. No comparative studies are available.

Inflammation and Mild Suppuration of the Gums

➤ **Tincture *Rx*:** Tinct. Sanguinariae 3.0,, Tinct. Myrrhae, 20.0.
  - *Dosage and administration*: Apply 1 tsp of the mixture diluted in 4 ounces of water to the gums, 2 to 3 times a day.
  - *Clinical value*: Good alternative to synthetic drugs.

Persistent "Lump" in the Throat or Need to Clear the Throat

➤ **Century herb**, **bogbean**, and **gentian root**. Prepare an infusion using one or more (equal parts) of these herbal remedies, or use the following tincture.
  Tincture *Rx*: Tinct. Resina myrrhae 10.0.
  - *Dosage and administration*: Add 1 teaspoon tincture to a glass of water, or 1 to 2 teaspoons tea mixture to 1 liter of water. Rinse the mouth or gargle, several times a day.
  - *Clinical value*: Comparable treatment regimens with synthetic drugs and/or chemical remedies do not exist.

Dryness of the Mouth and Sicca Syndrome

➤ Same as for lump in throat sensation (above).
  - *Action*: Bitters stimulate the remaining intact mucous glands.
  - *Clinical value*: Alternative to artificial saliva.

Herpes Simplex Labialis

➤ Apply externally on the lesions either lemon balm leaf dry extract in creme base, or St. John's wort oil.
  - *Dosage and administration*
    - Apply 10–20 mg of the creme per cm^2 of affected skin, 2 to 4 times of day.
    - *St. John's wort oil:* Apply 1–2 ml of the oil to the affected area, several times daily.
  - *Clinical value*: Useful alternatives to the synthetic counterparts; however, no convincing clinical studies to test this have been published.
  - St. John's wort oil has demonstrated anti-inflammatory and antiviral properties and may help reduce pain and inflammation.
  - ◉ *Note:* It is important to start treatment early, that is, as soon as the first signs appear.

Clinical Considerations

➤ **General comments**
  – Appetite is defined as an instinctive desire for food. It has a specific control mechanism that is mainly localized in the hypothalamus and an unspecific control mechanism in the limbic system. Hence, appetite is essentially subject to emotional control.
  – The gustatory nerves (vagus nerve) in the mouth trigger the production of saliva and gastric juices.
➤ **Herbal and general treatment measures:** Pleasant-tasting bitters can be used to stimulate the appetite and the production of gastrointestinal juices. The patients generally become accustomed to the prescribed herbs or herb preparations within a few weeks, so the herbal remedies soon lose their initial efficacy. This makes it necessary to periodically switch to different herbal preparations to maintain treatment efficacy.
➤ **Clinical value of herbal medicine:** Bitters used to stimulate the appetite are a prime example of the usefulness of herbal remedies because, in this case, no comparable synthetic alternatives are available.

Recommended Herbal Remedies (Overview)

➤ **Classification:** Bitters are divided into the following four groups: **tonic bitters** (tonic substances), **astringent bitters** (tannins), **aromatic bitters** (essential oils), and **acrid bitters** (pungent substances).
➤ **Tonic bitters** (amara tonica): **Centaury leaf** (Centaurii herba, see p. 84); **artichoke leaf** (Cynarae folium, see p. 36); **cinchona bark**; **gentian root** (Gentianae radix); **horehound herb** (Marrubii herba, see p. 76); **bogbean leaf** (Menyanthidis folium); **dandelion root** and **herb** (Taraxaci radix cum herba, see p. 54); **chicory leaf** and **root** (Cichorii herba et radix).
➤ **Astringent bitters** (amara adstringentia): Condurango bark (Condurango cortex, see p. 52 –use only in combination with other herbal remedies); **cinchona bark** (Chinchona cortex).
➤ **Aromatic bitters** (amara aromatica): **Wormwood herb** (Absinthii herba, see p. 129); **bitter orange peel** (see p. 39 Aurantii pericarpium–use only in combination with other herbal remedies); **calamus root** (Calami rhizoma, see p. 44); **angelica root** (Angelicae radix, see p. 33); **blessed thistle** (Cnici benedicti herba); **yarrow herb** and **flower** (Millefolii herba et flos, see p. 131).
➤ **Acrid bitters** (amara acria): **Cinnamon bark** (Cinnamomi cassiae or ceylanici cortex); **galangal root** (Galangae rhizoma); **ginger root** (Zingiberis rhizoma, see p. 70).
➤ **Contraindications**
  – *Gentian:* Should not be used by individuals with gastric or duodenal ulcers.
  – *Wormwood:* Should not be used during pregnancy.
  – *Calamus* (sweetflag): Should not be used during pregnancy or by children under 12 years of age.
➤ **Action**
  – Bitters initially stimulate the secretion of saliva. Once they reach the stomach, they stimulate the release of gastrin, thus enhancing upper gastrointestinal motility. Bitters also stimulate the secretion of bile, pancreatic juices, and pepsinogen.

- Bitters stimulate the appetite of patients who lack gastric juices (achylia, owing, for example, to chronic atrophic gastritis.
- Bitters do not stimulate the appetite of healthy individuals.
- Overdosage can lead to a digestion-suppressive effect.
- Bitters are usually not effective in treating cancer-related anorexia. Nonetheless, one should try the various preparations.

➤ **Side effects**
- Although rare, headaches may occur in sensitive individuals.
- Angelica root can cause photosensitivity. Individuals using it should avoid extensive sun exposure.

➤ **Dosage and administration**
- Bitters should be taken 15 to 30 minutes before meals and administered at doses large enough to be effective.
- Bitters should be briefly retained in the mouth before swallowing.

Range of Applications

To Stimulate the Appetite in Functional Achylia (lack of gastric juices) Secondary to an Acute Infection

➤ **Gentian root**; **centaury herb**; **bogbean**.
- *Dosage and administration*
  - *Gentian root:* Steep 1 teaspoon of the finely chopped herb in 1 cup of water for 5 minutes.
  - *Centaury herb:* Steep 1 to 2 teaspoons in 1 cup of boiled water for 15 minutes.
  - **Tea *Rx*:** Centaurii herba, Menyanthidis folium, Calami rhizoma, aa 20.0. Simmer 1 tablespoon in 1 liter of water for 15 minutes. Single dose 1 cupful. Heat before use.
  - *Gentian extract:* 0.5 – 2.0 g herbal preparation , 2 times a day, e. g., in pill form.
  - *Century extract:* 1 – 2 g, several times a day, e. g., in pill form.
  - *Bogbean leaf tincture:* 20 to 40 drops in $^1/_2$ glass of water; sip slowly.
  - *Gentian tincture:* 20 to 40 drops in 1 glass of water before each meal (very potent).
  - ◉ *Note:* Bitter teas, extracts, and tinctures should be taken before each meal.
- *Clinical value*: There are no synthetic drugs with comparable effects. Bog bean tea has an especially potent effect. Swallowing bitter preparations in capsules is less effective than use of preparations where the bitter flavor is tasted in the mouth.

Anorexia in Generalized Fatigue or Exhaustion

➤ **Additional indication:** For general roborant and stimulant effects after surgery.
- **Tincture *Rx*:** Tinct. Cinchonae comp. (described below), Tinct. Rhei vinosae aa 25.0.
- *Dosage and administration*: 1 teaspoon, 30 minutes before meals, 3 times day.
- *Clinical value*: Comparably pleasant taste, low-potency treatment.

Anorexia in Vegetative and Constitutional Weakness

▶ **Combined Cinchona Tincture** containing 6 parts cinchona bark, 2 parts bitter orange peel, 2 parts gentian root, and 1 part cinnamon.
- *Dosage and administration*: 20 drops in a glass of lukewarm water, 30 minutes before each meal. Long-term use is recommended.
- *Clinical value*: Easy to use, relatively good taste.

Gastric Anacidity, Achylia, and Anorexia (in the elderly)

▶ **Tea *Rx***: Absinthii herba, Menthae piperitae folium, aa 30.0.
- *Dosage and administration*: Steep 1 teaspoon in 1 cup of water for 10 minutes and strain. Take 1 cup, before meals, 2 times a day. Sip slowly.
- *Clinical value*: This is a rather effective remedy, but is soon rejected by many patients because of its bitter taste.

Anorexia (early stages)

▶ **Yarrow herb**; **peppermint leaf**; **centaury herb**; **calamus root**.
- *Dosage and administration*: Take 30 minutes before meals.
- **Tea *Rx***: Centaurii herba, Millefolii herba, Menthae piperitae folium, aa 20.0. Steep 1 teaspoon in 1 cup of boiled water. Drink, cold or lukewarm, before meals.
- *Calamus tincture:* 5 to 10 drops in a glass of water, 3 times a day.
- *Clinical value*: The effectiveness of these uses has not been documented in clinical studies. Calamus tincture should not be administered to children, or during pregnancy.

Lack of Appetite and Functional Upper Abdominal Complaints (in cases where carminative, cholagogue, and mild antispasmodic effects are desired)

▶ **Angelica root**; **blessed thistle herb**.
- *Dosage and administration*: These teas, extracts, and tinctures should be taken 30 minutes before meals.
- *Angelica root:* Steep 1 teaspoon in 1 cup of boiling water. Take 1 cup, 3 times a day.
- *Blessed thistle herb:* Steep 2 teaspoons in 1 cup of boiled water for 30 minutes. Take 2 to 3 cups a day, before meals.
- *Angelica tincture (1 : 5):* 20 to 30 drops in a glass of water.
- *Blessed thistle tincture (1 : 5):* 10 to 30 drops in a liqueur glassful of water.
- *Clinical value*: These herbs are useful in these indications as they have a beneficial effect on upper abdominal complaints.

Lack of Appetite and Insufficient Peristalsis

▶ **Ginger root** (see p. 70).
- *Dosage and administration*: Ginger tea or tincture should be taken 15 to 30 minutes before meals.
- *Dried ginger root:* Pour 1 cup of hot water onto 1 teaspoon of the coarsely powdered herb, then cover and steep for 5 to 10 minutes.
- *Ginger tincture (1 : 5):* 10 to 20 drops in $1/2$ to 1 glass of water. Useful alternative remedy.

- *Clinical value*: Rather well tolerated. Large interindividual differences in the efficacy of these remedies can be observed.

Anorexia in Severe Organic Diseases (Cancer)

➤ **Calamus root**.
- *Dosage and administration*: Calamus tincture: 20 to 30 drops in a glass of water, 15 to 30 minutes before meals, 3 times a day.
- *Clinical value*: Herbs that stimulate the appetite are not very effective for this indication.

Clinical Considerations _____

▶ **General comments**
- Reflux is characterized by the symptomatic backward flow of the stomach contents (especially gastric acid) into the esophagus owing to weakness (insufficiency) of the gastroesophageal sphincter.
- Acute stomach diseases (acute gastritis) can be caused by a variety of factors, such as simple overeating, stress, alcohol, medications, acids, alkaline substances, and bacterial infections. Acute stomach diseases can become chronic. The upper layers of the gastric mucosa are affected.
- *Symptoms:* Upper abdominal pain, anorexia, nausea, vomiting, bleeding.
- *Gastroduodenal ulcers* occur when there is an imbalance of protective and aggressive factors. Erosions extending into the deep layers of the stomach wall can be found on the mucous membrane of the stomach and/or duodenum.
- Functional stomach disorders (diagnosis of exclusion) play a very important role, as they are found in 30–50 % of all patients with upper abdominal complaints.
- Nervous disorders are suspected if no organic changes can be detected. It is difficult to distinguish nerve-related disorders from common upper abdominal complaints following meals (dyspeptic syndrome). The stomach and duodenum (nausea, belching, upper abdominal discomfort) as well as the small and large intestine (flatulence, cramplike abdominal pain, diarrhea) can be involved.
- *Ulcer-like dyspepsia:* Nocturnal pain, episodic pain, pinpoint pain.
- *Dysmotility dyspepsia:* Nausea or vomiting, premature satiation, belching, gas, upper abdominal tension, flatulence.
- *Reflux dyspepsia:* Heartburn.
- *Aerophagia:* Flatulence and belching.

▶ **Clinical value of herbal medicine and herbal treatment measures**
- *Reflux:* Herbal remedies are used for adjunctive treatment only.
- *Gastritis*
  - The effectiveness of herbal remedies for autoimmune gastritis (type A) is still unclear.
  - Treatment for *Helicobacter pylori*-related gastritis (type B) consists of eradicating the pathogen by way of acid blockade and antibiotic treatment. Herbal remedies can be prescribed as adjuvant measures.
  - Drug-induced gastritis (type C) caused by salicylates, nonsteroidal antiinflammatory drugs, and other medications responds well to mucoprotective herbal remedies. Their use is, however, limited to adjuvant therapy.
- *Ulcers:* Antacids, mucoprotective drugs, and antisecretory drugs (e.g., H_2-antagonists and proton pump inhibitors) are normally used. In this case, herbal remedies are limited to adjuvant therapy.
- *Non-ulcer-related dyspepsia:* A variety of herbal remedies are used to treat dyspeptic syndrome.

6.3 Reflux, Gastritis, Gastroduodenal Ulcers, Dyspepsia ■■

Recommended Herbal Remedies (Overview) ——————————

Antiphlogistics

➤ **Chamomile flower** (Matricariae flos, see p. 47); **peppermint leaf** (Menthae piperitae folium, see p. 102); **balm leaf** (Melissae folium, see p. 84); **licorice root** (Liquiritiae radix, see p. 85); **fennel seed** (Foeniculi fructus, see p. 65).
- *Action*: Anti-inflammatory. Aromatic herbs also have bacteriostatic effects and increase the local blood circulation.
  - *Chamomile flower*: Chamomile alone is not a very effective ulcer treatment. Because of its general efficacy and virtual lack of side effects, it is still commonly recommended for adjunctive treatment at the onset of and during acute ulcer episodes. The greatest strength of chamomile lies in prevention.
  - *Licorice root*: Because of its antiphlogistic effects, the herb is mainly prescribed for treating ulcer-related conditions, but is also indicated in gastritis and dyspeptic syndrome.
- *Contraindications*
  - *Licorice root*: Cholestatic liver diseases, cirrhosis of the liver, hypertension, hypokalemia, severe liver failure, and pregnancy.
  - *Chamomile flower*, dried and in alcoholic extracts: Known allergy to chamomile.
  - Peppermint leaf and its preparations: Reflux.
- *Dosage and administration*: Licorice preparations should not be used for more than 4–6 weeks at a time unless directed by a physician. Standardized licorice root extracts made with diluted ethanol and containing no less than 4.0% and no more than 6.0% glycyrrhizin should preferably be used.
  - Deglycyrrhinated licorice extract (DGL) is very commonly recommended and available in capsules or tablets in North America. The preparation is nearly as effective as whole licorice, but with fewer side effects. The daily dosage is based on the equivalent to 200–600 mg glycyrrhizin.
- *Side effects:* Undesirable mineralocorticoid effects occur after a weekly dose of ≥3.5 g glycyrrhizin (from licorice root). Rare cases of myoglobinuria have also been reported.

Demulcents

➤ **Flaxseed** (Lini semen, see p. 66).
- *Action*: Soothing.
- *Contraindications*: Bowel obstruction.
- 👁 *Important:* Flaxseed may impair the absorption of other drugs. The patient using flaxseed should drink plenty of fluids, at least 150 ml after taking the herb.

Anticholinergics

➤ **Belladonna** (Atropa belladonna).
- *Action*: Parasympatholytic. Alkaloids of the atropine group inhibit vagus nerve activity, reduce gastric juice secretion, and diminish intestinal motility. They are therefore used to relieve spasms, gastrointestinal colic, and gallbladder colic.

- *Contraindications*: Narrow-angle glaucoma, mechanical gastrointestinal tract stenosis, benign prostatic hypertrophy with residual urine formation, acute pulmonary edema, and tachycardiac arrhythmias.
- *Dosage and administration*
  - *Belladonnae radix:* Single dose 0.05 g; maximum single dose 0.1 g (equivalent to 0.5 mg total alkaloids). Maximum daily dose 0.3 g, equivalent to 1.5 mg total alkaloids calculated as L-hyoscyamin.
- *Belladonna extract:* Single dose 0.01 g; maximum single dose 0.05 g, equivalent to 0.73 mg total alkaloids calculated as L-hyoscyamin.
- ◉ *Note:* Belladonna is dispensed by prescription only.
- *Side effects*: Dose-dependent side effects, such as dry mouth, blurring of vision, micturition disorders, headaches, and stupor.

Range of Applications in Acute Clinical Pictures

Acute Gastritis and Esophagitis (in viral infection)

▶ **Chamomile**.
- *Dosage and administration*
  - *Special chamomile therapy:* The patient should drink 2 to 3 cups of fresh, hot chamomile tea (see p. 47), then lie on the back, left side, stomach, and right side for 5 minutes each. As an alternative to the tea, this therapy can also be performed using 30 to 50 drops of chamomile fluid extract or an appropriate commercial preparation, taken in a glass of hot water. The tea or diluted extract should be taken on an empty stomach in the morning.
- ◉ *Important*
  - This therapy should be continued for a few days after the symptoms have ceased.
  - Recovering alcoholics should not use chamomile extract because it contains alcohol.
- *Clinical value*: Useful and effective treatment measure without side effects.

Ulcers with Nocturnal Pain and Localized Epigastric Hunger Pain

▶ **Chamomile**; **licorice root**.
- *Dosage and administration*
  - *Chamomile:* see Acute Gastritis and Esophagitis.
  - *Licorice root fluid extract* (with 4–6% glycyrrhizinic acid): 1 teaspoon diluted in a small quantity of water, up to 4 times daily.
  - Deglycyrrhizinated licorice (DGL) chewable tablets. Take 2 to 4 380 mg chewable tablets before meals for acute symptoms, 1 to 2 tablets as a maintenance dose.
- ◉ *Note:* Should be taken under medical supervision and for no more than a few weeks.
- *Clinical value*: For adjunctive treatment.

Gastric Colic (Ulcerlike Pain without an Organic Finding)

➤ **Belladonna** (Atropa belladonna).
  – *Dosage and administration*
    • **Tincture *Rx***: Tinct. Belladonnae with 0.02 – 0.03 % total alkaloid content
      Tinct. Valerianae, Spir. Menthae pip., aa ad 30.0. Take 8 to 10 drops
      water, 3 times a day.
  – *Clinical value*: Useful for alleviating pain.

Range of Applications in Chronic Esophageal and Gastric Diseases

Chronic Esophagitis

➤ **Flaxseed.**
  – *Dosage and administration*: Grind flaxseed before use. Place 2 tablespoon
    of flax seed in ¹/₂ liter of water and bring to a boil. Strain and drink the liqui
    The use of commercial products is recommended. Take 3 to 4 sips of th
    gruel, several times a day.
  – *Clinical value*: For adjunctive treatment.

Chronic Gastritis

➤ **Fennel seed**; **peppermint leaf**; **lemon balm leaf**; **calamus rhizome** (Calan
  rhizoma, see p. 44).
➤ **Tea *Rx*:** Foeniculi fructus, Menthae piperitae folium, Melissae folium, Calan
  rhizoma, aa 20.0.
➤ **Flaxseed** (see p. 66).
  – *Dosage and administration*
    • *Tea mixture:* Steep 1 teaspoon in a cup of boiled water for 10 minute
      Take 1 cup, 2 to 3 times a day. Sip slowly while hot.
    • *Flaxseed gruel:* Soak 1 to 2 tablespoons ground flaxseed (daily portion
      in ¹/₄ to ¹/₂ liter of water overnight in the refrigerator. Drink lukewar
      before breakfast or in portions distributed throughout the day.
  – *Clinical value*: For adjunctive treatment.

Chronic Gastritis in Very Underweight or Weak Patients

➤ **Olive oil**; **flaxseed** (see p. 66).
  – *Dosage and administration*
    • *Olive oil:* Sip 1 tablespoon slowly each morning.
    • *Flaxseed:* see above
  – *Clinical value*: For adjunctive treatment.

Non-Ulcer-Related Dyspepsia (cf. Dyspeptic Symptom Complex, p. 174

➤ **Licorice root** (see p. 85).
  – *Dosage and administration*
    • *Dried licorice root*: Chop and steep ¹/₂ teaspoon in 1 cup boiled water fo
      15 minutes. Take 1 cup, 3 to 4 times a day. Can be taken for severa
      months because the glycyrrhizinic acid content is very low.
    • *Licorice fluid extract* (4 – 6 % glycyrrhizinic acid): 1 teaspoon in 1 cup wa
      ter, 3 to 4 times a day.
    • Deglycyrrhizinated licorice (DGL) chewable tablets: take 1 – 2 befor
      meals.

- ⊙ *Note:* The use of licorice fluid extract and commercial licorice products should be medically supervised. These preparations should not be taken for more than a few weeks at a time.
- *Clinical value*: For adjunctive treatment.

6.4 Dyspeptic Syndrome

Clinical Considerations

➤ **General comments**
  – *Dyspeptic syndrome* is the generic term for all types of upper abdominal and retrosternal pain, abdominal discomfort, heartburn, nausea, vomiting, and other gastrointestinal symptoms.
  – It is characterized by prolonged upper abdominal problems due to an underlying functional disorder with or without an additional psychovegetative component. The symptoms occur in the intestinal lumen without significant intestinal wall involvement. The following types can be distinguished:
    • Epigastric meteorism with distended abdomen (most common type). The stomach and intestine are often jointly involved.
    • Arteriosclerosis of gastrointestinal arteries: Characterized by deficient absorption of intestinal gases and flatulence.
    • Cholecystopathies (latent or manifest), food intolerance, the characteristic symptoms of which are distension of the stomachal region with bloating and belching.
    • Dysmotility type: Abdominal distension and bloating, premature feeling of satiation, diffuse abdominal pain in daytime only, nausea, food intolerance, vomiting, aversion to food, and constant discomfort.

➤ **Herbal treatment measures**
  – Herbal remedies can be used for trial treatment (for 14 days) or symptomatic treatment.
  – *Symptomatic herbal therapy*
    • *Dyspepsia with motor disorders:* Bitters can be used to counteract motor disorders of the upper gastrointestinal tract, e. g., a large flaccid stomach or motor disorders related to bile and pancreatic juice secretion. If the problem is already long-standing, treatment must usually be continued for several weeks before the preparations become effective. A high-fiber diet is also recommended.
    • *Meteorism:* Carminatives are used to treat meteorism (see below). They are sometimes combined with bitters, antiphlogistics, and/or tannin-containing herbs, depending on the symptoms involved.

➤ **Clinical value of herbal medicine**
  – Herbal remedies permit differentiated treatment according to the type and severity of the predominant symptoms.
  – Synthetic drugs and chemical remedies (e. g., prokinetic drugs) are used when there is positive evidence of organic disease or if the patient fails to respond to trial herbal therapy.

Recommended Herbal Remedies (Overview)

Carminatives

➤ **Caraway seed** (Carvi fructus, see p. 46); **fennel seed** (Foeniculi fructus, see p. 65); **aniseed** (Anisi fructus, see p. 34).
  – *Action*: When taken orally, carminatives induce a feeling of warmth and facilitate eructation and the passage of gas after meals. They contain essential oils that either induce spasmolysis or promote bowel motility and probably also have antibacterial effects. They are not as potent as the specific anti

biotics or antispasmodics. The most potent carminative is caraway, followed by fennel and aniseed.

– *Contraindications*: Patients with gallstones should not use carminatives unless directed by a physician.
– *Side effects*: Carminatives reduce the pressure in the esophageal sphincter and can therefore cause heartburn.

Bitters

▸ **Wormwood** (Absinthii herba, see p. 129); **angelica root** (Angelicae radix, see p. 33); **gentian root** (Gentianae radix); **chicory herb** and **root** (Cichorii herba et radix); **bogbean leaf** (Menyanthidis folium); **dandelion root** and **herb** (Taraxaci radix cum herba, see p. 54); **blessed thistle** (Cnici benedicti herba); **yarrow herb** (Millefolii herba, see p. 131).

– *Action*: Stimulate gastrointestinal motility.
– *Contraindications*: (cf. Anorexia, p. 165):
  • Patients prone to gallstones should not use bitters unless directed by a physician.
  • *Gentian root:* Ulcer-related dyspepsia, acute gastritis.
  • *Yarrow:* Known allergy to composite plants.
  • *Dandelion:* Biliary tract obstruction, gallbladder empyema.
  • *Wormwood:* Pregnancy.
– *Side effects*: See Anorexia p. 166.

Aromatic Herbs

▸ **Aniseed** (Anisi fructus, see p. 34); **calamus root** (Calami rhizoma, see p. 44); **caraway seed** and **oil** (Carvi fructus et aetheroleum, see pp. 45, 46); **cinnamon bark** (Cinnamomi cassiae cortex, C. zeylanici cortex); **turmeric root** (Curcumae longae rhizoma, C. xanthorrizae rhizoma, see p. 121); **bitter orange peel** (Aurantii pericarpium, see. p. 39); **coriander** (Coriandri fructus, see p. 365); **fennel seed** (Foeniculi fructus, see p. 65); **chamomile flower** (Matricariae flos, see p. 97); **balm leaf** (Melissae folium, see p. 84); **peppermint leaf** (Menthae piperitae folium, see p. 102); **rosemary leaf** (Rosmarini folium, see p. 112).

– *Action*: Antispasmodic and antibacterial; increases peristalsis.
– *Contraindications*
  • *Turmeric:* Should not be used by patients with biliary tract occlusion or gallstones.
  • *Anise:* Known allergy to anise or anethole.
  • *Calamus:* Should not be used by children under 12 years of age or during pregnancy or breast feeding.
  • *Chamomile:* Known allergy to chamomile.
  • *Menthol:* Biliary tract obstruction, gallstones, gallbladder inflammation, severe liver damage.
– *Side effects*: (Cf. Anorexia, p. 166):
  • *Anise:* Although rare, allergic reactions of the skin, respiratory tract, and gastrointestinal tract may occur.
  • *Turmeric:* May irritate the gastric mucosa if used for extended periods or overdosed.

Other Herbs

➤ **Galangal root** (Galangae rhizoma); **papaya peel** (Caricae papayae fructus, **pineapple** (Ananas comosus); **artichoke leaf** (Cynarae folium, see p. 36).
- *Action*: Used to treat enzyme deficiencies. Galangal bark stimulates the secretion of pancreatic enzymes. Papaya and pineapple contain digestive enzymes.

Range of Applications in Bloating and Meteorism

Mild Pain and Meteorism

➤ **Caraway; aniseed; fennel; balm; peppermint; wormwood** (see p. 129).
- *Dosage and administration*
  • **Tea Rx:** Carvi fructus, Foeniculi fructus, aa 20.0; Menthae piperitae folium, Melissae folium, aa 30.0. Steep 1 teaspoon in 1 cup of boiled water for 15 minutes. Take 1 cup of the tea while hot, 3 to 6 times a day.
  • **Tincture Rx:** Ol. Carvi 5.0, Tinct. Absinthii, Tinct. Foeniculi Compos., aa 20.0. Take 20 to 30 drops in water, 3 times a day.
  • *Aniseed:* Pour 1 cup of boiled water onto 1 heaped teaspoon of the freshly crushed or coarsely powdered herb, then cover and steep for 10 to 1 minutes. Take 1 cup, 3 to 5 times a day.
  • *Anise oil:* 3 drops on a cube of sugar, several times a day.
  • *Commercial products:* Take as directed on the product label.
- *Clinical value*: All of these remedies are generally recognized in Europe as safe and effective. Hence, they can be selected according to the taste preference of the patient.

Mild Gastrointestinal Pain, Bloating, and Meteorism

➤ **Caraway; fennel; wormwood** (see p. 129); **yarrow.**
- *Dosage and administration*
  • **Tea Rx:** Carvi fructus, Foeniculi fructus, Absinthii herba, Millefolii herba aa 25.0. Steep 1 teaspoon in 1 cup of boiled water for 15 minutes. Take cup of the hot tea before each meal.
- *Clinical value*: Effective and well-recommended tea formulation, owing to inclusion of wormwood, the duration of application should be limited.

Severely Distended and Painful Stomach

➤ **Caraway; olive oil; fennel; aniseed.**
- *External remedies: Dosage and administration*
  • **Liniment Rx:** Ol. Carvi 10.0, Ol. Olivinarum ad 100.0. Apply 10 to 1. drops onto the stomach in a circular pattern, 2 to 3 times a day. Can also be used in small children.
- *Internal remedies: Dosage and administration*
  • **Tea Rx:** Carvi fructus (crushed), Foeniculi fructus (crushed), Anisi fructus (crushed), aa 20.0. Steep 1 teaspoon in 1 cup of boiled water for 20 minutes. Drink a cup of the warm tea after each meal.
  • *Caraway oil:* 2 to 3 drops in a small amount of water at meal time.
  • *Caraway seed:* Pour 1 cup of boiled water onto 1 teaspoon of the freshly crushed seeds, then cover and steep for 5 minutes. Take 1 cup at or after meals.

– *Clinical value*: These herbal remedies, especially caraway oil, have good effects in this indication according to clinical experience in Europe.

ostprandial Bloating and Meteorism

Caraway; **fennel**; **wormwood herb** (see p. 129); **yarrow herb**; **turmeric root**; **artichoke leaf**.
– *Dosage and administration*
  • **Tea *Rx*:** Carvi fructus, Foeniculi fructus, Absinthii herba, Millefolii herba, aa 25.0. Pour 1 cup of boiled water onto 1 teaspoon of the tea mixture, then cover and steep for 15 minutes. Take 1 cup of the hot tea before each meal.
  • Turmeric root, artichoke leaf: Use commercially available preparations

eteorism and Cramping with Inflammation and Diarrhea

Caraway; **fennel**; **chamomile**.
– *Dosage and administration*
  • **Tea *Rx*:** Carvi fructus, Foeniculi fructus, aa 20.0; Matricariae flos, ad 100.0. Steep 1 to 2 teaspoons in 1 cup of boiled water for 10 minutes and sip slowly while hot.
– *Clinical value*: Effective and well-tolerated remedies.

oating and Meteorism with Cramplike Gallbladder Pain

Gentian root; **wormwood herb** (see p. 129); **peppermint leaf**; **belladonna**.
– *Dosage and administration*
  • **Tincture *Rx* 1:** Tinct. Gentianae, Tinct. Absinthii, aa 20.0; Tinct. Menthae Piperitae 10.0. Take 30 drops in a glass of water, shortly before meals, 3 times a day.
  • **Tincture *Rx* 2:** Tinct. Belladonnae 2.0, Tinct. Menthae Piperitae 10.0; Tinct. Gentianae 20.0. Take 10 to 15 drops in a glass of water shortly before meals, 3 times a day.
  ◉ *Note:* Pharmacists are required to standardize belladonna tincture with respect to its alkaloid content. The use of belladonna tincture for more than 3 weeks is not recommended.
– *Clinical value*: Effective and safe for short-term use.

ore Severe Colics and Meteorism

Peppermint leaf; **aniseed**; **calamus root**; **blessed thistle**; **wormwood**.
– *Dosage and administration*
  • **Tea *Rx* 1:** Menthae piperitae folium, Anisi fructus, Calami rhizoma, aa 20.0. Steep 1 tablespoon in 1 liter of water for 1 hour. Warm and drink 1 cup before each meal.
  • **Tea Rx 2:** Cnici benedicti herba, Absinthii herba (see p. 129), Melissae folium, aa 20.0. Steep 1 teaspoon in 1 cup of boiled water for 20 minutes. Take 1 cup, 3 times a day.
– *Clinical value*: Large interindividual differences in the effects of these remedies can be observed.

6.4 Dyspeptic Syndrome

Range of Applications in Functional Epigastric Complaints

Spastic Functional Epigastric Syndrome

➤ **Peppermint leaf**; **belladonna**; **wormwood** (see p. 129); **caraway seed**; **valerian root** (see p. 125).
  – *Dosage and administration*
    • *Peppermint leaf*: Pour 1 cup of hot, not boiling water onto 1 to 2 teaspoons of the herb, then cover and steep for 10 to 15 minutes. Take 1 cup after or between meals. The tea should be drunk slowly while warm.
    • *Peppermint tincture*: 5 drops in half a glass of water. Gives two doses daily. Preferably used for acute symptoms only.
    • **Tincture *Rx*:** Ol. Carvi 3.0, Tinct. Belladonnae, Tinct. Absinthii, Tinct. Carminativa, aa 10.0; Tinct. Valerian. Aeth., ad 50.0. Take 30 drops in water after meals, 3 times a day.
    ◉ *Warning:* The latter formulation contains belladonna and should not be used for more than 3 weeks (see p. 171).
  ◉ *Note:* Antacids can dissolve the enteric coating of some tablets, leading to stomach upset.
  – *Clinical value*: Large interindividual differences in the effects of these remedies can be observed.

Roemheld's Complex
(Spastic Functional Epigastric Syndrome with Severe Meteorism)

➤ **Galangal root**.
  – *Dosage and administration*
    • *Dried herb:* Pour 1 cup of boiled water onto 1 teaspoon of the finely chopped or coarsely powdered herb, then cover and steep for 5 to 10 minutes. Take 1 cup, 15 to 30 minutes before each meal.
    • *Tincture (1 : 10):* Take 10 drops in lukewarm water, 15 minutes before meals, 3 times a day.
  – *Clinical value*: Large interindividual differences in the effects of these remedies can be observed.

Roemheld's Complex with Poor Evacuation of the Bowels

➤ **Caraway**; **fennel**; **senna leaf** (see p. 436).
  – *Dosage and administration*
    • **Tea *Rx*:** Carvi fructus, Foeniculi fructus, aa 20.0; Menthae piperitae folium, Sennae folium, aa 30.0. Steep 1 to 2 teaspoons in 1 cup of boiling water for 20 minutes. Take 1 cup in the morning and evening.
    ◉ *Warning:* This formulation contains senna and should not be used for more than one month at a time.
  – *Clinical value*: Effective, but duration of use is restricted.

Dyspepsia Associated with Enzyme Deficiencies

➤ **Papaya peel**; **pineapple**, or their derivatives, papain and bromelain.
  – *Dosage and administration*
    ◉ *Note:* See p. 416 for side effects.
    • *Papain, bromelain, pancreatin, trypsin, chymotrypsin:* Commercial tablets are widely used.

- ◉ *Warning:* Allergic reactions, ranging from mild reactions to anaphylactic shock, can occur. Bloating, flatulence and occasional nausea can occur when administered at high doses.
- ◉ *Warning:* Bromelain can increase the potency of antibiotics and anticoagulants. Other side effects include harmless changes in the consistency, color, and smell of stools.
- *Contraindications*: Severe congenital or acquired coagulopathies, known hypersensitivity to any of the ingredients. Should not be used before surgery.
- *Clinical value*: Large interindividual differences in the effects of these remedies can be observed.

6.5 Chronic Hepatitis and Cirrhosis of the Liver

Clinical Considerations

➤ **General comments**
  – Chronic viral hepatitis is caused by infection with hepatitis B, C, or D viruses.
  – Toxic liver damage is caused by alcohol, drugs, or chemicals.

➤ **Herbal and general treatment measures**
  – Artichoke leaf extracts have antioxidant effects and stimulate choleresis. Clinical studies on the efficacy of artichoke leaf extract in hepatitis or liver cirrhosis are not available.
  – Commercial milk thistle fruit products are used to treat toxic liver damage and chronic hepatitis. They are also used for adjunctive treatment of cirrhosis of the liver.
  – Use only standardized products that do not contain alcohol. The efficacy of many polypharmaceutical combinations containing milk thistle is rather controversial.

➤ **Clinical value of herbal medicine**
  – Despite the considerable research effort, synthetic remedies for viral hepatitis and toxic liver disease often do not achieve satisfactory results.
  – Herbal remedies also cannot be expected to achieve curative results.
  – Studies on the use of herbal remedies for treatment of chronic autoimmune hepatitis, primary biliary cirrhosis, and metabolic diseases that cause cirrhosis of the liver exist but are not very conclusive in showing efficacy.

Recommended Herbal Remedies (Overview)

➤ **Milk thistle fruit** (Cardui mariae fructus, see p. 93); **artichoke leaf** (Cynarae folium, see p. 36).
  – *Artichoke leaf:* Has membrane-protective and antioxidant effects.
  – *Milk thistle fruit:* The herb and silymarin, a compound in it, are reported to have hepatoprotective, antioxidant, and proregenerative effects when administered by the oral route. A cholagogue effect has also been demonstrated.
  – *Standardized milk thistle extracts:* The silymarin content comprises no less than 30 % silybinin, the actual active constituent. Commercial products usually contain up to 80 % total silybinin and related compounds. Silybinin stimulates the entire process of cellular protein synthesis, resulting in regenerative effects. Its primary target organ is the liver, where silybinin primarily accumulates due to its marked enterohepatic circulation.
  – *Contraindications:* Artichoke leaf should not be used by individuals with known allergy to artichoke or other composite plants or by patients with biliary tract obstruction, and should be used with caution in gallstone disease.
  – *Side effects:* All of these preparations have a mild laxative effect.

Range of Applications

Beginning Stages of Liver Damage Associated with Dyspepsia, Sensations of Pressure and Fullness in the Right Upper Quadrant and Decreasing Physical Exercise Capacity.

➤ **Milk thistle fruit**; **artichoke leaf**; **peppermint leaf** (Menthae piperitae folium, see p. 102).
  – *Dosage and administration*
  • Add 2 to 3 mL of milk thistle tincture to 1 cup of peppermint leaf tea. Drink one cup three or four times daily.
  • *Standardized milk thistle extract* (70–80% silymarin, 140 mg tablets or capsules): take 1 to 2, twice daily with meals.
  • *Artichoke leaf extract:* Many commercial products available.

Chronic Infectious Hepatitis, Toxic Liver Damage, Cirrhosis of the Liver

➤ **Milk thistle fruit**.
  – *Dosage and administration:* Numerous standardized extract products available.
  – *Clinical value:* Clinical studies on the efficacy of milk thistle in these indications are available.

Clinical Trials

➤ A few studies since 1989 involving groups of patients with chronic liver diseases have yielded good results, demonstrating enhanced immune functions, an antioxidant and free-radical scavenging effect in the liver, enhanced liver function, reduced liver enzymes, and relief of symptoms such as tiredness, abdominal pressure, poor appetite, nausea, and itching.
➤ Good, high-quality studies with large enough groups of patients to really prove effectiveness or no effectiveness have not yet been funded or performed.

✣ **Literature**
  – Allain H et al.: Aminotransferase levels and silymarin in de novo tacrine-treated patients with Alzheimer's disease. Dement Geriatr Cogn Disord 10(3) (1999), 181–185; Bunout D et al.: Controlled study of the effect of silymarin on alcoholic liver disease. Rev Med Child 120(12) (1992),1370–1375; Buzzelli G et al.: A pilot study on the liver protective effect of silybin-phosphatidylcholine complex (IdB1016) in chronic active hepatitis. Int J Clin Pharmacol Ther Toxicol 31(9) (1993), 456–460; Chan MK et al.: Hepatitis B infection and renal transplantation: The absence of anti-delta antibodies and the possible beneficial effect of silymarin during acute episodes of hepatic dysfunction. Nephrol Dial Transplant 4 (1989), 297–301; Ferenci P et al.: Randomized controlled trial of silymarin treatment in patients with cirrhosis of the liver. J. Hepatol. 9 (1989), 105–113; Lang I et al.: Immunomodulatory and hepatoprotective effects of in vivo treatment with free radical scavengers. Ital J Gastroenterol 22(5) (1990), 283–287.

6.6 Diseases of the Gallbladder and Biliary Tract ▰▰▰▰▰

Clinical Considerations

➤ **General comments**
  – So-called functional disorders such as gallbladder dyskinesia and post-cholecystectomy syndrome are often seen in general practice.
  – The symptoms include indefinite complaints in the right upper quadrant that radiate to the back or to the right shoulder. This may progress to mild colic.
  – These symptoms are sometimes associated with irritable colon. The etiology is still unclear.

➤ **Herbal treatment measures**
  – Cholagogues are remedies with biliary-stimulating action. They are commonly used in the above indications. Pungent herbs remedies such as caraway, pepper, and ginger root as well as bitters and antispasmodics also are commonly used. Since most of these patients also suffer from constipation herbal laxatives are often helpful.
  – When using commercial products, only those containing no more than six different herbal components should be selected. Teas and tinctures with a strong aroma should preferably be used.
  – Fixed combinations with laxatives should be avoided.
  – All gallbladder teas can be sweetened with sugar, honey, or artificial sweeteners.

➤ **Clinical value of herbal medicine:** Cholagogues are not suitable for treating cholelithiasis, cholangitis, or intrahepatic cholestasis. In many cases, they are even contraindicated.

Recommended Herbal Remedies (Overview)

Choleretics

➤ **Boldo leaf** (Boldo folium); **milk thistle fruit** (Cardui mariae fructus, see p. 93); **turmeric root** (Curcumae longae rhizoma, C. xanthorrizae rhizoma, see p. 121); **artichoke leaf** (Cynarae folium, see p. 36); **fumitory** (Fumariae herba, see p. 68); **yarrow herb** and **flower** (Millefolii herba et flos, see p. 131); **radish root** (Raphani radix); **dandelion root** and **herb** (Taraxaci radix et herba, see p. 54).
  – *Action:* Stimulate the flow of bile and induce spasmolysis.
  – *Contraindications*
    • *Boldo leaf:* Biliary obstruction, severe liver disease. Should be used with caution in patients with gallstones.
    • *Artichoke, turmeric, dandelion:* Liver disease. Should not be used concomitantly with hepatotoxic medications.
    • *Yarrow:* Hypersensitivity to yarrow and other composite plants.
  – *Side effects*
    • *Radish:* Can upset the stomach and cause heartburn and belching.
    • *Dandelion:* Can upset the stomach by causing hyperacidity.

Cholegogues

➤ **Peppermint oil** (Menthae piperitae aetheroleum, see p. 103); **peppermint leaf** (Menthae piperitae folium, see p. 102); **radish**; **fumitory** (Fumariae herba, see p. 68); **dandelion herb** (Taraxaci herba, see p. 54).

- *Action*: These herbal remedies have specific antispasmodic effects and stimulate exocrine pancreatic juice secretion. They are variably effective in increasing the secretion and release of bile (choleresis).
- *Contraindications*
  - *Peppermint oil:* Biliary tract obstruction and jaundice. Should be used with caution by patients with gallstones.
- *Side effects*
  - *Peppermint oil:* Stomach problems. Gastroesophagealreflux.

Range of Applications in Acute Clinical Pictures

Sudden and Severe Flatulence

➤ **Wormwood** (see p. 129); **belladonna** (see p. 170); **caraway**; **valerian root**.
  - *Dosage and administration*
    - **Tincture *Rx*:** Ol. Carvi 5.0, Tinct. Absinthii, Tinct. Carminativa, aa 10.0; Tinct. Belladonnae 10.0; Tinct. Valerianae aeth. 15.0. Take 30 drops after meals, 3 times a day.
  - *Clinical value:* See Epigastric Complaints, p. 174.

Biliary Dyskinesia

➤ **Wormwood** (see p. 129).
  - *Dosage and administration*
    - *Dried herb:* Steep 1 teaspoon of the finely chopped herb or a commercial tea bag in 1 cup of water for no more than 5 minutes. Drink 1 cup, 3 times a day.
    - *Tincture:* 10 to 30 drops in a relatively small amount of water, 3 times a day.
    - ◉ *Note:* The bitter taste is absolutely essential. Not to be used during pregnancy or lactation. Teas are safer: avoid using alcoholic preparations for more than 1 week.
  - *Clinical value:* Large interindividual differences in the effects of these remedies can be observed.

Gastrointestinal Spasms with Gallbladder Dyskinesia

➤ **Boldo leaf** (Boldo folium); **turmeric root** (Curcumae longae rhizoma); **fumitory** (Fumariae herba, see p. 68).
  - *Dosage and administration*
    - *Boldo leaf:* Steep 2 teaspoons of the finely ground herb in 1 cup of boiled water for 10 minutes. Take 1 cup, 2 to 3 times a day.
    - *Turmeric root:* Pour 1 cup of boiled water onto 1 to 2 teaspoons of the finely chopped root, then cover and steep for 5 minutes. Drink 1 cup before meals.
    - *Fumitory:* Steep 2 teaspoons of the herb in 1 cup of boiled water for 10 minutes. Drink 1 cup with meals, 3 times a day.
    - ***Rx* 1** Turmeric *tincture (1 : 10):* 10 to 15 drops in a small amount of water, 3 times a day.
    - **Tincture *Rx* 2:** Ol. Menthae Piperitae 1.0; Tinct. Belladonnae 4.0; Tinct. Cardui Mariae, aa ad 30.0. Take 40 drops in water, 3 times a day.
    - ◉ *Note:* The duration of use should be limited to 3 to 4 weeks. If no improvement after 3 to 4 weeks, seek alternative therapy.

– *Clinical value*
  • *Fumitory:* Relatively strong antispasmodic.
  • *Boldo leaf:* Mild antispasmodic.
  • *Turmeric root:* Cholecystokinetic agent.
  • Tinctures of peppermint oil, belladonna: Relatively strong effects.
  • Interindividual differences in effects can be observed. The remedy should be selected according to the individual preferences of the patient.

Range of Applications in Chronic Clinical Pictures

Reduced Bile Flow (with or without lack of appetite)

➤ **Wormwood**; **peppermint leaf**; **dandelion root**; **milk thistle fruit**; **blessed thistle**.
  – *Dosage and administration*
    • **Tea *Rx*:** Cnici benedicti herba, Absinthii herba, Menthae piperitae folium, Cardui mariae fructus, Taraxaci radix cum herba, aa ad 100.0. Steep 1 teaspoon in 1 to 2 cups of boiled water for 20 minutes. Take 1 cup, 3 times a day, for a duration of 3 to 4 weeks.
    • **Tincture *Rx*:** Tinct. Cardui Mariae, Tinct. Absinthii, aa 15.0; Spir. Menthae Piperitae 20.0. Take 20 drops in water shortly before meals, 2 times a day.
  – *Clinical value:* For medium-strength treatment.

Chronic Biliary Dyskinesia with Frequent Dyspepsia and Constipation

➤ **Radish**; **caraway**; **fennel**; **peppermint leaf**; **yarrow**; **senna leaf**; **wormwood**; **frangula bark**.
  – *Dosage and administration*
    • *Black or white radish juice:* Peel and chop or grate the radish, then extract the juice (preferably with a vegetable juicer). Refrigerate for a few hours. Add sugar, honey, or flaxseed meal or gruel before use. Drink 100–150 mL of the juice, divided into small portions, for 4 to 5 consecutive days, then take a break for 2 to 3 days.
    ◉ *Note:* Can upset the stomach (see p. 182).
    • **Tea *Rx* 1:** Carvi fructus, Foeniculi fructus, aa 10.0; Menthae piperitae folium 30.0, Millefolii herba, Lavandulae flos, aa 20.0; Sennae folium 15.0. Steep 1 to 2 teaspoons in 1 cup of boiled water for 15 minutes. Take 1 cup each morning and evening.
    ◉ *Note:* This tea can be used for several weeks at a time.
    • **Tea *Rx* 2:** Carvi fructus 10.0; Menthae piperitae folium, Absinthii herba, aa 30.0; Frangulae cortex, Sennae folium (chopped), aa 15.0. Steep 1 to 2 teaspoons in 1 cup of boiled water for 10 minutes. Take 1 cup each morning and evening.
    ◉ *Note:* This rather potent tea should not be used for more than 1 to 2 weeks.
  – *Clinical value:* Large interindividual differences in effects can be observed.

Chronic Biliary Dyskinesia with Dyspepsia and Lack of Appetite

➤ **Dandelion root**; **belladonna**; **fennel**; **wormwood**; **milk thistle fruit**; **chamomile flower**.
  – *Dosage and administration*
    • *Dandelion root:* Place 1 to 2 teaspoons of the finely chopped herb in 1 cup of cold water, bring to a boil, remove from heat and allow to steep for 15 minutes. Take 1 cup each morning and evening for a period of 4 to 6 weeks.
    • **Tincture *Rx*:** Tinct. Belladonnae, Tinct. Absinthii, Tinct. Cardui Mariae, Tinct. Foeniculi Comp, Tinct. Chamomillae, aa 10.0. Take 20 drops in water after the noon and evening meal for no more than 3 to 4 weeks.
    • *Commercial dandelion juice:* Adults take 1 tablespoon after meals, 2 to 3 times daily. Children take 1 teaspoon after meals, 2 to 3 times daily.
    • *Commercial dandelion coated tablets:* Take 1 to 2 tablets with water or allow to dissolve in water and drink.
      ◉ *Note:* Can upset the stomach (see p. 182).
  – *Clinical value*: These remedies are helpful in many patients.

Diseases and Dysfunctions of the Digestive Organs

3

Diseases and Dysfunctions of the Digestive Organs

6.7 Diseases of the Rectum and Colon

Clinical Considerations

➤ **General comments**
- *Acute proctitis:* Symptoms range from mild to severe rectal pain, mucous and/or bloody discharge, and tenesmus. The main pathogens involved are *Herpes simplex virus, Cytomegalovirus, Gonococcae, Chlamydia, Yersinia, Isospora, Treponema pallidum,* and various amebae.
- *Chronic inflammatory bowel disease:* Proctitis associated with such diseases as ulcerative colitis must be differentiated from idiopathic ulcerative proctitis.
- *Radiation proctitis:* Often does not occur until several months or years after abdominal radiotherapy.
- *Hemorrhoids:* Hemorrhoids are a common problem. Habitual sitting activity, chronic constipation, and familial disposition promote their development. Mild hemorrhoids respond well to conservative therapy.
- ◎ *Important:* The possibility of a carcinoma must always be ruled out when hemorrhoidal bleeding is found.

➤ **Herbal treatment measures**
- Herbs with anti-inflammatory, mucilaginous, astringent, vulnerary, and venotonic effects are used for local treatment.
- Antispasmodic, anti-inflammatory, and laxative herbs are used internally.
- A variety of active principles can be used. External and internal remedies can be combined as needed.

➤ **Clinical value of herbal medicine**
- Herbs are not suitable for causal treatment of these diseases.
- Herbal remedies are suitable for adjunctive treatment of acute proctitis.
- Herbal remedies are suitable for adjunctive treatment of proctitis associated with chronic inflammatory bowel disease or radiation proctitis.
- Herbal remedies can be used to treat mild hemorrhoids and to prevent their recurrence.

Recommended Herbal Remedies (Overview)

Antiphlogistics

➤ **Arnica flower** (Arnicae flos, see p. 35); **chamomile flower** (Matricariae flos, see p. 47); **witch hazel leaf** and **bark** (Hamamelidis folium et cortex, see p. 128).
- *Action:* For local treatment of inflammation.
- *Contraindications:* Arnica and chamomile flower should not be used by individuals with a known allergy to composite plants.

Astringents

➤ **Witch hazel leaf** and **bark** (Hamamelidis folium et cortex, see p. 128); **oak bark** (Quercus cortex, see p. 99); **mallow flower** and **leaf** (Malvae flos et folium, see p. 89); **horse chestnut seed** (Hippocastani semen, see p. 77).
- *Action*
  - *Topical application:* Slight coagulation and drying of the superficial cell layers, formation of a protective barrier against bacteria, alleviation of inflammation-related complaints, relieves itching.
- *Contraindications:* Oak bark should not be used by patients with extensive skin damage at the site of application.
- *Side effects:* None known to occur after external application.

Hemostyptics

➤ **Alchemilla** (Alchemillae herba); **yarrow herb** (Millefolii herba, see p. 131).
  - *Action*: Hemostyptic.
  - *Contraindications*: None known.
  - *Side effects*: None known.

Demulcents

➤ **Mallow leaf** (Malvae flos, see p. 89); **flaxseed** (Lini semen, see p. 66).
  - *Action:* When applied externally, the mucilage in these herbs relieves irritation by covering nerve endings.
  - *Contraindications:* None known.
  - *Side effects*: None known.

Vulnerary agents

  - **St. John's wort oil** (Oleum Hyperici, see p. 115).
    • *Action*: Promotes wound healing when applied topically.
    • *Contraindications*: None known.
    • *Side effects*: None known.

Laxatives

➤ **Indian plaintain seed** and **husk** (Plantaginis ovatae semen et testa, see p. 106).
  - *Action:* Softens the stools, making it easier to have a bowel movement. For internal use only.
  - *Contraindications:* Bowel obstruction, abdominal pain of unknown origin, pathological narrowing of the gastrointestinal tract, refractory diabetes mellitus.
  - *Side effects:* If gastrointestinal inflammation exists, the herbal remedy can cause additional irritation and cramps; constipation may also occur.

Tonics

➤ **Calamus root** (Calami rhizoma, see p. 44).
  - *Action:* Stimulates the secretion of mucus and improves intestinal smooth muscle tone. For internal use only.
  - *Contraindications:* Should not be applied during pregnancy or by children under 12 years of age.
  - *Side effects:* None known.

Range of Applications in Acute Clinical Pictures _____

Acute Proctitis

➤ **St. John's wort**; **chamomile**; **mallow**; **flaxseed**.
  - *Dosage and administration*
    • *Retained enema:* Inject twice daily with an irrigator.
    • *Irrigation:* Flush the colon with an infusion made of chamomile flower, mallow flower or flaxseed (1 teaspoon of either herb in 150 mL of water).
  - *Clinical value:* For adjunctive treatment.

6.7 Diseases of the Rectum and Colon

Acute Hemorrhoidal Inflammation

➤ **Chamomile**; **arnica**; **oak bark**; **witch hazel**.
  – *Dosage and administration*
    • *Chamomile fluid extract:* 1 teaspoon in 500 mL of water.
    • *Arnica tincture:* 1 to 2 teaspoons in 500 mL of water.
    • *Oak bark:* Boil one small handful in 1 liter of water for 1 minute, then allow to cool to room temperature and use to prepare wet compresses. The compresses should be applied for at least 1 hour in the morning and evening (and at noon, if necessary): The infusion can also be used for a sitz bath. Apply witch hazel ointment immediately after the treatment and after each bowel movement.
  – *Clinical value:* Effective treatment measures.

Range of Applications in Chronic Diseases

Subacute and Chronic Proctitis

➤ **Tormentil**; **chamomile flower**; **calamus root**.
  – *Dosage and administration*: Inject either of the two solutions below into the colon using an irrigator.
    • *Tormentil tincture:* 1 teaspoon in 1 cup of chamomile tea.
    • *Calamus root:* 2 teaspoons in 150 mL of water.
  – *Clinical value*: Useful alternative to synthetic drugs.

Chronic hemorrhoids

➤ **Internal: Chamomile**; **calamus root**; **fennel seed**; **senna leaf**; **frangula bark**. **External: Witch hazel**.
  – *Internal dosage and administration*
    • **Tea Rx:** Matricariae flos, Calami rhizoma, Foeniculi fructus, Sennae folium, Frangulae cortex, aa ad 100.0. Steep 1 to 2 teaspoons in 1 cup of boiled water for 10 minutes. Drink 1 cup each morning and evening for no more than 1 to 2 weeks.
    • *Commercial product:* Stir 1 teaspoon of the blend in plenty of water and take 2 to 6 times daily. Other medications should not be taken until 30 to 60 minutes later.
  – *External dosage and administration*
    • *Witch hazel ointment:* Gently apply a thin layer several times a day, as needed.
    • *Witch hazel suppositories:* Use 1 to 2 suppositories per day.
    • *Commercial products:* Many commercial products are available.
    ◉ *Note:* We recommend combining the internal and external remedies.
  – *Clinical value*: These remedies are effective alternatives to synthetic drugs.

Anal Fissures

➤ **Horse chestnut**; **belladonna**.
  – Dosage and administration
    • *Horse chestnut:* creams, standardized extract in capsules or tablets
    • **Ointment Rx:** Extr. Myricae 5.0, Extr. Belladonnae 0.5, Unguentum Molle, ad 50.0. For topical application as needed.

– *Clinical value*: Effective treatment measures that quickly alleviate the problems associated with anal fissures. Should not be used for extended periods.

6.8 Acute and Chronic Diarrhea

Clinical Considerations

➤ **General comments**
  – Diarrhea is defined as the passage of pasty or watery stools more than 3 times a day.
  – It is the cardinal symptom of infectious diseases and viral enteritis.
  – Other causes of diarrhea include functional bowel disorders with hypermotility and hypersecretion (especially, in the small intestine), allergic enteropathy, ulcerative colitis, hyperthyroidism, and chronic alcoholism.

➤ **Herbal treatment measures:** Blackberry root, white oak bark tea (1 to 4 g/day), bilberry standardized extract (25% anthocyanidins) in capsules or tablets (80 mg, 3 times aday).
  – Bilberry is especially suitable for pediatric use. Astringent teas and tinctures contain tannins that seal the surface of the intestinal mucosa, thereby reducing the escape of fluids.

➤ **Clinical value of herbal medicine**
  – Herbal antidiarrheal agents can be used as a part of dietary therapy or for purely symptomatic treatment. They are especially useful in cases where synthetic drugs cannot or should not be used. Hence, the herbs are used in subacute cases of enteritis and enterocolitis as well as in summer diarrhea and, with certain restrictions, functional diarrhea.
  – Antibiotics are the first-line drugs for treatment of severe bacterial enterocolitis.

Recommended Herbal Remedies (Overview)

Astringents

➤ **Blackberry root** as a tea (2–4 g/day); **bilberry fruit** (Myrtilli fructus); **black currant** (Ribes nigrum); **blackberry** (Rubi fructicosi folium, Rubi fructicosi radix); **oak bark** (Quercus cortex, see p. 99); tormentil root see p. 121 (Tormentillae rhizoma)
  – *Action:* Seal the surfaces of the intestinal mucosa.
  – *Contraindications:* None known.
  – *Side effects:* Oak bark and tormentil root may upset the stomach of sensitive individuals.

Laxatives

➤ **Psyllium** (Psylli semen, see p. 106); **blond psyllium** (Plantago ovatae semen, see p. 106).
  – *Action:* Psyllium helps to regulate the bowels and bind excess fluids.
  – *Contraindications:* See p. 107.
  – *Side effects:* See p. 107.

Antiphlogistics

➤ **Oak bark** (Quercus cortex, see p. 99).
  – *Action:* Anti-inflammatory.
  – *Contraindications:* None known.
  – *Side effects:* May upset the stomach of sensitive patients.

Immunostimulants

➤ **Dry yeast** (*Saccharomyces boulardii*).
  – *Action:* Dry yeast antagonizes a number of intestinal pathogens and temporarily fortifies the overall immune system by unspecific stimulation of humoral and cellular immune defenses. It colonizes the small intestine and is lysed in the colon by bacteria that are resident there.
  – *Contraindications:* None known.
  – *Side effects:* None known.

Range of Applications in Acute Diarrhea _____

Acute Diarrhea of Any Origin

➤ **White oak bark**; **bilberry**; **blackberry leaf and root**; **oak bark**; **black currant**.
  – *Dosage and administration*
    • *White oak bark:* Place 1 teaspoon of the chopped herb in 1 cup of cold water and bring to a short boil. Take 1 cup, 3 times a day.
    • *White oak bark tincture 1 : 10:* Take 10 to 30 drops in a liqueur glassful of water several times daily or, for acute conditions, hourly.
    • **Tincture *Rx*:** Tinct. Cortex Quercus albae, Tinct. Carminative, aa 25.0. Take 30 to 40 drops in warm chamomile tea, 3 to 5 times a day.
    • *Dried bilberries:* Simmer 3 tablespoons in $^{1}/_{2}$ liter of water for 30 minutes. Take 1 cup, 3 to 5 times a day. Heat each portion before use. Alternatively, take 2 capsules of standardized bilberry extract.
    • *Blackberry leaves:* Steep 1 teaspoon of the finely chopped herb in 1 cup of boiled water for 10 to 15 minutes. Drink 1 cup between meals, 3 to 5 times a day.
    • *Oak bark:* Place $^{1}/_{2}$ teaspoon of the finely chopped bark in 1 cup of cold water, bring to a boil and steep for 5 minutes. Take 1 cup, 30 minutes before each meal.
    • *Black currant juice:* Drink 1 glass, 3 to 5 times a day.
    • *Blackberry or raspberry leaf, or blackberry root powder Rx*: Folia Rubi idaei, Folia Rubi fruticosi, or Radix Rubi fruticosi (finely powdered) 100.0. Take 1 coffee spoonful, 3 to 5 times a day.
  – *Clinical value*
    • *Black currant:* For mild action.
    • *Tormentil tincture:* For mild action.
    • *Bilberry and blackberry:* Medium-strength remedies.
    • *Tormentil root:* Relatively strong action.
    • *Oak bark:* Potent remedy.

Gastroenteritis with Torpidity

➤ **Tormentil root**; **wormwood**; **gentian root**.
  – *Dosage and administration*
    • **Tincture *Rx*:** Tinct. Tormentillae 30.0; Tinct. Absinthii, Tinct. Gentiana, ad 50.0. Take 30 drops in water, 3 times daily.
    ◎ *Note:* Should not be used for more than a few days at a time.
  – *Clinical value*: Relatively potent remedies.

3

Infant Dyspepsia (Infantile Dystrophy)

➤ **Bilberry**; **chamomile**; **fennel**.
   – *Dosage and administration*
     • Add contents of 1 capsule of standardized bilberry extract to water or chamomile tea.
     ◉ *Note:* This is a very low-calorie preparation.
     • *Fennel seed:* Pour 1 cup of boiled water onto 1 teaspoon of the crushed seeds, then cover and steep for 5 minutes. Take 1 to 2 cups, 5 times a day.
     • *Fennel oil:* Take 2 to 4 drops in a small quantity of water, 5 times a day. Dose: 150–200 g/kg per day.
   – *Clinical value*
     • *Bilberry:* Effective remedy, even in infantile vomiting and diarrhea-related diaper rash.
     • *Fennel:* For mild action.

Acute Diarrhea in Small Children

➤ **Bilberry**; **chamomile**.
   – *Dosage and administration:* Suspend the finely ground and sieved dried bilberry fruit in water or chamomile tea to yield a 10–20% suspension, boil for 3 minutes, then bind with 15% rice flour. Take 3 to 5 teaspoons, 3 to 5 times a day.
   – *Clinical value:* Well tolerated and effective remedy.

Range of Applications in Chronic Diarrhea _____

Chronic Enteritis

➤ **Fennel**; **balm**; **calamus root**; **peppermint leaf**.
   – *Dosage and administration*
     • **Tea *Rx*:** Foeniculi fructus, Menthae piperitae folium, Melissae folium, Calami rhizoma, aa 20.0. Steep 1 teaspoon in 1 cup of boiled water for 10 minutes. Take 1 cup, 2 to 3 times a day. The tea should be sipped slowly while hot.
   – *Clinical value*: This formulation is suitable for long-term use.

Abnormal Bacterial Flora

➤ **Chamomile**.
   – *Dosage and administration*
     • 1 cup of strong chamomile tea, sweetened with 1 to 2 teaspoons of lactose (milk sugar), 3 to 4 times a day.
   – *Clinical value:* For adjuvant therapy.

Recurrent Diarrhea

➤ **Psyllium seed and husk**.
   – *Dosage and administration:* Take 2 teaspoons, 3 times a day for 1 to 3 days. Afterwards, take 3 times daily as needed.
   ◉ *Note:* After taking psyllium seed, the patient should wait for 30 to 60 minutes before taking other medications.
   – *Clinical value:* For adjuvant therapy.

Preternatural Anus

➤ **Psyllium seed and husk**.
  – *Dosage and administration:* Swallow 1 to 2 teaspoons whole, with at least 1 glass of water.
  – 👁 *Note:* After taking psyllium seed, the patient should wait for 30 to 60 minutes before taking other medications.
  – *Clinical value:* For adjuvant therapy.

Crohn's Disease

➤ **Psyllium seed and husk**.
  – *Dosage and administration:* Psyllium seed: Swallow 1 to 2 teaspoons whole, with at least 1 glass of water. Granulated psyllium husks: Take 1 teaspoon or 1 packet, mixed with a glass of water, 2 to 6 times daily.
  – 👁 *Note:* After taking psyllium seed, the patient should wait for 30 to 60 minutes before taking other medications.
  – *Clinical value:* For adjuvant therapy.

6.9 Irritable Bowel Syndrome

Clinical Considerations _____

➤ **General comments**
  - Irritable bowel syndrome (irritable colon) is an intestinal dysfunction of unknown etiology. It is characterized by chronic, often agonizing abdominal pain with bowel irregularities and flatulence.
  - Painless diarrhea as well as spastic colon with sheep-dung stools are common symptoms.
  - Direct questioning of the patient often reveals a connection between the occurrence of symptoms and personal crises, stress, and so forth. This makes it easier to differentiate between these cases and irritable colon of organic origin. Irritable bowel syndrome is a diagnosis of exclusion.

➤ **Herbal and general treatment measures**
  - Dietary measures are extremely important. The patient should avoid all foods known to cause problems.
  - Wet hot compresses or a hot water bottle can be recommended for more severe complaints.
  - Bulk laxatives and swelling agents are the mainstay of herbal treatment. Demulcents should preferentially be used because of their high water-binding capacity but relatively low potential for gas formation.
  - Relaxants that primarily target the smooth muscle of the colon (e. g., peppermint oil in enteric-coated capsules) can be very useful.
  - Herbal carminatives can be used for adjunctive treatment. Digestive enzymes should not be used.

➤ **Clinical value of herbal medicine**
  - Conventional treatment regimens for these conditions often are not very effective.
  - Anticholinergic agents do nothing to improve the subjective symptoms.
  - Herbal remedies are often able to achieve clear improvement of symptoms.

Recommended Herbal Remedies (Overview) _____

Demulcents

➤ **Psyllium seed** (Psyllii semen, see p. 106); **psyllium seed and husk** (Plantaginis ovatae semen, see p. 106).
  - *Action:* Improve bowel regularity.
  - *Contraindications:* See p. 107.
  - *Side effects:* Cf. p. 107. Preexisting complaints such as flatulence and bloating may worsen during the first few days of treatment, but subside during the further course of treatment. Hypersensitivity reactions occur in isolated cases.
  - *Interactions:* Should not be taken concomitantly with other antidiarrheal drugs that affect intestinal motility. May delay the uptake of medications administered by the intestinal route.

Relaxants

➤ **Peppermint oil** (see p. 103).
  - *Action:* When used in enteric-coated capsule form, the menthol in peppermint oil is released into the colon. It blocks calcium channels of the nifedipine type in the smooth muscle, thereby exerting a spasmolytic effect on

the colon. The menthol does not enter into the circulation owing to a high first-pass effect.

– For further details, see p. 103. A recent metaanalysis of available clinical trials showed some efficacy over 4 to 6 weeks.

Range of Applications in Irritable Bowel Syndrome

➤ **Psyllium seed; psyllium seed and husk**
  – *Dosage and administration*
  – *Clinical value:* Long-term use is required for successful treatment.

Metaanalysis of Clinical Trials

  – Pittler MH, Ernst E: Peppermint oil for irritable bowel syndrome: a critical review and metaanalysis. Am J Gastroenterol 93(7) (1998), 1131–1135.

Diseases and Dysfunctions of the Digestive Organs

Clinical Considerations

➤ **General comments**
- Acute constipation usually has an identifiable organic cause.
- Chronic constipation is due to functional causes in 80–90 % of cases. Lack of exercise, unhealthy eating habits, suppression of the urge to defecate, and pseudoconstipation play an important role.
- Acquired diverticulosis is characterized by the presence of multiple pseudodiverticula (circumscribed mucosal protrusions through gaps in the muscle layer). They develop when the intraluminal pressure becomes abnormally elevated owing to a low-fiber diet, chronic constipation, and weakness of the muscle and fibrous tissue in the intestinal wall (sigmoid colon in two-thirds of all cases).

➤ **Herbal and general treatment measures:** The primary goal of treatment is to eliminate the functional causes of constipation or colonic diverticulosis. Herbal laxatives should be used primarily for supportive treatment.

➤ **Clinical value of herbal medicine**
- Bulk laxatives have a very low incidence of side effects and are therefore an excellent choice for long-term treatment, especially in patients with chronic constipation.
- Stimulant laxatives should not be employed before all other measures have failed. They should not be used for more than 1 to 2 weeks without medical supervision. Stimulant laxatives can be used in combination with bulk laxatives in the transitional period.

Recommended Herbal Remedies (Overview)

Antiabsorptive and Hydragogue Laxatives (Anthranoid Drugs)

➤ **Rhubarb root** (Rhei rhizoma); **senna leaf and fruit** (Sennae folium et fructus); **frangula bark** (Frangulae cortex, see p. 67); **buckthorn fruit** (Rhamni cathartici fructus, see p. 42).
- *Action:* Almost all herbal stimulant laxatives are anthracene derivatives. They develop therapeutic action by stimulating local receptors after coming into contact with the intestinal mucosa. They effect an increase in propulsion and a decrease in intestinal passage time. The impairment of ion pumps leads to a loss of water and electrolytes in the intestinal lumen and impedes absorption, hydrating the fecal mass. The bacterial flora in the colon releases anthrones, the actual active principles, from the pharmacologically inert anthranoid drugs.
- *Contraindications:* Pregnancy (may induce abortion), appendicitis, gastrointestinal bleeding or stenosis, bowel obstruction, acute inflammatory diseases of the bowel, severe water and mineral imbalances. Should not be used by children under 12 years of age. Should not be used by women nursing a baby unless the expected benefits clearly outweigh the potential risks.
- *Side effects*
  - Excessive laxative action can lead to diarrheal stools, often in combination with abdominal pain. Cramplike gastrointestinal pain can occasionally occur, in which case the herbal remedy should be discontinued.
  - Triggers an increase in blood flow in the abdominal arteries, especially in the uterus and adnexa.

3

- Long-term use can affect the water and mineral balance, leading to potassium deficiencies, especially when taken together with diuretics or adrenal steroids. These laxatives can therefore amplify the effects of cardiac glycosides.
- May cause reversible pigmentation of the intestinal mucosa and reddish-brown discoloration of the urine.
- When administered intermittently and at low doses, side effects such as hypokalemia, damage to the renal tubules, and worsening of constipation are not to be expected.

Bulk Laxatives

➤ **Psyllium seed and husk** (Plantaginis ovatae semen, see p. 106); **psyllium seed** (Psylli semen, see p. 106); **flaxseed** (Lini semen, see p. 66).
  - *Action:* For mild laxative and mechanical stimulatory action. Bulk-forming agents absorb large quantities of fluids, thereby increasing the volume of the feces. This results in enlargement of the colon (stretch reflex) and increased intestinal peristalsis.
  - *Contraindications:* Esophageal stenosis, gastrointestinal stenosis, imminent or existing bowel obstruction, refractory diabetes mellitus.
  - *Side effects*: Hypersensitivity reactions have been reported in isolated cases.
  - *Interactions*
    - May delay the absorption of concomitant medications. Other medications should therefore be taken no sooner than 30 to 60 minutes after the laxative.
    - It may be necessary to reduce the insulin dose in insulin-dependent diabetics.

Range of Applications in Acute Clinical Problems _____

Mild Constipation during Pregnancy and in Cases where Softening of the Stools is Medically Indicated

➤ **Psyllium seed** (see p. 106); **psyllium seed and husk** (see p. 106).
  - *Dosage and administration*
    - Commercial products containing psyllium seed: see recommendations noted on labels.
    - Commercial products containing psyllium husks: see recommendations noted on labels.
  - *Clinical value:* These herbal remedies provide a mild and well-tolerated laxative for adults and children over 12 years of age. They can be safely used for extended periods.

Moderate Constipation

➤ **Caraway seed** (see p. 46); **fennel seed** (see p. 65); **peppermint leaf** (see p. 102); **senna leaf** (see p. 436); **frangula bark** (see p. 67); **rhubarb root.**
  - *Dosage and administration*
    - **Tea *Rx***: Carvi fructus, Foeniculi fructus, Menthae piperitae folium, Sennae folium, aa ad 100.0. Steep 2 to 3 teaspoons in 250 mL of boiling water for 15 minutes. Drink 1 to 2 cups of the tea in the evening, as directed.

- **Tea *Rx*:** Carvi fructus 20.0, Menthae piperitae folium 30.0, Sennae folium 10.0, Frangulae cortex 30.0. Steep 1 teaspoon in 1 cup of boiling water for 10 minutes. Take 1 cup each evening.
- *Dried rhubarb root:* Steep 1 teaspoon of the coarsely powdered root in 1 cup of boiling water for 10 minutes. Sweeten to taste with honey, a little licorice, or other sweetener. Take 2 cups each evening.
- *Clinical value:* These teas have medium potency and should not be used for more than 1 to 2 weeks at a time.

Severe Constipation

➤ **Senna leaf** (see p. 436).
  - *Dosage and administration:* For oral administration, preferably in the evenings.
  - *Clinical value:* Senna leaves have moderate to strong therapeutic action. Should not be taken for more than 1 to 2 weeks without medical supervision. Should not be administered to children under 12 years of age.

Severe Bowel Irritation and Severe Constipation

➤ **Senna leaf** (see p. 436).
  - *Dosage and administration:* Steep 1 teaspoon of the finely chopped leaves in 1 cup of cold water for 1 hour, then drink. For evening use only.
  - *Clinical value:* Medium-strength remedy. Should not be used for more than 1 to 2 weeks at a time.

Chronic Constipation

➤ **Chamomile flower** (see p. 47); **fennel seed** (see p. 65); **frangula bark** (see p. 67); **senna leaf** (see p. 436); **rhubarb root**.
  - *Dosage and administration*
    - **Tea *Rx*:** Matricariae flos, Foeniculi fructus, Frangulae cortex, Sennae folium, aa ad 100.0. Steep 1 to 2 teaspoons in 1 cup of boiling water for 10 minutes.
    - *Frangula fluid extract:* 20 to 40 drops each evening.
    - *Rhubarb tablets:* 2, 4, or 6 tablets each evening, depending on the severity of constipation.
  - *Clinical value:* Since these remedies are relatively mild, they are especially suitable for elderly patients with arteriosclerosis and gastrocardiac symptom complexes. Habituation is rarely observed.

Spastic Constipation

➤ **Belladonna** (see p. 170); **frangula bark** (see p. 67).
  - *Dosage and administration*
    - ***Rx*:** Extr. Belladonnae, standardized to 0.5 % total alkaloids; the average dose is about 0.5 mg alkaloids, 3 times a day. 0.3 – 0.5 Extr. Frangulae Fluid. ad 30.0. Take 20 to 40 drops in water in the evenings.
  - *Clinical value:* Should not be taken for more than 1 to 2 weeks at a time.

Range of Applications in Chronic Disease _____

Chronic Constipation

▶ **Flaxseed; psyllium seed** (see p. 106).
  – *Dosage and administration*
    • ***Rx:*** Lini semen (crushed or coarsly-ground) 200.0. Take 2 to 4 table-spoons mixed with stewed fruit, hot cereal, etc., 1 to 3 times a day.
    ◉ *Note:* Crushed flaxseed should be refrigerated and consumed within a week before the oil becomes rancid. Linseed has a high caloric and fat content. People with weight problems should therefore swallow the herbal remedy whole without chewing it, since the bulk-forming muci-lages are located in the epidermis of the seed husks.
    • *Psyllium seed:* Use commercial products as directed on the label.
  – *Clinical value:* These products are suitable for long-term or continuous use. Flaxseed takes at least 3 days to take effect. Mild to strong effects.

Diverticulosis

▶ **Psyllium seed and husk** (Plantaginis ovatae semen).
  – *Dosage and administration*
    • *Psyllium seed:* Take 2 teaspoons with at least 1 glass of water 1 hour be-fore retiring. If necessary, take an additional dose of 1 teaspoon before breakfast.
    • *Psyllium husks:* Use commercial products as directed on the label.
  – *Clinical value:* Low to medium strength remedy suitable for extended use.

Anal Fissures

▶ See Diverticulosis.

7.1 Urinary Tract Infections

Clinical Considerations

➤ **General comments**
  - Acute and chronic infections of the urogenital tract and bladder are more common in women than in men owing to differences in the pelvic anatomy. As in irritable bladder (see p. 204), increased urinary frequency and painful urination are the typical presenting symptoms.
  - Urine tests for identification of the bacterial pathogen facilitate the differential diagnosis and selection of an appropriate antibiotic.

➤ **General and herbal treatment measures**
  - The adequate intake of fluids (at least 2 liters per day) plays an essential role in the elimination of urinary tract infections.
  - Herbal teas can be used to dilute the urine. Warm sitz baths and graduated footbaths can enhance the effects of herbal teas.
  - *Warning:* Therapy with herbal diuretics (also called aquaretics) is contraindicated in patients with edema due to heart or kidney failure.

➤ **Clinical value of herbal medicine**
  - In urinary tract infection (UTI) without kidney involvement, herbal diuretics are administered for increased urinary excretion of the causative organisms.
  - Herbal diuretics help to eliminate water and harmful substances, such as bacteria. Some diuretic herbs (goldenrod, for example) have additional spasmolytic and/or analgesic effects.
  - UTI with kidney involvement requires primary antibiotic treatment. However, antibiotics are often unable to eliminate the infection completely, and many patients develop recurrences or antibody resistance, resulting in chronic disease. In these cases, herbal diuretics can be a useful adjunctive treatment measure.
  - Considering their effectiveness and very low rate side effects, the administration of diuretic herbs is very helpful in chronic urinary tract infection. We recommend the use of effective herb combinations.

Recommended Herbal Remedies (Overview) and Range of Applications

Arbutin-containing Herbs

➤ **Bearberry leaf** (Uvae ursi folium, see p. 123).
  - *Action:* In alkaline urine, arbutin is metabolized to the bacteriostatic substance hydroquinone.
  - *Indications:* For increased urinary excretion in cases of acute urinary tract infection.
  - *Contraindications*
    • Pregnancy and breast feeding. Should not be used by children under 12 years of age.
    • Arbutin-containing products should not be used for more than 1 week at a time or more than 5 times a year. Hence, they are not suitable for treatment of chronic disease.
  - *Dosage and administration:* Commercial bearberry leaf teas and medicaments should be taken as recommended by the manufacturer, usually 3 to 5 times a day. When using bearberry leaves alone, the tea should be

prepared as a cold infusion (see p. 123) to minimize the amount of tannins extracted. Owing to its strong taste, we recommend mixing bearberry leaves with other herbal diuretic herbs.

- *Side effects:* The tannins in bearberry leaf can cause stomach irritation.
- *Interactions:* Bearberry leaf should always be taken with foods (tomatoes, potatoes, fruit, etc.) or chemicals (e. g., sodium bicarbonate) that alkalinize the urine.
- Commercial products are readily available standardized to 20 % arbutin. Many brands of unstandardized tinctures in 30-mL dropper bottles are available, as is the bulk herb to make tea.
- **Tea *Rx*** for supportive treatment of acute inflammations of the lower urinary tract: Species Urologicae DAB 6/NRF: Uvae ursi folium 20 g, Orthosiphonis folium 10 g, Equiseti herba 20 g; Betulae folium 20 g, bean pods 20 g, Mate leaves 10 g. Pour 150 mL of hot water onto 1 teaspoon of the herbs, then cover and steep for 5 to 10 minutes. Take 1 cup, 6 times a day.

Other Herbal Diuretics

▶ **Birch leaf** (Betulae folium, see p. 39); **goldenrod herb** (Solidaginis virgaurea herba, see p. 63); **orthosiphon leaf** (Orthosiphonis folium, see p. 79); **stinging nettle herb** (Urticae herba, see p. 78); **horsetail herb** (Equiseti herba, see p. 97); **parsley root** (Petroselini radix, see p. 101); **dandelion root** and **herb** (Taraxaci radix cum herba, see p. 54).

- *Action:* These herbal remedies have diuretic effects owing to their content of essential oils, saponins, and flavonoids. The diuretic effect of some (especially dandelion leaf) may be due to potassium salts with osmotic effects.
- *Indications:* Acute and chronic urinary tract infections.
- *Contraindications:* Medications containing alcohol should not be used together with these herbal remedies. Do not use during pregnancy.
- *Dosage and administration:* Commercial teas and medications should be taken as recommended by the manufacturer, generally 3 to 5 times a day.
- *Side effects:* Individuals with edema due to heart or kidney failure should not use herbal diuretics.

7.2 Dysuria

Clinical Considerations

➤ **General comments:** Dysuria is a generic term referring to all conditions asso ciated with painful or difficult urination. This includes mild to moderate ur nary tract infection and stone-related urinary retention.
➤ **General and herbal treatment measures**
  – Herbal diuretics are used for increased urinary excretion of harmful chem icals and organisms. This form of diuretic therapy is contraindicated i patients with edema due to heart or kidney failure.
➤ **Clinical value of herbal medicine:** Herbal diuretics promote the urinary ex cretion of harmful substances and organisms. Unlike chemical diuretics, diu retic herbs do not attack the renal tubules, but increase the filtration rate an primary urine volume through increased blood flow and osmosis.
  🔘 *Warning:* The patient should consult a physician at the first signs of bloo in the urine or fever and/or if the general symptoms persist despite trea ment.

Recommended Herbal Remedies (Overview) and Range of Applications

➤ **Aromatic Herbs**
➤ **Juniper berry** (Juniperi fructus, see p. 80); **lovage root** (Levistici radix, se p. 88); **parsley** (Petroselini herba, see p. 101).
  – *Action:* Increase the urinary excretion of harmful bacteria, thus reducing th symptoms of chronic urinary tract disorders.
  – *Indications:* Dysuria.
  – *Contraindications:* Nephritis, pregnancy.
  – *Dosage and administration*
    • *Tea:* 1 cup, 3 to 5 times a day.
    • Commercial products should be used in these indications. They shoul be taken as recommended by the manufacturer, generally 3 to 5 times day.
  – *Side effects*
    • *Juniper berries:* Can cause albuminuria when overdosed or used for mor than 4 weeks.
    • *Parsley:* Kidney irritation or damage to the kidneys; photosensitizatio
    • *Lovage:* Photosensitization.
  – *Interactions:* None known.
➤ **Flavonoid-containing herbal remedies**
➤ **Goldenrod** (Solidaginis virgaureae herba, see p. 63); **birch leaf** (Betula folium, see p. 39); **horsetail** (Equiseti herba, see p. 97); **stinging nettle lea** (Urticae herba, see p. 97); **orthosiphon leaf** (Orthosiphonis folium, see p. 79
  – *Action:* See Urinary tract infection.
  – *Indications:* Dysuria.
  – *Contraindications:* None known.
  – *Dosage and administration:* Tea: 1 cup, 3 to 5 times a day, drink warm. Com mercial products should be administered as recommended by the manu facturer, generally 3 to 5 times a day.
  – *Side effects:* None known.

Diuretic Tea to Eliminate Urinary Tract Infection and Prevent Renal Gravel

▸ **Tea *Rx*:** Juniperi fructus, Solidaginis virgaurea herba, Levistici radix, Liquiritiae radix ad 25 g. Pour 150 mL of boiling water onto 1 teaspoon of the herbs, then cover and steep for 5 to 10 minutes. Take 1 cup, 3 to 5 times a day.

7.3 Irritable Bladder

Clinical Considerations

➤ **General comments**
  – Irritable bladder is a problem that primarily affects women. It is characterized by an increased urge to urinate with pollakisuria and burning during urination.
  – Harmful organisms in the urine generally are not found in irritable bladder.
  – Nonbacterial (fungal) infections, menopausal disorders (estrogen deficiency), and metabolic diseases (diabetes mellitus) have been implicated as etiological factors.
➤ **General and herbal treatment measures:** See Urinary Tract Infection, p. 200
➤ **Clinical value of herbal medicine:** Herbs that increase the excretion of urine (diuretics) can improve the symptoms of irritable bladder. If psychovegetative stress also plays a role, it can be helpful to combine the diuretics with stress-relieving herbs such as valerian, St. John's wort and/or hops.

Recommended Herbal Remedies (Overview) and Range of Applications

Diuretics

➤ **Birch leaf** (Betulae folium, see p. 39); **goldenrod leaf** (Solidaginis virgaureae herba, see p. 63); **orthosiphon leaf** (Orthosiphonis folium, see p. 79); **stinging nettle herb** (Urticae herba, see p. 97); **horsetail herb** (Equiseti herba, see p. 78); **parsley root** (Petroselini radix, see p. 101); **dandelion root and herb** (Taraxaci radix cum herba, see p. 54); **pumpkin seed** (Cucurbitae peponis semen, see p. 108).
  – *Action:* See Urinary Tract Infection, p. 200 ff. Anti-inflammatory herbs used for prostatic hyperplasia (see p. 207) have also proved to be helpful in irritable bladder.
  – *Indications:* Irritable bladder.
  – *Contraindications:* All of these herbs, except dandelion, nettle herb, and pumpkin seed, are contraindicated in pregnancy because they contain essential oils and are irritants or, in the case of horsetail, contain known toxic compounds. In North America, dandelion and nettle herbs are universally considered safe in pregnancy. Most of these herbs are sold in alcoholic tincture form in North America: people with preexisting liver disease should avoid these herbs and use them only in consultation with a qualified health care provider.
  – *Dosage and administration:* Commercial products should be administered as recommended by the manufacturer, generally 3 to 5 times a day.
  – *Side effects:* None known.

linical Considerations

- **General comments**
  - Urinary stones are classified as oxalate stones, calcium stones, urate stones, cystine stones, and phosphate stones according to the substances contained in them. Making the appropriate dietary changes is generally a sufficient prophylactic measure.
  - Around two-thirds of all urinary stones are small enough to be passed spontaneously.
- **General and herbal treatment measures**
  - Stone patients should receive diuretics to promote the urinary excretion of substances responsible for urolithiasis.
  - A fluid intake of 2–2.5 liters per day is also recommended to dilute the urinary concentration of stone-forming salts.
  - 👁 *Warning:* Herbal diuretic therapy is contraindicated in patients with edema due to heart or kidney failure.
- **Clinical value of herbal medicine**
  - Herbal diuretics increase the urinary excretion of stone-forming substances. Unlike chemical diuretics, they do not attack the renal tubules, but increase the filtration rate and primary urine volume by means of osmosis and circulatory stimulation.
  - In times of stone passage, analgesics and spasmolytics are required along with the diuretics.
  - 👁 *Warning:* The patient should consult a physician at the first signs of blood in the urine or fever and/or if the general symptoms persist despite treatment.

Recommended Herbal Remedies (Overview) and Range of Applications

Aromatic Herbs

- **Lovage root** (Levistici radix, see p. 88); **parsley herb** (Petroselini herba, see p. 101).
  - *Action:* See Dysuria, p. 202.
  - *Indications:* For increased urinary excretion in cases of urolithiasis.
  - *Contraindications:* Pregnancy.
  - *Dosage and administration:* Tea: 1 cup, 3 to 5 times a day.
  - *Side effects*
    - *Parsley:* Kidney irritation and damage; photosensitization.
    - *Lovage:* Photosensitization.

Flavonoid-bearing Herbal Remedies

- See Dysuria, p. 202.
  - *Action:* See Dysuria, p. 202.
  - *Indications:* For increased urinary excretion in cases of urolithiasis.
  - *Contraindications:* None known.
  - *Dosage and administration*: Tea: 1 cup, 3 to 5 times a day. Commercial products should be administered as recommended by the manufacturer, generally 3 to 5 times a day.
    - *Side effects:* None known.

3

7.4 Urolithiasis

For Prevention of Renal Gravel
➤ See Dysuria, p. 202.

Clinical Considerations

➤ **General comments**
- The prevalence of benign prostatic hyperplasia increases with age. About 55% of all men between 50 and 60 years of age are already affected.
- Symptoms do not manifest until significant prostate enlargement has occurred. A distinction is made between obstructive symptoms (delayed start of urination, diminished urinary stream, leakage of urine) and irritative symptoms (increased frequency of urination, nocturia, perception of residual urine).
- *Vahlensieck's classification*
  - *Stage I:* Unimpaired urination with or without a diminished urinary stream and without residual urine.
  - *Stage II:* Intermittent difficulty in urinating with or without small quantities of residual urine; mild bladder trabeculation.
  - *Stage III:* Constant difficulties in urination, bladder enlargement, obstruction of the upper urinary passages due to occlusion of the urethra, >50 mL of residual urine.
  - *Stage IV:* Constant difficulties in urination, bladder enlargement, obstruction of the upper urinary passages due to occlusion of the urethra, >100 mL of residual urine, progressive renal insufficiency.
- Multifactorial events, especially hormonal changes in advancing age, have been implicated as the cause of prostatic hyperplasia.
- Noninfectious prostate inflammation and recurrent urinary tract infections are responsible for the recurrent irritative symptoms.

➤ **General treatment measures**
- The possibility of urinary obstruction or malignant disease must be ruled out before starting any treatment measures, conventional or herbal.

➤ **Clinical value of herbal medicine**
- Herbal remedies are often used to treat stage I/II benign prostatic hyperplasia because they improve the irritative symptoms. The organ size is not affected.

Recommended Herbal Remedies (Overview) and Range of Applications

Herbal Remedies

➤ **Saw palmetto fruit** (Sabal fructus, see p. 116); **stinging nettle root** (Urticae radix, see p. 98); **pumpkin seed** (Cucurbitae peponis semen, see p. 108).
- *Action*
  - *Saw palmetto fruit:* Oily extracts of the herbal remedy were found to inhibit 5α-reductase and 3α-hydroxysteroid oxidoreductase as well as to inhibit the synthesis of prostaglandins and leukotrienes that promote inflammation and edema formation. They were also found to have antiandrogenic and antiestrogenic effects in humans.
  - *Stinging nettle root:* Water–ethanol extracts of the herbal remedy contain phytosterols, polysaccharides, lectins, and other important compounds. Stinging nettle has anti-inflammatory and immunomodulatory effects, inhibits cell growth, and modifies steroid metabolism. The herbal remedy reduces the frequency of nocturnal voiding. It also reduces the

3

residual urine volume while increasing the maximum urinary flow and urine volume.

- *Pumpkin seed:* The fatty oil in the herbal remedy is reported to be anti-bacterial, diuretic, and anti-inflammatory.

– *Indications:* Benign prostatic hyperplasia.

– *Contraindications:* None known.

– *Dosage and administration*: The use of commercial products is recommended since teas prepared from the herbs are not sufficiently potent. All of the commercial preparations are taken orally, as recommended by the manufacturer (generally 1 to 3 times a day).

– *Side effects*
- *Saw palmetto fruit:* Can upset the stomach in rare cases.
- *Stinging nettle root:* Occasionally causes nausea, bloating, heartburn, diarrhea, and flatulence.

Clinical Considerations

▶ **General comments**

- Around 20–30% of the population is affected by sleep disorders, and the frequency of these disorders increases with age.
- Alternation between different depths of sleep is essential for restful sleep. Mental performance and general well-being are also greatly dependent on restful sleep.
- A progressive sleep deficit (insomnia) due to deficient quality and/or quantity of sleep is classified as a manifest disease when the difficulties in falling asleep or staying asleep and general poor quality of sleep persist for more than one month, recur at a rate of at least three times a week, and have a negative effect on the patient's daytime well-being.
- Primary insomnia is a separate entity characterized by disturbances in the rhythmic change between sleep and wakefulness. Melatonin and various neurotransmitters play a role in the complex control mechanisms underlying these changes. The production of melatonin, the substance that synchronizes the sleeping–waking rhythm, slackens with age.
- Secondary insomnia may occur due to organic causes (e. g., restless legs syndrome) or psychiatric diseases as well as due to the consumption of alcohol, drugs, or medications.

▶ **General and herbal treatment measures**

- So-called sleep hygiene measures and behavioral therapy play an important role in the treatment of sleep disorders. Pharmaceutical agents should not be used unless these measures have failed.
- Herbal sleep aids should be taken orally. They are mainly used for treatment of nervous sleep disorders.
- Certain herbal baths also promote sleep. See Herbal Hydrotherapy, p. 285.

▶ **Clinical value of herbal medicine:** In light of the known side effects and danger of habit formation of benzodiazepine tranquilizers and other synthetic and chemical tranquilizers, herbal sedatives containing valerian, hops, passion flower, and lemon balm are becoming increasingly important in the treatment of mild to moderate sleep disorders.

Recommended Herbal Remedies and Range of Applications

▶ **Valerian root** (Valerianae radix, see p. 125); **hop cones** (Lupuli strobulus, see p. 75); **balm leaf** (Melissae folium, see p. 84); **passion flower herb** (Passiflorae herba, see p. 101); **lavender flower oil** (Lavandulae flosoleum. see p. 59)

- *Action*
  - *Valerian root:* The most important constituents in valerian root are the essential oil, valepotriates, and amino acids, which were shown to have overall central sedative and muscle relaxant effects in animals. No study data are available on their absorption, distribution and excretion in humans. Recent clinical studies in insomnia patients demonstrated that valerian root was able to normalize the sleep profile while improving the quality of sleep as well as the patient's daytime well-being. However, it took several days for the herbal remedy to take effect.
  - *Hop cones:* Oxidation products of the bitter principles humulone and lupulone as well as flavonoids are assumed to be responsible for the sleep-promoting effect of the herb. Hop cones are generally used in combina-

tion with other herbal remedies. In one clinical study, a mixture of ho
cones and valerian root was shown to improve the sleep pattern, de
crease the sleep induction time, and improve the patients' ability t
sleep through the night.

- *Passion flower herb:* The constituents responsible for the rather mil
sedative effects of the herb still have not been identified. Passion flowe
is almost always used in combination with other herbal remedies.
- *Balm leaf:* Balm leaf oil has calming and central sedative effects as wel
as spasmolytic, carminative, and antibacterial actions. This herb is par
ticularly useful in patients who find it difficult to fall asleep owing t
nervous heart and gastrointestinal problems.
- *Lavender flower:* Lavender flower oil has a weak calming effect and mit
igates nervous gastrointestinal complaints.
- *Chamomile:* Chamomile flower is mildly calming and promotes sleep a
a tea before bedtime. Chamomile tea is generally considered one of th
safest teas for children and mothers, and during pregnancy.

– *Contraindications:* Because of the lack of study data, valerian should not b
used during pregnancy and lactation or in children under 12 years of age
Patients with impaired liver function, epilepsy, or brain damage should no
use preparations containing alcohol.

– *Dosage and administration*
- **Sedative tea *Rx* 1:** Valerianae radix 40 g, Lupuli strobulus 20 g, Melissa
folium 15 g, Menthae piperitae folium 15 g, Aurantii pericarpium 10 g
Pour 1 cup of water onto 1 teaspoon of the herbs, then cover and stee
for 5 to 10 minutes. Take 2 to 3 cups during the day and 1 cup befor
retiring.

  ◉ *Note:* This tea is known for its pleasant taste.
- **Sedative tea *Rx* 2:** Valerianae radix, Lupuli strobulus, Melissae folium
Lavandulae flos, aa ad 100 g. Pour 1 cup of boiling water onto 1 teaspoo
of the herbs, then cover and steep for 5 to 10 minutes. Take 2 to 3 cup
during the day, and 1 cup before retiring.

– *Side effects* and drug interactions: Not known.
– *Clinical value:* These herbal treatments are a very good alternative to syn
thetic tranquilizers that are potentially habit-forming.

Clinical Considerations

➤ **General comments**
  – The frequency of nervous disorders and stress intolerance increases with age. These problems often affect people in poor social conditions, menopausal women, and aging smokers.
  – "Burnout" is caused by intense mental strain. The initial symptoms include listlessness, tiredness, and lack of motivation. These can later progress to dizziness, heart pains, gastrointestinal problems, sleep disorders, tensed back muscles, and low resistance to infections.

➤ **General and herbal treatment measures**
  – Stress intolerance and nervous disorders should be treated using a holistic strategy that includes exercise, relaxation, reduction of dietary fats and meats, and herbal treatment measures.
  – Standardized kava root extract (*Piper methysticum*) is an increasingly popular remedy for anxiety and tension.
  – Lemon balm oil is another safe and effective alternative treatment.
  – Unlike their synthetic counterparts, herbal tranquilizers are not habit-forming and they do not affect the patient's mental alertness or reaction time when taken short-term.

➤ **Clinical value of herbal medicine:** The growing number of clinical studies demonstrating beneficial effects and vast amounts of empirical data indicate that herbal remedies play an increasingly important role in these indications.

Recommended Herbal Remedies (Overview)

➤ **Kava rhizome** (Piperis methystici rhizoma, see p. 82); **balm leaf** (Melissae folium, see p. 84); **valerian root** (Valerianae radix, see p. 125); **passion flower herb** (Passiflorae herba, see p. 101); **lavender flower** (Lavandulae flos, see p. 59); St. John's wort (Hyperici herba, see p. 115).
  – *Action, dosage, and administration*
    • *Kava*
      – Kava extract contains anxiolytic substances called kavapyrones. Dopaminergic, glutamatergic, and serotoninergic mechanisms and inhibition of monoamine oxidases A and B may play a role in their therapeutic action. Only low-level binding of kava pyrones with the $GABA_A$-benzodiazepine receptor complex can be observed.
      – The herbal remedy induces relaxation without significant sedation. It also improves the anxiety, hot flushes, sleep disorders, and vertigo associated with menopausal syndrome.
      – Evidence suggests that kava also has a neuroleptic component.
      – Kava extracts are taken orally. Fundamentally, no rebound effects should occur when a patients is switched from benzodiazepines to kava. Moreover, one report shows that no rebound effects were observed after 24-week treatment with kava root extract was discontinued, and improvement of clinical symptoms was observed after only one week of treatment. Owing to the lack of sufficient clinical study data, kava cannot be recommended for treatment of panic attacks, phobias, compulsive disorders, or generalized anxiety disorders.
    • *Valerian and passion flower extracts*

- Counteract daytime nervous unrest and related concentration difficulties.
- The most important constituents in valerian root are the essential oil, valepotriates, and amino acids, which were shown to have overall central sedative effects and muscle relaxant effects in animals.
- No study data are available on their absorption, distribution, and excretion in humans.
- The constituents responsible for the rather mild sedative effects of passion flower herb still have not been identified. Passion flower is almost always used in combination with other herbal remedies.
  - *Balm leaf oil* relaxes tension and reduces sympathetic muscle tone.
  - *Lavender flower oil* has a weak sedative effect.
  - *St. John's wort:* See Psychovegetative Syndrome, p. 214.
- *Contraindications:*
  - *Kava:* Owing to the lack of sufficient study data, pregnant and nursing women, children under 12 years of age, and patients with endogenous depression should not use kava. Kava should also not be used by people with preexisting liver disease, or if taking potentially hepatotoxic pharmaceutical drugs, or if using alcohol regularly, without the advise of a qualified health care practitioner.
  - See Psychovegetative Syndrome, p. 214.
- *Side effects*
  - *Kava:* Although rare (1–3%), gastrointestinal complaints, headaches, or general allergic reactions can occur. Extrapyramidal side effects have also been reported. Patients with a history of liver damage and elderly individuals, especially those with Parkinson's disease, should use the herbal remedy with caution and medical supervision.
    ◉ *Warning:* See also p. 82.
- *Interactions:* Kava has potential for interacting with substances with central nervous system effects, e. g., alcohol, sleeping pills, and psychoactive drugs.

Range of Applications in Disorders of the Nervous System ____

Tension, Anxiety, Nervous Unease

➤ **Kava root**
- *Dosage and administration:* Oral daily dose: 60–120 mg of kava pyrones. Some researchers used as much as 210 mg of kava lactones per day in their clinical studies.
- *Clinical value:* Kava root is a safe and effective herbal alternative to potentially habit-forming synthetic tranquilizers.

Tension and Unease

➤ **Balm leaf** (see p. 84); **valerian root** (see p. 125); **passion flower herb** (see p. 101); **lavender flower** (see p. 59).
- *Dosage and administration*
  - *Balm spirit:* 2 teaspoons in 150 mL of water each day.
  - When using commercial products, they should be taken as recommended by the manufacturer. The recommended herbal remedies should be taken each day for a period of several weeks.
  - *Lavender flower oil:* Use in a vaporizer, 1 to 2 times daily.

- *Clinical value:* The recommended herbal remedies are good alternatives to synthetic tranquilizers, which can be habit-forming.
- ◉ *Note:* There is a lack of adequate proof of efficacy for most of the herbal remedies except valerian root and balm leaf oil.

8.3 Psychovegetative Syndrome

Clinical Considerations

➤ **General comments**
  - Psychovegetative syndrome is the generic term for all functional health disorders caused by stress or mental strain.
  - The typical patient has alternating symptoms (e.g., headache, stomach ache, heart problems, fatigue, and dizziness) without any pathophysiological or organic causes being detectable.
  - Around 25 % of the population is affected, especially women and individuals from poor social backgrounds.[1] The peak occurrence is in 20- to 40-year-olds.

➤ **Herbal treatment measures**
  - St. John's wort, either alone or in combination with valerian root extract (see Sleep Disorders, p. 209, and Depression and Mood Swings, p. 216) is the mainstay of herbal treatment.
  - The combination of St. John's wort extract with valerian root is thought to be more effective in psychovegetative syndrome.

➤ **Clinical value of herbal medicine:** Considering their low rate of side effects, herbal treatments should preferably be used instead of conventional psychoactive drugs.

Recommended Herbal Remedies (Overview)

➤ **Valerian root** (Valerianae radix)**:** For drug action, see Sleep Disorders, p. 209.
➤ **St. John's wort** (Hyperici herba, see p. 115)
  - *Action*: The literature currently shows that multiple mechanisms of action and substances are responsible for the therapeutic action of St. John's wort extract.
    • Hyperforin is said to be responsible for the herb's inhibition of synaptosomal norepinephrine, serotonin, dopamine, GABA, and glutamate uptake.
    • Another constituent, hypericin, may contribute to the herb's antidepressant effect by inhibiting dopamine β-hydroxylase.
    • Extracts of the herb contain flavonoids and flavonols, which are reported to up-regulate the density of HT_2 receptors and down-regulate beta receptors.
    • The herb inhibits the release of interleukin-6, the substance that increases cortisol secretion by activating the thyroid gland.
    • When tested in healthy volunteers, the herb was found to increase the release of interleukins from monocytes and to increase melatonin secretion, which may have a sleep-promoting effect.
  - *Contraindications:* Pregnant and nursing women should not use St. John's wort owing to the lack of adequate study data.
  - *Dosage and administration*
    • The recommended commercial products, which are generally standardized for hypericin, and increasingly hyperforin, are taken orally.
    • St. John's wort must be taken for at least 10 to 14 days before the effects become noticeable. A minimum three months of treatment is generally

---

1   WHO: The World Health Report 1998: Life in the 21st century. A vision for all. WHO, Geneva (1998). ISBN 92 4 156189 0.

recommended. Once the symptoms have improved, the herbal remedy should be gradually discontinued. Abrupt discontinuation is not recommended. Evidence shows that satisfactory effects can be achieved using low doses of the herbal remedy in long-term therapy.

– *Side effects*
  • The possibility of high-dose St. John's wort administration causing photo-sensitization in fair-skinned individuals cannot be ruled out. Until now, only few cases have been observed during postmarketing surveillance studies.
  • Gastrointestinal complaints, nausea, allergic skin reactions, and vertigo are rare side effects.
– *Interactions:* As St. John's wort mediates induction of the cytochrome P450 enzyme complex and induces the P-glycoprotein drug transporter, it can dampen the effects of numerous drugs such as cyclosporin, indinavir, and other protease inhibitors used in treatment of HIV or digoxin. It has also been found to counteract the effect of coumarin-type anticoagulants and of hormonal contraceptives.

Range of Applications in Psychovegetative Syndrome

➤ **St. John's wort** (see p. 115); **valerian root** (see p. 125).
  – *Dosage and administration*
    • *St. John's wort:* Recommended oral daily dose 900 mg standardized extract (corresponding to a minimum of 2 g St. John's wort per day).
  – *Valerian:* Commercial products should be taken as recommended by the manufacturer.
  – St. John's wort and valerian root are used either alone or in combination.
  – *Clinical value*: St. John's wort is rapidly gaining significance as a remedy for psychovegetative syndrome but, controlled studies on St. John's wort and/or valerian for this use are still not available.

8.4 Depression and Mood Swings

Clinical Considerations

➤ **General comments**

- Depression of variable severity occurs at a prevalence of over 15 %. This makes depression one of the most common diseases of our time. Women of various cultural groups are affected almost twice as often as men. Around 20–30 % of all individuals over 65 develop elderly-onset depression.
- Depression is almost always accompanied by sleep disorders, which can occur even before depression becomes clinically manifest. Patients with severe depression typically have difficulty going back to sleep and experience the lowest mood levels in the morning. Over half of these patients also suffer from some type of anxiety disorder.
- Although extensively researched, the cause of depression still is not fully understood. Recent studies on conventional antidepressants have, however, provided important new insights.
- Antidepressants increase the concentrations of norepinephrine, dopamine, and serotonin in the synaptic clefts of neuron complexes in the brain by inhibiting the enzymes that break down these substances and/or by promoting the reabsorption of neurotransmitters. It takes around 2 weeks for the adaptive changes in beta receptor sensitivity (beta down-regulation) to take effect. This coincides precisely with the time required for the drugs to take therapeutic effect. A regulatory increase in the number of alpha receptors in the brain also occurs, whereas the HT_2 receptor density decreases.
- Glutamatergic and GABAergic receptor systems are also believed to play an important role, because chronic administration of antidepressants leads to down-regulation of $GABA_A$ receptors. Depressive suicide victims have significantly higher densities of these receptors than normal subjects. Antidepressant and antimaniacal drugs induce a regulatory increase in $GABA_B$ receptors.

➤ **Herbal treatment measures:** Oral St. John's wort extracts are recommended for mild to moderate depression.

➤ **Clinical value of herbal medicine**

- Since conventional antidepressants, especially tricyclic drugs, are known to cause unpleasant and sometimes serious side effects, many patients and physicians refuse to use them.
- In recent years, high-dose St. John's wort extract has become an established alternative treatment for depression in Europe, and increasingly in North America and other countries. A number of efficacy studies have shown that the herbal remedy is just as effective as conventional antidepressants in mild to moderate depression. As for drug tolerance, that of St. John's wort was clearly superior to that of its conventional counterparts.
- St. John's wort extract does not have sedative effects. Moreover, it does not cause habituation or dependency and does not affect the patient's mental alertness or reaction time.
- Extracts made from St. John's wort can be prescribed for mild affective disorders, menopause-related depressive complaints, winter depression, and burnout syndrome and to help patients through a period of mourning.

Recommended Herbal Remedies and Range of Applications _____

➤ **St. John's wort**.
- *Action, contraindications, side effects:* See p. 115.
- *Dosage and administration:* See p. 115.
- *Bipolar affective disorders:* No evidence of a prophylactic effect has been found.
- *Severe depression:* St. John's wort should not be used to treat severe depression.
- The patient should be switched to a synthetic antidepressant if, after 4 to 6 weeks of treatment with St. John's wort extract, the symptoms fail to improve or worsen, especially if there is a risk that the patient may commit suicide.
- If the patient must be switched from St. John's wort to a synthetic antidepressant, the herbal remedy should not be discontinued until the synthetic drug has begun to take effect and, then, only gradually discontinued.
- ◉ *Note:* The available study data are not sufficient for an assessment of combined therapy with St. John's wort and synthetic antidepressants.

8.5 Primary Headache Disorders

Clinical Considerations

➤ **General comments**
  – Headaches are extremely common: 2.4 million Germans and as many as 45 million Americans are chronic headache sufferers.
  – Around 90 % of all headaches are either tension or migraine headaches.
  – *Tension headaches* are described as a radiating or dull pain or sensation of pressure of mild to moderate intensity that is felt throughout the entire head region. Tension headaches are usually episodic, but may become chronic. Their prevalence increases with age. Muscle tensions of physical or psychosomatic origin have been implicated as the probable cause of tension headache.
  – *Migraine headaches* are characterized by a sudden and severe onset of pain, usually only on one side of the head, that is often accompanied by nausea, vomiting, photophobia, phonophobia, and/or neurological deficits. When a migraine headache occurs, the cerebral blood vessels first contract, then undergo massive dilation. The latter phenomenon is responsible for the sensations of pain.
  ◉ *Note:* Headaches caused by permanent use of analgesics should be considered in the differential diagnosis.

➤ **General and herbal treatment measures**
  – *Tension headaches:* Physical measures are generally effective. Relaxation exercises are also useful if the problem is aggravated by emotional stress.
  – Peppermint oil relieves muscle pain and tension. It is applied topically to tender muscles or, in the case of tension headache, to the temples.

➤ **Clinical value of herbal medicine**
  – Many patients use OTC analgesics without medical supervision, although these drugs frequently cause side effects. Herbal remedies such as peppermint oil and guarana seed (*Paulina cupana*) are well-tolerated alternatives.
  – *Butterburr* contains petasin, a substance suitable for long-term management of migraine headaches.
  – Both guarana and butterburr are effective remedies for mild migraine headaches.

Recommended Herbal Remedies (Overview)

➤ **Butterbur root** (Petasitidis radix, see p. 107).
  – *Action:* Petasin has relatively strong spasmolytic and analgesic action.
  – *Contraindications:* Should not be used by pregnant and nursing women or by children under 12 years of age. The use of the herb is contraindicated in patients with preexisting liver conditions, unless pyrrolozidin-free extracts are used.
  – *Dosage and administration:* Recommended dose should be followed.
  – *Side effects:* None known.

➤ **Peppermint oil** (Menthae piperitae aetheroleum, see p. 103).
  – *Action:* Together with its main constituent, menthol, peppermint oil is readily absorbed by the skin. The analgetic action of the oil is presumably due to local stimulation of cold receptors, inhibition of nociceptors, and central stimulation. Peppermint oil also has muscle relaxant and vasodilatory effects.

– *Contraindications:* Should not be applied to or near the face of infants and small children.
– *Side effects:* Rare cases of type IV allergic reactions have been observed after topical administration.
– For details, see p. 103.

➤ **Guarana seed** (Paulinae cupanae semen).
– *Action:* Mother tinctures prepared from the roasted and ground seeds of *Paulina cupana* contain caffeine, theobromine, tannins, essential oil, saponins, and resins. The mode of action and active constituents of the herbal remedy have not yet been identified.
– *Contraindications:* Should not be used by pregnant and nursing women or by children under 12 years of age. Excessive or long-term use of any caffeine-containing herb can contribute to high blood pressure, nervousness, and insomnia.
   ◉ *Warning:* see p. 388.
– *Side effects:* None known.

Range of Applications

Migraine and Tension Headaches

➤ **Butterburr**; **guarana seed**; **peppermint oil**.
– *Dosage and administration*
   • *Migraine headaches:* Butterburr: Take 1 to 3 capsules, 3 times a day, as needed. To prevent new attacks, take 2 capsules twice daily for a period of 4 months.
   • *Tension or migraine headaches:* Guarana. For acute attacks, take 5 to 10 drops every 30 minutes. The single doses can be increased to as much as 20 drops if necessary. For chronic pain, take 5 to10 drops, 3 times a day. The single doses can be increased to as much as 20 drops if necessary.
   • *Tension headaches:* Massage a few drops of peppermint oil into the skin of the temples and the neck.
– *Clinical value*
   • *Butterburr extract:* Clinical studies demonstrate positive proof of efficacy of the herbal remedy in migraine headaches.
   • *Peppermint oil:* Clinical studies have demonstrated that the herbal remedy is a safe and effective alternative remedy for tension headaches.
   • *Guarana:* Postmarketing surveillance studies on guarana have been conducted for different types of headache. Guarana was not able to prevent migraine attacks.

Vertigo

➤ See Cardiovascular Diseases: Vertigo and Tinnitus, p. 142.

Dementia

➤ See Cardiovascular Diseases: Dementia, p. 143.

9.1 Non-age-related Debility

Clinical Considerations

➤ **General comments:** States of organic or functional debility can occur owing to various diseases, organ damage, surgery, or emotional strain. These problems are usually temporary.

➤ **Herbal treatment measures**
- These conditions are traditionally treated with tonics, roborants and analeptics, most of which target a particular organ, as well as adaptogenic drugs (alterants), which can also be recommended in phases of increased physical stress.
- Bitters are used to alleviate anorexia caused by severe disease, vegetative dysfunction, general asthenia, and reduced digestive enzyme function. They also help to speed up recovery from illness.
- Adaptogenic drugs are mainly used to counteract non-infection-related stressors. Immunostimulatory, nootropic, and anabolic affects have also been observed. These drugs have, in particular, been found to stimulate the cerebral metabolism as well as corticoid synthesis in the adrenal gland and DNA and protein synthesis in various organs.

➤ **Clinical value of herbal medicine**
- Herbal remedies are traditionally used in these indications.
- No comparable chemical medications are available. Anabolic drugs are associated with numerous side effects.

Recommended Herbal Remedies (Overview)

➤ **Tonic bitters: Centaury herb** (Centaurii herba, see p. 84); **cinchona bark** (Cinchonae cortex); **artichoke leaf** (Cynarae folium, see p. 36); **gentian root** (Gentianae radix); **horehound herb** (Marrubii herba, see p. 76); **bogbean leaf** (Menyanthidis folium, use only in combination with other herbal remedies); **dandelion leaf** and **root** (Taraxaci radix cum herba, see p. 54); **chicory herb** and **root** (Cichorii herba et radix).

➤ **Astringent bitters: Condurango bark** (Condurango cortex, see p. 52): to be used only in combination with other herbs.

➤ **Aromatic bitters: Wormwood** (Absinthii herba, see p. 129); **bitter orange peel** (Aurantii pericarpium, use only in combination with other herbal remedies); **calamus root** (Calami rhizoma, see p. 44); **angelica root** (Angelica radix, see p. 33); **blessed thistle herb** (Cnici benedicti herba); **yarrow herb** and **flower** (Millefolii herba et flos, see p. 131).

➤ *Acrid bitters:* **Cinnamon bark** (Cinnamomi cortex from *Cinnamomum cassiae* or *C. ceylanici*); **galangal root** (Galangae rhizoma); **ginger root** (Zingiberis rhizoma, see p. 70).

➤ **Adaptogenic herbal remedies: Siberian ginseng root** (Eleutherococcus radix, see p. 58). For further details, see Adaptogens, p. 227.

➤ **Other herbal remedies: Milk thistle fruit** (Cardui mariae fructus, see p. 93); **garlic bulb** (Allii sativi bulbus, see p. 70).
- *Action:* See Anorexia, p. 165; Immunodeficiency Diseases, p. 226; Chronic Hepatitis and Cirrhosis of the Liver, p. 180.
- *Contraindications:* Cf. pp. 93 and 70.
  - *Milk thistle:* Should not be used by children under 12 years of age.

- *Side effects:*
  - *Side effects:* Mild laxative effects, nervousness, and intolerance reactions have been observed in isolated cases.
  - *Garlic:* Gastrointestinal disturbances and allergic reactions have been reported as rare side effects of garlic, especially when fresh.
  - There is a slight possibility of interaction with blood-thinning medications such as dicoumarol.
  - ◉ *Warning:* Avoid garlic use for approximately 1 week before and after major surgery.

Range of Applications

Postflu Asthenia

➤ **Wormwood** (see p. 129).
  - *Dosage and administration*
    - *Tea:* Steep 1 teaspoon of the finely chopped herb in 1 cup of boiling water for no more than 5 minutes.
    - Commercial tea bags can also be used.
    - ◉ *Note:* The herbal remedy should not be taken for more than 3 to 4 weeks at a time.
  - *Clinical value*: Wormwood is very effective in stimulating the appetite.

Convalescence

➤ **Black currant** (see p. 350).
  - *Dosage and administration:* Black currant juice should be diluted with hot water. Drink 1 glass at noon and in the evening.
  - *Clinical value:* Completely safe household remedy.

Postsurgical and Postinfective Conditions

➤ **Wormwood herb** (see p. 129); **Siberian ginseng root** (see p. 58); **milk thistle fruit** (see p. 93); **garlic bulb** (see p. 70).
  - *Wormwood:* See tea preparation instructions listed above (Postflu Asthenia).
  - *Siberian ginseng, milk thistle, garlic:* Commercial products are recommended for these indications. They should be administered as recommended by the manufacturer.
  - *Clinical value:* These medications are well tolerated during periods of recovery, but clinical studies are not sufficient.

9.2 Adaptive and Functional Disorders of Aging ▬▬▬

Clinical Considerations _____

➤ **General comments**
  – *Dementia syndrome:* Dementia syndrome is usually caused by Alzheimer's disease (about 80 %); vascular causes are less common (about 10 %). The typical complaints include memory and concentration disorders, depressive mood, buzzing or ringing in the ears, and headaches.
  – *Arteriosclerotic cardiovascular diseases*
    • Includes heart failure (NYHA II) and "senile heart." In senile heart, the patient often suffers from objectively mild yet subjectively very disturbing cardiac arrhythmias and other diffuse cardiac complaints in the absence of any concrete anomalies.
    • Other typical age-related disturbances that respond to herbal remedies are mild arterial occlusive disease as well as tinnitus, sudden hearing loss (chronic), and generalized arteriosclerosis, including anginal complaints. Herbal remedies are generally administered as an adjunctive treatment measure.
  – *Anorexia and poor digestion:* Inappetence in this patient group is generally caused by troublesome changes in the masticatory apparatus and, less commonly, by reduced sensitivity of the taste receptors. Diminished gastrointestinal secretion and peristalsis result in impaired digestion.
  – *Respiratory tract diseases:* Latent damage caused by smoking and poor air quality tend to become more openly manifest as lung function decreases with age. The lungs can no longer clear themselves as well, resulting in low resistance to infections and chronic problems associated with coughing and expectoration (see Bronchitis, p. 154).
  – *Urological diseases:* Older men generally begin to experience problems associated with benign prostatic hyperplasia during the course of aging. The frequency of urinary tract infection increases in both men and women owing to unfavorable anatomic and hormonal changes (see Urinary Tract Infection, p. 200).
  – *Degenerative diseases and related pain:* Almost all elderly individuals experience temporary or chronic pain due to degeneration of supporting and connective tissues. These ailments have a decisively negative impact on the quality of life (see Rheumatic Diseases, p. 231).
  – *Psychiatric diseases:* States of restlessness and/or agitation and sleep disorders are very common in the elderly population. Depression can occur without many noticeable symptoms, and apathy is frequently the main complaint. These diseases can have a considerable to severe impact on the overall quality of life.
  – *General debility and convalescence:* Owing to the decreasing capacity of the immune defenses, elderly individuals generally have longer recovery periods, during which recurrence of the primary disease or a new disease can often occur.
➤ **Herbal treatment measures**
  – *Geriatric preparations*
    • Geriatric herbal preparations are preparations designed to improve age-related losses of function or vitality of the individual organ systems.
    • Lower-potency herbal preparations should always be used first. If the treatment results are unsatisfactory, more potent preparations can be

recommended later. Prolonged use should always be considered carefully.

◉ *Note:* When treating diseases characteristic of or caused by aging, the therapist should bear in mind that the bioavailability and pharmacokinetics of the active constituents also change as the body ages.

– *Nootropic preparations*
  • Nootropic herbal preparations are used to treat dementia syndrome.
  • They take effect in the brain and are reported to improve higher integrative cerebral functions such as memory, learning, cognition, thinking, and concentration capacities. Standardized ginkgo biloba leaf extracts can be used when a nootropic preparation is desired.

– *Senile heart*: The symptoms associated with this condition are often unresponsive to synthetic antiarrhythmic drugs. Standardized hawthorn extracts are used in this indication. They should be administered for at least 6 weeks. Three-month interval therapy is recommended.

– *Inappetence and poor digestion*
  • This is a classical indication for the geriatric use of bitters. The bitter taste stimulates specific taste buds of the tongue and, through them, a number of reflexes that increase the secretion of saliva and gastric juices. This, in turn, increases the secretion of enzymes and digestive juices, improves the utilization of nutrients, and stimulates motility throughout the entire gastrointestinal tract. It is not always necessary to start treatment with the most potent herbal remedy. Bitters are not suitable for long-term use.
  • Nausea, a common problem in the elderly, can be treated using standardized artichoke leaf extracts (see p. 36). They have cholagogue and antidyspeptic effects. Bile secretion can be stimulated using the herbal choleretics fumitory and celandine (see p. 68). Dandelion herb acts as a cholagogue (see p. 182).

➤ **Clinical value of herbal medicine:** Herbal preparations can be used in the field of holistic gerontotherapeutics, that is, therapeutic management designed to retard the sudden drop in performance that may occur after the sixth decade of life. Because patients tend to accept herbal remedies more readily than their synthetic alternatives, they are an excellent choice for treating the above-mentioned adaptive and functional disorders of aging.

Recommended Herbal Remedies (Overview)

Nootropic Preparations

➤ **Standardized ginkgo biloba leaf extract** (Ginkgo bilobae folium, see p. 71).

– *Action:* Treatment is designed to improve the memory, learning, cognition, thinking, and concentration capacities of patients with dementia-related diseases. Ginkgo presumably does this by stimulating the adaptive capacity of the still-intact neuron complexes. By various mechanisms (calcium antagonism, gene induction to promote stress hormone production), it also protects neurons from injurious effects of energy metabolism and transmitter metabolism or damage due to a deficient blood supply. Good treatment results can most easily be achieved in patients with mild to moderate dementia-related diseases, primary degenerative dementia, vascular dementia, and mixed forms of these diseases.

9.2 Adaptive and Functional Disorders of Aging

- *Contraindications:* Should not be used by children under 12 years of age.
- *Side effects:* Although very rare, gastrointestinal disturbances, allergic skin reactions, and headaches can occur.
- For further details on ginkgo, see Circulatory Disorders, p. 141.

Geriatric Preparations

➤ **Arteriosclerotic cardiovascular diseases: Hawthorn leaf** and **flower** (Crataegi folium cum flore, see p. 74); **lily-of-the-valley herb** (Convallariae herba, see p. 86); **garlic bulb** (Allii sativi bulbus, see p. 70); **ginkgo leaf extract** (Ginkgo bilobae folium, see p. 71); **artichoke leaf extract** (Cynarae folium, antilipemic effect, see p. 36).

➤ **Inappetence and poor digestion** (see p. 165 ff.): **Gentian root** (Gentianae radix); **centaury herb** (Centaurii herba, see p. 84); **bogbean leaf** (Menyanthidis folium); **dandelion root** and **herb** (Taraxaci radix cum herba, see p. 54); **calamus root** (Calami rhizoma, see p. 44); **angelica root** (Angelicae radix, see p. 33); **blessed thistle herb** (Cnici benedicti herba); **yarrow herb** and **flower** (Millefolii herba et flos, see p. 131); **artichoke leaf** (Cynarae folium, see p. 36); **fumitory herb** (Fumariae herba, see p. 68).

➤ *Respiratory tract diseases, urological diseases, degenerative diseases, psychiatric diseases:* The reader should refer to the chapter on the specific organ in question, since no particular differences are to be expected when treating elderly patients.

➤ **Panasthenia, convalescence: Ginseng root** (Ginseng radix, see p. 37); **Siberian ginseng root** (Eleutherococci radix, see p. 58). See also Conditions Related to Acquired Immunodeficiency, p. 226.

➤ **Other herbal remedy groups**
- *Bitters,* see p. 165.
- *Antilipemic herbal remedies,* see p. 144.
- *Antiatherosclerotic herbal remedies,* see p. 144.

Range of Applications in Dementia Syndrome

➤ **Ginkgo leaf.**
- *Dosage and administration:* The duration of treatment is determined in accordance with the severity of disease. In the above indications, treatment should be continued for no less than 8 weeks. After 3 months of treatment, the patients should be given a questionnaire to help the therapist determine and document whether continuation of treatment is justifiable.
- 💿 *Note:* The recommended dosage for all ginkgo products is 120–240 mg dry extract per day (in conformity with monograph specifications, see p. 72), to be administered as 2 to 3 divided doses.
- *Clinical value:* See Cardiovascular Diseases: Circulatory Disorders, p. 141.

Range of Applications in Cardiovascular Disease

For Heart Failure (NYHA II) and Senile Heart

➤ For details, see Heart Failure, p. 132.
➤ **Hawthorn**; **lily-of-the-valley**.
💿 *Important:* Lily-of-the-valley should not be used by individuals with hypokalemia or concomitant digitalis medications. It is dispensed by prescription only.

- *Clinical value:* Clinical studies comparing the effectiveness of hawthorn with synthetic drugs in treating heart failure stage NYHA II have been conducted and show improvement of capacity.

In Early Stages of Arterial Occlusive Disease

➤ For details, see Circulatory Disorders, p. 141.
➤ **Ginkgo biloba**.
  - *Dosage and administration:* See p. 71.
  - *Clinical value:* The chosen preparation should be administered on an interval therapy schedule. Studies comparing ginkgo with synthetic drugs are available.

For Tinnitus and Sudden Hearing Loss

➤ For details, see Vertigo and Tinnitus, p. 142.
➤ **Ginkgo biloba extract** (GBE), standardized (in conformity with monograph specifications, see p. 71).
  - *Dosage and administration:* GBE should be administered on an interval therapy schedule using commercial ginkgo products (see p. 71).
  - *Clinical value:* Studies comparing GBE with synthetic drugs are available.

Atherosclerosis

➤ For details, see Atherosclerosis, p. 144.
➤ **Artichoke leaf** (standardized extract); **garlic**.
  - *Clinical value:* These herbal remedies are primarily used for preventive purposes. They can also be used for maintenance therapy. Garlic was reported to have antiarteriosclerotic effects.

Range of Applications in Gastrointestinal Diseases

Lack of Appetite and/or Poor Digestion

➤ For details, see Anorexia, p. 165.
➤ *Clinical value:* The recommended bitters and cholegogues are based on many years of empirical experience.

Clinical Trials

- Rietbrock N, Hamel M, Hempel B, Mitrovic V, Schmidt T, Wolf GK: Actions of standardized extracts of Crataegus berries on exercise tolerance and quality of life in patients with congestive heart failure. Arzneimittelforschung 51(10) (2001), 793–798; Zapfe G Jr: Clinical efficacy of crataegus extract WS 1442 in congestive heart failure NYHA class II. Phytomedicine. 8(4) (2001), 262–266.

10.1 Conditions Related to Acquired Immunodeficiency ■

Clinical Considerations

➤ **General comments**
- Immune defenses can be diminished as a result of alcoholism, old age, primary cardiopulmonary disease, infectious diseases, and leukoses or lymphomas.
- Many top athletes also experience problems with immunodepression, presumably because their immune cells work overtime in eliminating damaged cells from muscle tissues.

➤ **General and herbal treatment measures**
- The basic goal of therapy is to strengthen the immune defenses through prophylactic measures. These include eating healthy foods, getting enough sleep, learning to relax, avoiding stress, and building up one's resistance to disease (e. g., through cold baths or showers, temperature stimulation, alternating hot-and-cold showers, regular sauna use).
- Supplements providing vitamin E, vitamin C, and trace elements can also be recommended.
- Immunomodulators can stimulate or diminish immune responses, independently of the mode of administration and concentrations used. For therapeutic purposes, however, the optimal concentration must be known. Plant-derived immunomodulators work unspecifically; that is, they activate specific immune system function via the release of mediators and cytokines through their polysaccharide or lectin constituents. This is said to increase the readiness of the immune system.
- Herbal treatments with adaptogenic effects (Siberian ginseng root, ginseng root) are indicated during periods of convalescence. They help the patient better cope with stress and overcome fatigue.

➤ **Clinical value of herbal medicine**
- Herbal immunomodulators (Echinacea, Ginseng root, Siberian ginseng root) can be recommended for adjunctive treatment of risk patients (e. g., in those receiving antibiotics or chemotherapy) as prophylactic or supportive measures.
- Most of the available pharmacological and clinical study data pertain to Purple echinacea. The herbal remedy was found to have a beneficial effect on the severity and course of catarrhal disorders and seems to be successful in fighting concomitant infections during chemotherapy.
- Recent studies have demonstrated that combinations of remedies from medicinal plants (*Echinacea purpurea*, *Baptisia tinctoria*, *Thuja occidentalis*; see Colds and Flu, p. 150) are superior to single-preparation products as a result of synergism.
- *Ginseng root:* A number of studies using various stress models in experimental animals, isolated organs, and cultured mammalian cells have shown that the herb improves the resistance to stressors. Ginseng root contains a large number of compounds, and those responsible for the individual therapeutic effects have not yet been identified. Clinical studies have shown that treatment is able to improve psychophysical performance and various parameters of cardiovascular and pulmonary function. These effects persist for days after discontinuation of treatment.
- *Siberian ginseng root:* Because of its performance-enhancing and fatigue-fighting effects, Siberian ginseng root is classified as both adaptogenic and

immunostimulant. Polysaccharides in the herb have immunomodulatory effects. Siberian ginseng was found to improve the stress resistance of experimental animals. Extracts of the herb have hormonelike effects that beneficially modulate the axis of the adrenal cortex and anterior pituitary lobe. In human subjects, the herb was found to improve performance levels, and the number of immunocompetent cells was increased after four weeks of treatment.

◉ *Note:* In severe disease, the patient's immune status should be determined before starting immunostimulatory therapy.

Recommended Herbal Remedies (Overview)

Immunostimulants

➤ **Purple echinacea herb** (Echinacea purpureae herba, see p. 56); **pale-flowered echinacea root** (Echinacea pallidae radix, see p. 56); **Siberian ginseng root** (Eleutherococci radix, see p. 58).
– *Action:* Extracts prepared from the aerial parts of flowering *Echinacea purpurea* or the root of *Echinacea pallida* are mainly used to treat respiratory and urinary tract infections. These herbal remedies have immunomodulatory and antiviral effects and inhibit bacterial hyaluronidase.
– For details, see Colds and Flu, p. 150.

Adaptogens

➤ **Ginseng root** (Ginseng radix, see p. 37); **Siberian ginseng root** (Eleutherococci radix, see p. 58).
– *Action*
  • Confers strength and fortification in fatigue and asthenia, decreased mental performance and concentration, exhaustion, and during convalescence.
  • Improves the resistance to stressors.
– *Contraindications:* None known.
– *Side effects:* None known.

Range of Applications in Chronic Infections

Chronic, Recurrent Respiratory Tract and Urinary Tract Infections

➤ **Purple echinacea herb** (see p. 56); **pale-flowered echinacea root** (see p. 56).
– *Dosage and administration*
  • *Liquid forms:* Take 30 to 40 drops, 3 to 4 times a day. Solid forms (lozenges, tablets, capsules): Take 1 to 2 single doses, 3 times a day or as directed by the manufacturer.
  • According to the latest findings, Echinacea is best administered at the first signs of disease for at least 6 days to no more than 14 days. The study findings on longer terms of treatment are still unclear. Alcohol-based extracts are reputed to be especially effective.
– *Clinical value*
  • Comparable chemical and synthetic drug products do not exist.
  • Use of oral dosage forms should be supervised by a physician.
  • The products can also be administered concomitantly with antibiotics.

10.1 Conditions Related to Acquired Immunodeficiency ■

As an Adjunct to Antibiotic Therapy, Chemotherapy, or Radiotherapy

➤ **Purple echinacea herb** (see p. 56).
  – *Indications:* Chronic, recurrent respiratory tract or urinary tract infections.
  – *Clinical value:* The herbal remedy may shorten the duration of illness and reduce both the number of symptoms and the frequency of recurrence. There are no restrictions on use.

Range of Applications in Fatigue-related Immunodeficiency _____

Immunodeficiency due to Excessive Athletic Training

➤ **Purple echinacea** (see p. 56).
  – *Dosage and administration:* Oral administration is recommended. See Chronic Infections, p. 56.
  – *Clinical value*
    • Some studies have shown that the herbal remedy shortens the duration of respiratory infections.

Exhaustion, Convalescence, Subjective Fatigue and Debility, Decreased Mental Performance and/or Decreased Concentration Capacity

➤ **Ginseng root** (see p. 37); **Siberian ginseng root** (see p. 58).
  – *Dosage and administration (commercial products)*
    • *Ginseng:* 1–2 g herb per day. Treatment should be restricted to a period of no more than 3 months. The herbal remedy can be continued after a break in treatment (the optimal length of the treatment-free interval is not known).
    ◉ *Note:* Many ginseng products are adulterated. Therefore, only high-quality, standardized products or whole roots (for tea) should be purchased.
    • *Siberian ginseng root (oral products):* Fluid extract: 3 to 5 drops in a glass of water, 3 to 5 times a day. Commercial products are recommended for these indications. They should be administered as recommended by the manufacturer.
  – *Clinical value:* The therapeutic range of the herbal remedy has, in part, been verified in clinical studies.

Clinical Considerations

➤ **General comments**
  – Second only to cardiovascular disease, cancer is a leading cause of death in industrialized nations (ca. 33 %).
  – The most common triggers are exogenous factors (physical, chemical, and biological noxae) that damage the genetic material, causing mutations. When the endogenous control system (immune system) is unable to respond adequately to the pathological proteins produced by the mutated cells, the mutated cells multiply freely at the expense of the total organism. Tumors and other neoplastic diseases then develop.

➤ **Herbal treatment measures:** In Germany, subcutaneous administration of mistletoe is generally recommended by the manufacturers. Most qualified health care practitioners prefer to inject the herbal remedy into the upper arm or leg. Injection into irradiation fields or areas proximal to the tumor should be avoided.

➤ **Clinical value of herbal medicine**
  – Surgery, chemotherapy, and radiotherapy, the three standard arms of conventional cancer therapy, are able to cure cancer or achieve long-term remission in around 45 % of all cases. Temporary remission or alleviation of symptoms (palliative therapy) is all that can be achieved in the remaining patients.
  – Researchers are showing increasing interest in biological therapy, which is designed to enhance the endogenous immune defenses. Secondary plant chemicals such as conjugated isoflavones from soybeans or phytoestrogens may soon play an important role.
  – Herbal medicine has played an undisputed role in palliative medicine. Wraps, compresses, baths, and inhalations prepared using herbal extracts can help cancer patients feel better and improve their quality of life.
  – Herbal preparations are useful for treatment of concomitant symptoms, such as anxiety, sleep disorders, and depression (see corresponding sections of the book).
  – Mistletoe extract regimens have a special status and were originally developed as a part of anthroposophic medicine. The herbal remedy is reported to enhance the body's immune defenses.
  – Clear proof of clinical efficacy is lacking for both anthroposophic and conventional mistletoe preparations. Most of the available clinical studies do not conform with modern scientific standards. Moreover, the researchers tended to use different methods of manufacture and dilution and use material obtained from different host trees, making it impossible to compare the data. Extensive clinical studies are therefore being conducted to assess the effects of mistletoe extract on tumor progression and recurrence, metastatic spread, cytostatic-induced side effects, and quality of life.

Range of Applications of Conventional Phytopharmaceuticals

➤ In Germany, **mistletoe** administered intravenously or subcutaneously (Visci herba, see p. 64). In North America, a **1 : 10 mistletoe tincture** (20 to 40 drops, 3 times a day) is recommended by herbal and naturopathic practitioners, though no clinical trials showing efficacy are available.

- *Action*
  - Aqueous mistletoe extracts contain a variety of low and high molecular weight (HMW) compounds. High-molecular weight mistletoe lectins, especially mistletoe lectin 1 (ML-1), were found to exert immunomodulatory effects on humoral and cellular components of the immune system in a number of in vitro studies. Researchers have therefore developed extracts standardized for ML-1.
  - The literature also provides evidence that lectin-free mistletoe extracts may have immunomodulatory properties.
- *Contraindications:* Pregnancy and lactation, hypersensitivity to proteins, chronic progressive infections (e. g., tuberculosis). Owing to the lack of adequate study data, mistletoe extracts should not be used by children under 12 years of age.
- *Side effects:* Local reddening at the injection site, increase in body temperature by 0.5–1 °C, anginal complaints, orthostatic hypotension, allergic reactions.
- *Dosage and administration*
  - In Germany, mistletoe extracts are administered parenterally, either by the subcutaneous or the intravenous route. Liquid oral preparations are commonly recommended by herbalists and naturopaths in North America for similar purposes because injectable preparations are not approved in North America.
  - A dose window of 0.5–2 ng/kg has been established for preparations standardized for ML-1. Higher doses of 2.5–5.0 ng/kg tend to have immunosuppressive effects. The optimal dosage scheme is 0.5–1.0 ng of ML-1 per kilogram body weight, 1 to 2 times a week, for a period of 3 months, followed by a 4- to 8-week break in treatment. Treatment is then repeated in cycles.
  - Total treatment period: 5 years or the usual time for recurrence of the individual tumor in question.

  ◉ *Important:* The preparation should not be injected into inflamed skin or radiation fields.

Range of Applications of Anthroposophic Phytopharmaceuticals

➤ **Mistletoe herb** (see p. 64).

- *Action:* Immunomodulation.
- *Contraindications:* Hypersensitivity to proteins, chronic progressive infections (e. g., tuberculosis), high fever, acute inflammations. Should not be used during the first trimester of pregnancy unless the expected benefits clearly outweigh the potential risks.
- *Dosage and administration:* The herbal remedy preparations should be administered subcutaneously, with the doses individualized according to the dosage guidelines specified by the manufacturer.

  ◉ *Important:* If there is a tendency to develop phlebitis, the preparation should not be injected in regions of predisposition.

- *Side effects*
  - *Local administration:* Reddening, increase in body temperature by 0.5–1 °C, regional lymph node enlargement (rare).
  - *Parenteral administration:* Chills, drop in blood pressure, shortness of breath, and shock have been observed.

Clinical Considerations

▶ **General comments**

– Rheumatic disease is the generic term for degenerative (arthrosis) and inflammatory diseases (e. g., rheumatoid arthritis) of the supporting and connective tissues. The exact etiology is rarely identifiable.

– In rheumatoid arthritis, elevated levels of proinflammatory cytokines TNF and IL-1β can be detected in synovial fluid. These substances maintain joint inflammation and promote the production of enzymes that destroy the cartilage. Inflammatory processes also occur in arthrosis, but are induced by mechanical irritations due to malposition.

– It is impossible to predict the course of the disease over time. In many cases, improvement or worsening cannot be reliably attributed to any definite therapeutic measure.

– Curative treatment of rheumatic diseases is not possible. Most treatment strategies still do not achieve very satisfactory long-term results, especially in rheumatic inflammatory diseases.

▶ **General and herbal treatment measures**

– The goal of traditional rheumatism treatments is to stimulate metabolic and excretory (hepatic and renal) processes.

– Recent studies have shown that herbal remedies can alleviate pain and inhibit the endogenous production of tissue hormones (prostaglandins and leukotrienes) involved in the development of rheumatoid inflammation.

– *Essential oils* for rheumatic complaints (e. g., peppermint, camphor, eucalyptus, rosemary) are applied topically. After transdermal absorption, viscerocutaneous reflexes convey the effects of the oils to the internal organs. *Arnica flower* is an effective antiphlogistic remedy.

– *Cayenne fruit* contains capsaicin, a substance that works by local irritation, causing skin reddening and warming. This helps to alleviate muscle tension and postherpetic neuralgia. Powdered mustard seed and ginger root have a similar mechanism of action.

– Inactive arthrosis is treated using *grass flower pillows*. These are pillows filled with dried flowers of hay, commercially available in Germany. In North America, the closest approximation to this is *Avena* flower. In North America, baths with ginger tea added to the bathwater and, as topical treatment, ginger compresses are used instead. Also, adding *essential oils* (conifer oil) to the bathwater is a possible treatment.

▶ **Clinical value of herbal medicine**

– Herbal remedies are suitable for adjunctive treatment of rheumatoid diseases.

– Nonsteroidal antirheumatic pharmaceutical drugs tend to cause a number of side effects, especially in the gastrointestinal tract. Adjunctive treatment with the recommended herbs makes it possible to reduce the dose frequency and level of nonsteroidal antirheumatics.

– Similar to the herbal remedies used for primary treatment, oral phytomedicines take several weeks to become fully effective.

– Further intensive research is required to adequately document the efficacy of so-called antidyscratics (e. g., dandelion root, stinging nettle leaf, birch leaf) in rheumatic diseases and to analyze their active principles.

11.1 Rheumatism and Pain

External Remedies That Work by Stimulating Skin Receptors

Local Irritants

➤ **Cayenne fruit** (Capsici fructus, see p. 46); **white mustard seed** (Sinapis alba semen, see p. 127); **ginger root** (Zingiberis rhizoma, see p. 70).
  – *Action:* Local irritants work by stimulating pain and heat receptors on the skin, causing counterirritation. This helps to lessen pain and inflammation.
  – *Contraindications:* These herbal remedies should not be applied to open wounds or to broken or diseased skin.
  – *Side effects:* High-dose exposure can cause blistering or necrosis of the skin.

Other External Remedies

➤ **Peppermint oil** (Menthae piperitae oleum, see p. 103).
  – *Action:* Stimulates cold receptors on the skin, thereby increasing the blood flow.
  – For further details, see Respiratory Tract Diseases, p. 148 ff.

Aromatic Herbs for External Use

➤ **Conifer oils** (see p. 157); **camphor** (Cinnamomi camphorae aetheroleum, see p. 45).
  – For further details, see Respiratory Tract Diseases, p. 148 ff, and Herbal Hydrotherapy, p. 284 ff.

Other External Remedies

➤ **Grass flowers** (Graminis flos); **arnica flower** (Arnicae flos, see p. 35).
  – *Action:* See Herbal Hydrotherapy, p. 286, and Skin Diseases, p. 276.

Herbal Remedies that Modulate Prostaglandin and Leukotriene Synthesis

Salicylate-containing Herbs

➤ **Willow bark** (Salicis cortex); **aspen leaf** and **bark** (Populi tremulae folium cortex).
  – *Action:* Relieves pain when administered internally or externally. Various compounds in willow bark, ash bark, and aspen leaf and bark have antipyretic, antiphlogistic, and/or analgesic effects. Salicin is converted in vivo to salicylic acid, a substance that mainly inhibits cyclooxygenase and reduces the prostaglandin concentration in inflamed tissues without causing gastrointestinal side effects. Other still unknown ingredients are also involved.
  – *Contraindications:* Hypersensitivity to salicylates.
  – *Side effects:* Gastrointestinal complaints can occur in rare cases.

Other Herbal Remedies

➤ **Indian frankincense** (*Boswellia serrata*) (Boswelliae resina); **devil's claw root** (Harpagophyti radix, see p. 54); **stinging nettle leaf** (Urticae folium, see p. 97); **licorice root** (Liquiritiae radix, see p. 85); **bittersweet stems** (Dulcamarae stipites, see. p. 40).

– *Action:* Stinging nettle leaf extract inhibits prostaglandin and leukotriene synthesis and acts as a cytokine antagonist. This helps to protect cartilage and connective tissues from the destructive effects of cytokines. Indian frankincense is an inhibitor of 5-lipoxygenase and cyclooxygenase, which are key enzymes for tissue hormones involved in inflammatory processes (prostaglandins and leukotrienes). The herbal remedy also has an analgesic effect. The root of the devil's claw plant contains harpagoside, a substance that inhibits prostaglandin synthesis. Licorice root and bittersweet have cortisone-like effects.

– *Contraindications:* None known for stinging nettle leaf extract. See p. 85 for licorice root, p. 54 for devil's claw.

– *Side effects:* None known for stinging nettle leaf extract, bittersweet, or devil's claw. See p. 85 for licorice root.

Herbal Remedies with Diuretic, Choleretic, or Mild Laxative Effects (so-called antidyscratic herbal remedies)

▶ **Dandelion root** and **herb** (Taraxaci radix cum herba, see p. 54); **birch leaf** (Betulae folium, see p. 39); **goldenrod herb** (Solidaginis virgaureae herba, see p. 63);

– *Action*: Reputed to improve metabolism in connective tissues.

– *Contraindications*
  • *Dandelion:* Biliary tract obstruction, bowel obstruction. Gallstone patients should not use the herbal remedy unless instructed by a qualified health care practitioner.
  • *Birch leaf:* Patients with edema due to impaired heart or kidney function should not use birch leaf or other diuretics.

Range of Applications in Rheumatic Diseases

Rheumatoid Arthritis

▶ **Devil's claw root**; combinations of **aspen bark** and **leaf**, **ash bark** and **goldenrod herb**; **stinging nettle leaf**.

– *Clinical value*: A few clinical studies have been conducted, especially on devil's claw, willow bark, and the above-mentioned combination which show some efficacy, but further research will be necessary. The analgesic effects of these well-tolerated remedies are comparable to those of low-dose nonsteroidal antirheumatic drugs.

Clinical Trials

– Leblan D, Chantre P, Fournie B: *Harpagophytum procumbens* in the treatment of knee and hip osteoarthritis. Four-month results of a prospective, multicenter, double-blind trial versus diacerhein. Joint Bone Spine 67(5) (2000), 462–467.

General Rheumatic Complaints

▶ Combinations of **ash bark**, **aspen bark**, **aspen leaf**, and **goldenrod herb**; **willow bark**, **devil's claw root**.

– *Antirheumatic tea:* Pour 2 cups of boiling water onto 1 tablespoon of finely chopped devil's claw root, allow to steep at room temperature for 8 hours,

then strain. Divide into 3 portions, to be warmed and taken shortly befor meals.
   - *Clinical value*: The analgesic effects of these well-tolerated remedies ar comparable to those of low-dose nonsteroidal antirheumatic drugs.

Osteoarthritis and Arthrosis

➤ **Internal: Devil's claw**; combinations of **aspen**, **ash bark**, and **goldenrod**.
➤ **External: Conifer oil**; **camphor**; **grass flower** (see Herbal Hydrotherapy **powdered mustard seed**; **ginger root** (see Section 4).
   - *Dosage and administration:* Same as in rheumatoid arthritis.
   - *Clinical value*: The analgesic effects of these well-tolerated remedies ar comparable to those of low-dose nonsteroidal antirheumatic drugs.

Range of Applications in Pain Management

For Muscle Pain and Tension, Sore Muscles, Pulled Muscles and Contusions, Massages after Sports, and Connective Tissue Massages

➤ **Conifer oils** in alcohol base (rubbing alcohol); **camphor, powdered mustar seed** (see Section 4); **grass flowers** (see Herbal Hydrotherapy); **arnica flower** (see Skin Diseases).
   - *Dosage and administration*
     • **Tincture *Rx*:** Tinctura aromaticae 0.4: Spiritus aetheris nitrosi 0.5, Tinctura rhatanhiae, 6 drops; ethanol (90 % by volume) 100.0, distilled wate ad 200.0.
     • *Spiritus vini gallici:* Rubbing alcohol with 48 % (v/v) pine needle oil.
     • For external use. Apply to the tender region up to 4 times a day.
   - *Clinical value:* Induces hyperemization in the sense of counterirritation, ar has antiphlogistic and analgesic effects. Effectively alleviates the abov complaints.

Tension Headaches

➤ **Peppermint oil.**
   - *Contraindications:* Should not be used by infants and small children.
   - *Dosage and administration*: Apply to the skin in the temple and forehea region. Repeat liberally until the pain subsides.
   - *Clinical value:* Peppermint oil is a safe and inexpensive alternative to or analgesics.

Clinical Trials

   - Leblan D, Chantre P, Fournie B: *Harpagophytum procumbens* in the treatment of knee and hip osteoarthritis. Four-month results of a prospectiv multicenter, double-blind trial versus diacerhein. Joint Bone Spine 67(5 (2000), 462–467; Schmid B, Ludtke R, Selbmann HK, Kotter I, Tschirdewah B, Schaffner W, Heide L: Efficacy and tolerability of a standardized willow bark extract in patients with osteoarthritis: randomized placebo-contro led, double blind clinical trial. Phytother Res 15(4) (2001), 344–350.

linical Considerations

- **General comments**
  - Three-quarters of all cases of gouty arthritis (uratic arthritis) are caused by deficient renal excretion of uric acid. The other quarter is caused by excessive purine body production. The main presenting symptom is a severe attack of arthritis, i.e., gout. Hyperuricemia is the most important finding.
  - In metabolic syndrome, the degree of hyperuricemia correlates with the degree of cardiovascular risk.
- **Herbal treatment measures:** Only commercially manufactured oral preparations are used.
- **Clinical value of herbal medicine:** Meadow saffron extract can be administered to determine, according to the therapeutic effect (ex juvantibus diagnosis), whether a previously unclear case of acute arthritis can be diagnosed as gout and treated accordingly.

Recommended Herbal Remedies and Range of Applications

- **Seeds** of **meadow saffron** (Colchici autumnalis semen).
  - *Action:* The herbal remedy contains colchicine, an alkaloid that inhibits the proliferation of inflammation-causing cells.
  - *Contraindications:* Should not be used by children and adolescents or by individuals with impaired liver function, abnormal changes in blood picture, known gastrointestinal disease, impaired cardiovascular function, poor general health, liver disease. Should not be used during pregnancy and lactation. Reliable contraception is required during treatment and up to 3 months after discontinuation of the herbal remedy.
  - *Dosage and administration:* Use only during attacks of gouty arthritis according to the recommendation of a qualified health care practitioner. Initial dose should be 1 mg colchicine, followed by 0.5 – 1.5 mg every 1 to 2 hours until the pain subsides. Do not administer more than 8 mg colchicine per day.
  - ⊙ *Note:* These medications are dispensed by prescription only.
  - *Side effects:* Diarrhea, nausea, vomiting, abdominal pain, occasionally leukopenia. Skin changes, agranulocytosis, aplastic anemia, alopecia, and myopathy have occasionally been observed in long-term use.

12.1 Disturbances of the Menstrual Cycle

Clinical Considerations

➤ **General comments:** The woman's menstrual cycle is in a delicate balance. Stress and various other factors can easily cause disturbances such as hormone- or function-related menstrual disorders, cycle irregularities, and dysmenorrheic complaints such as abdominal and back pain, headaches, circulatory problems, irritability, and lack of appetite.

➤ **Herbal treatment measures:** Hip baths and herbal wraps prepared using grape flowers (see p. 286), rosemary, or yarrow (see Herbal Hydrotherapy, p. 26) trigger cutivisceral reflexes that stimulate the blood flow and lead to a better function of internal organs. In folk medicine, silverweed and shepherd's purse are also used in these indications.

➤ **Clinical value of herbal medicine:** Compared to nonsteroidal antirheumatic drugs and hormone preparations, the recommended herbal remedies are very low in side effects.

Recommended Herbal Remedies and Range of Applications

➤ **Silverweed herb** (Anserinae herba, see p. 117); **shepherd's purse** (Bursae pastoris herba).

– *Action:* Silverweed contains phytosterols and flavonoids as well as high concentrations of tannins. The herbal remedy is astringent, analgesic, and spasmolytic. Shepherd's purse has flavonoids, saponins, and minerals. As a mild styptic agent, it is recommended for treatment of heavy menstrual bleeding.

– *Contraindications:* None known.

– *Dosage and administration:* We recommend commercial preparations which should be used as recommended by the manufacturer.

– *Side effects:* Silverweed can upset a sensitive stomach.

– *Clinical value:* Silverweed and shepherd's purse are gentle phytomedicines with few or no side effects. A case report on silverweed can be found in the literature.

Clinical Considerations

➤ **General comments**

- Psychovegetative and physical premenstrual complaints such as water retention, constipation, swelling and tenderness of the breasts, abdominal and/or back pain, mood swings, irritability, and restlessness can occur 7 to 10 days before the start of menstruation due to a relative preponderance of estrogens over progestins.
- Hyperactivity of dopamine, a neurotransmitter that releases the hormone prolactin from the anterior lobe of the pituitary gland, is another cause of premenstrual syndrome (PMS).

➤ **Clinical value of herbal medicine**

- *Chaste tree fruit* is a useful alternative to hormone preparations in individuals with mild to moderate premenstrual complaints, irregular menses, and premenopausal complaints. Chaste tree fruit extract has been investigated in clinical studies. Several studies show efficacy for relieving symptoms of breast tenderness.
- *Bugleweed* can alleviate pain and tension of the mammary glands in the second half of the menstrual cycle. It is also recommended for vegetative and nervous disorders associated with mild hyperthyroidism.

Recommended Herbal Remedies and Range of Applications

➤ **Chaste tree fruit** (Agni casti fructus, see p. 48); **bugleweed herb** (Lycopi herba).

- *Action*
  - *Chaste tree fruit* contains dopamine antagonists, i.e., chemicals that occupy dopamine receptors in the brain and anterior pituitary lobe, thus preventing dopamine from taking action.
  - *Bugleweed* contains hydroxycinnamic acid derivatives rosmarinic acid and caffeic acid, which are presumed to inhibit prolactin release from the anterior pituitary lobe. The herb also causes slight suppression of thyroid function.
- *Contraindications*
  - Alcohol-based preparations should not be used by individuals with a history of liver disease, epilepsy, alcoholism, or brain damage.
  - *Chaste tree fruit*: Pituitary tumors, breast cancer. Should not be used during pregnancy and lactation.
  - *Bugleweed:* Hypothyroidism, thyroid enlargement without dysfunction.
- *Dosage and administration*
  - *Chaste tree fruit:* The preparation should be administered orally for a period of at least 3 months. Ideally, treatment should be continued for at least 3 months after the herbal remedy has taken effect. The daily dose of 1 mL first thing in the morning is often recommended, but see instructions on the product label.
  - *Bugleweed herb:* The herbal remedy is administered orally and should be used as recommended by the manufacturer.
- *Side effects*
  - *Chaste tree fruit:* Skin rashes with blister formation are a rare side effect.

- • *Bugleweed:* Thyroid enlargement can occasionally occur when administered for extended periods and at high doses. Sudden discontinuation of the herbal remedy can aggravate the symptoms.
  - – *Interactions*
    - • *Chaste tree fruit:* Possible interaction with dopamine antagonists cannot be ruled out.
    - • *Bugleweed:* Should not be used by patients on thyroid hormones. Interferes with thyroid tests performed using radioactive material.
  - – *Clinical value:* See p. 237.
- ◉ *Important:* Patients with PMS problems should consult a qualified health care practitioner before using these products.

Clinical Considerations

▶ **General comments:** Painful menstruation in the absence of detectable changes in the reproductive organs (primary dysmenorrhea) mainly affects younger women and is probably caused by prostaglandins produced in the mucous membrane of the uterus.

▶ **General and herbal treatment measures**
   – Primary dysmenorrhea is generally treated by administering substances that inhibit prostaglandin synthesis 24 to 48 hours before the start of menstrual bleeding and during the first two days of the cycle. Ovulation inhibitors are sometimes used.
   – *Black cohosh root* is known to have a similar effect and can be used as an alternative.

▶ **Clinical value of herbal medicine:** See below.

Recommended Herbal Remedies and Range of Applications

▶ **Black cohosh root** (Cimicifugae rhizoma, see p. 41).
   – *Action:* The mechanisms of action of actein, cimifugoside, and formonetin, the primary constituents in black cohosh root, are not fully understood. The hypothesized estrogen-like effects of the herbal remedy on the mucous membrane of the uterus could not be confirmed.
   – *Contraindications:* Pregnancy, lactation, estrogen-dependent tumors. Alcohol-based preparations should not be used by individuals with a history of liver disease, epilepsy, alcoholism, or brain damage.
   – *Dosage and administration:* Liquid unstandardized tinctures and standardized powdered extracts in capsules and tablets are widely available. We recommend the use of commercial oral black cohosh root extracts as directed on the label. The herbal remedy should not be used for more than six months without medical supervision.
   – *Side effects:* Stomach upset and weight gain are occasional side effects.
   – *Clinical value:* Black cohosh can be used as an alternative to prostaglandin synthesis inhibitors, especially in patients with mild complaints.

12.4 Menopausal Complaints

Clinical Considerations

➤ **General comments**
  – Menopausal complaints start to develop after around the 45th year of li
    owing to the deterioration of ovarian function.
  – The resulting lack of estrogen may contribute to vegetative, functional ar
    emotional problems.
  – The most common symptoms are hot flashes, sweats, anxiety, insomni
    and depression.
  – Other typical symptoms that may occur include dryness of the skin and mu
    cous membranes, urinary incontinence, joint problems, bone loss, rap
    pulse, and weight gain.

➤ **Clinical value of herbal medicine**
  – Black cohosh root with or without the addition of St. John's wort is now pa
    of the standard phytotherapy regimen for menopause-related neurovege
    tative and emotional disorders in cases where hormone therapy is no
    appropriate or not yet necessary. This regimen is also useful in individua
    who refuse hormone replacement therapy. The patient must understan
    that it can take several weeks for these treatments to take effect.
  – Black cohosh root cannot prevent osteoporosis or reduce the menopause
    related risk of arteriosclerosis.
  – An unfavorable effect of black cohosh on estrogen-dependent tumors has bee
    suggested but not yet confirmed. Animal and human studies conflict, makin
    it difficult to determine the estrogenic effect of black cohosh in humans.

Recommended Herbal Remedies and Range of Applications

➤ **Black cohosh root** (Cimicifugae rhizoma).
  – *Action:* See Dysmenorrhea, p. 239.
    • Clinical studies demonstrated that black cohosh root has effects similar t
      those of low-dose estrogen preparations. The herbal preparation was abl
      to greatly reduce hot flushes, sweats, nervousness, and mood swing
      even during long-term treatment, in 60–70 % of the women studied.
  – *Contraindications:* See Dysmenorrhea, p. 239.
  – *Dosage and administration*
    • These herbal remedies are to be taken orally, as directed on the produc
      label.
    ◉ *Note:* It can take several weeks for the herbal remedy to take full effec
    • Black cohosh root should not be used for more than 6 months withou
      the supervision of a qualified health care practitioner.
  – *Side effects:* See Dysmenorrhea, p. 239. When used in combination with S
    John's wort, light sensitivity can occur in fair-skinned individuals.
  – *Clinical value:* Treatment of choice in patients with menopause-relate
    neurovegetative and emotional disorders (see above).

Clinical Trials

  – Liu Z, Yang Z, Zhu M, Huo J: Estrogenicity of black cohosh (*Cimicifuga race
    mosa*) and its effect on estrogen receptor level in human breast cancer MC
    7 cells. Wei Sheng Yan Jiu 30(2) (2001), 77–80; Zierau O, Bodinet C, Kolb
    S, Wulf M, Vollmer G: Antiestrogenic activities of *Cimicifuga racemos*
    extracts. J Steroid Biochem Mol Biol 80(1) (2002), 125–130.

Pediatric Diseases

Clinical Considerations _____

▶ Since herbal remedies have few or no side effects, they are especially suitable for pediatric use. Herbs with mild effects are more highly recommended, since the more potent ones generally are not as well tolerated.

▶ **Preferred herbal preparations**

◉ *Important:* Some commercial herbal products previously used by children in North America now bear the warning, "Should not be used by children under 12 years age." In many cases, the warning was added simply to point out the lack of sufficient study data on the safety and efficacy of the herbal remedy or herbal preparation in children, and does not usually indicate any existing reports or studies of actual side effects in children. This also applies to the recommended dosages, which are often established through empirical experience as opposed to scientific dose-finding methods.

– *External remedies:* Herbal inhalants, liniments, wraps, and baths are very effective in pediatric patients.

– *Internal remedies:* Teas, juices, and suppositories are recommended for pediatric use.

– *Side effects:* Herbal remedies have a typical profile of side effects and contraindications in children. This should always be taken into consideration. Medications containing alcohol, for example, should never be administered to infants or small children.

▶ **General dosage guidelines** (if none are provided by the manufacturer):

– *Ages 0 to 5 years:* Mean dosage approximately one-third of the recommended dose for adults.

– *Ages 6–9 years:* Approximately one-half of the recommended dose for adults.

– For further information, we recommend *Kinderdosierungen von Phytopharmaka*, edited by Kooperation Phytopharmaka, 1998; ISBN 3-929964-14-7., and *An Encyclopedia of Natural Healing for Children*, Mary N.D. Bove, McGraw-Hill, NY, 2001.

13.2 Acute Febrile Infections

Clinical Considerations

➤ **General comments**
- The common cold generally begins with a runny nose and a sore throat (rhinopharyngitis). In children, these symptoms are frequently, but not always, accompanied by a high fever.
- Pediatric febrile infections are usually viral. The range of pathogens involved (RS virus, rhinovirus, adenovirus, Coxsackie virus, ECHO virus, parainfluenza virus) differs significantly from that in adults. Bacterial infections (e. g., by streptococci, *Haemophilus influenzae*, pneumococci, etc.) are rare.
- Recurrent infections are common, especially in children, whereas primary immunodeficiencies are rare.
- Signs of the absence of immunodeficiency are normal thriving and recurrent infection involving only one organ.
- Anatomic and respiratory disorders of the upper respiratory tract, early weaning, failure to build up adequate resistance and insufficient immune training are common reasons for frequent infections.
- In early childhood, infections are primarily warded off through nonspecific mechanisms. The specific immune systems does not become fully developed until around the eleventh year of life.
- The functional capacity of both the nonspecific (phagocytes) and specific (T lymphocytes) immune systems is impaired in children with atopic dermatitis (neurodermatitis) or allergies.

➤ **Herbal treatment measures**
- If bacterial infection plays a role, adjunctive non-herbal measures to lower fever should be initiated as soon as possible to prevent the need for antibiotics. Calf wraps (only if the legs are warm), cooling baths (water temperature 1–2 °C less than the rectal temperature), and similar measures can be recommended.
- The preferred dosage forms for children are teas, plant juices, syrups and lozenges or, for external administration, liniments, inhalations, and baths.
- The goal of symptomatic treatment is to relieve the symptoms responsible for discomfort.
- Herbal diaphoretics (elder or linden flower) used to lower fever can also be combined with mild anti-inflammatory and analgesic drugs such as meadowsweet.
- A pleasant taste is extremely important in oral preparations for children. Bitter orange peel and peppermint leaf are effective taste enhancers.
- For runny nose and other respiratory tract problems, we recommend chamomile flower steam baths as well as the inhalation and topical application of peppermint oil, mint oil, pine oil, pine needle oil, and/or eucalyptus oil.
- ◉ *Note:* These applications should not be used in infants and small children.
- Aniseed and fennel preparations are used for catarrhal disorders of the upper respiratory tract.
- Sage leaf preparations contain tannins that help to alleviate mouth and throat inflammation. Chamomile flower extracts have anti-inflammatory properties and are used as gargles and mouthwashes.
- Mallow, marshmallow root, and Iceland moss sooth inflamed mucous membranes. They can also be used in addition to ribwort plantain to treat

dry coughs. Ribwort plantain has local anti-inflammatory and antiphlogistic effects.

– Sundew herb is used to treat paroxysmal or hacking cough.

– Mullein has high concentrations of saponins and mucilage and is therefore effective in alleviating subacute bronchial irritations.

– Thyme herb has antibiotic and bronchospasmolytic action. Camphor induces local hyperemization. White deadnettle flower, not available in North America, has mucilage and saponin components. Teas made from it are used to treat catarrhal disorders of the upper respiratory tract.

– Herbal immunomodulators such as preparations of *Echinacea purpurea* or *E. pallida* have unspecific immunomodulatory and antiviral properties, as was described in detail in the chapter on immunodeficiency diseases. These herbal remedies contain polysaccharides that stimulate specific immune system function via the release of mediators and cytokines.

• Most of the available pharmacological and clinical study data pertains to purple echinacea herb. The herbal remedy was found to have a beneficial effect on the severity and course of catarrhal disorders and seems to be successful in fighting concomitant infections during chemotherapy.

• More recent studies have demonstrated that combinations of medicinal herbs from *Echinacea purpurea* (Echinaceae purpureae herba), *Baptisia tinctoria*, and *Thuja occidentalis* (Thujae herba [Arbor vitae, see p. 119 regarding the extended use of preparations containing thujone]; see Colds and Flu, p. 150) are superior to single-herb products owing to synergism.

▶ **Clinical value of herbal medicine**

– Herbal medications can be highly recommended for symptomatic treatment of acute febrile infections in pediatric patients.

– Many antibiotics as well as chemical and synthetic febrifuges tend to suppress the immune system, thereby increasing the likelihood of recurrence of disease.

– For recurrent infections, we highly recommend Kneipp hydrotherapy measures as well as visits to spas by the sea or in the mountains. Herbal immunomodulators such as echinacea (*Echinacea purpurea*) can be administered at acute infection as an additional measure. Flavored liquid products that include glycerine instead of alcohol are popular for children.

Recommended Herbal Remedies (Overview)

▶ For details on the individual herbal preparations, see Respiratory Diseases, p. 148 ff, and Diseases of the Mouth and Throat, p. 161 ff.

Astringents and Antibiotics

▶ **Sage leaf** (Salviae folium, see p. 114); **thyme herb** (Thymi herba, see p. 120); **ribwort plantain herb** (Plantaginis lanceolatae herba, see p. 60).

Antiphlogistics

▶ **Meadowsweet flower** (Filipendulae ulmariae flos, see p. 92); **sage leaf** (Salviae folium, see p. 114); **chamomile flower** (Matricariae flos, see p. 47); **licorice root** (Liquiritiae radix, see p. 85).

13.2 Acute Febrile Infections

Demulcents and Antitussives

➤ **Marshmallow root** (Althaeae radix, see p. 91); **Iceland moss** (Lichen islandicus, see p. 79); **mallow flower/leaf** (Malvae flos and folium, see p. 89), **ribwort plantain herb** (Plantaginis lanceolatae herba, see p. 60); **white deadnettle flower** (Lamii albi flos, see p. 127); **sundew herb** (Droserae herba, see p. 118

Sweat-inducing Preparations (Diaphoretics)

➤ **Linden flower** (Tiliae flos, see p. 87); **elder flower** (Sambuci flos, see p. 62).

Expectorants and Secretolytics

➤ **Eucalyptus oil** (Eucalypti aetheroleum, see p. 61); **spruce needle oil** (Piceae aetheroleum); **pine needle oil** (Pini aetheroleum, see p. 104); **aniseed** (Anisi fructus, see p. 34); **fennel seed** (Foeniculi fructus, see p. 65); **thyme herb** (Thymi herba, see p. 120); **ivy leaf** (Hederae helicis folium, see p. 158); **cowslip root** (Primulae radix, see p. 105); **licorice root** (Liquiritiae radix, see p. 85); **mullein flower** (Verbasci flos, see p. 94); **white deadnettle flower**; Lamii albi flos, see p. 127); **elder flower** (Sambuci flos, see p. 62).

– *Contraindications*
  • *Camphor, eucalyptus, spruce and pine needle oil:* Bronchial asthma and whooping cough (can aggravate bronchospasms).
  • *Mint oil, peppermint oil, fennel:* Bronchial asthma. Should not be administered to infants and children under three years of age.
  • *All essential oils:* Should not be used topically by patients with exanthematous skin conditions or childhood diseases.
  • *Fennel seed:* Pregnancy and lactation.
  • *Mint oil and peppermint oil:* Gallstones, biliary tract obstruction, cholecystitis, and severe liver disease.
  • *Licorice:* high blood pressure.
– *Restrictions on use*
  • *Camphor and eucalyptus; spruce needle, pine needle, peppermint and mint oils:* Should not be applied to the face, especially the nose, of infants and small children or used for inhalation. Should not be applied directly onto or near the mucous membranes.
  • *Licorice root:* Should not be used for more than 4 to 6 weeks.
  • *Chamomile flower:* Do not use to treat the eyes.
– *Side effects*
  • *Fennel seed:* Allergic reactions involving the skin and mucous membranes can occur in isolated cases.
  • *Thyme herb:* Allergic exanthematous or urticarious skin changes can occur in isolated cases.
  • *Cowslip root:* Isolated cases of gastric discomfort and nausea as well as hypersensitivity reactions involving the skin, respiratory tract, and gastrointestinal tract can occur.
– *Interactions:* Local application of herbs containing mucilage can delay the absorption of other herbal preparations and synthetic drugs.

Cold Receptor Stimulators

➤ **Mint oil** (Menthae arvensis aetheroleum); **peppermint oil** (Menthae piperitae aetheroleum, see p. 103). For details, see p. 148.

Irritants

➤ **Camphor tree** (Cinnamomi camphorae aetheroleum, see p. 45). For details, see p. 148.
  – *Action*: Enhances the blood flow.
  – *Contraindications:* See Expectorants above.
  – *Side effects*: Contact eczema (rare).

Immunomodulators

➤ **Purple echinacea herb** (Echinacea purpureae herba, see p. 156); **pale echinacea root** (Echinacea pallidae radix, see p. 56).

Range of Applications _____

Acute Febrile Infections

Internal Remedies

➤ **Linden flower**; **meadowsweet flower**; **peppermint leaf**; **chamomile flower**; **thyme herb**; **aniseed**; **fennel seed**; **ivy leaf**; **Iceland moss**.
  – *Dosage and administration*
    • **Diaphoretic and febrifuge tea *Rx*** (for adults and children): Tiliae flos (chopped) 70.0, Spireae flos (chopped) 10.0, Menthae piperitae folium (chopped) 15.0, Aurantii pericarpium (chopped) 5.0. Steep 1 teaspoon in 150 mL of boiling water for 10 minutes. Works best when taken while hot.
    • **Tea *Rx*:** Tiliae flos 25.0, Sambuci flos 35.0, Cynosbati fructus 30.0, Liquiritiae radix 10.0. Steep 1 teaspoon in 150 mL of boiling water for 10 minutes. Works best when taken while hot.
    • Diaphoretic teas work best when taken in the afternoon after a warming bath supplemented with aromatic herbs or pure essential oils, which open up the respiratory passages.
    • *Other teas:* Take 1 cup, 3 times a day, sweetened to taste with honey.
    • **Iceland moss lozenges** (where available): Allow a lozenge to dissolve in the mouth. Repeat several times daily.
    • *For dry cough due to mouth and throat irritation:* English plantain juice (commercial product where available or fresh plant juice; see p. 60); teas made from marshmallow root, mallow, or plantain leaf. The remedies should be taken orally, 3 to 5 times daily (see teas for respiratory tract diseases, p. 156 ff).
  – *Clinical value:* A comparative study on the efficacy of linden flower tea in colds showed that the herbal treatment was significantly superior to antibiotics with respect to reducing the duration of infection and the rate of complications.

Acute Febrile Infections

External Remedies

➤ **Eucalyptus oil** (see p. 61); **spruce needle oil** (see p. 104); **pine needle oil** (see p. 104); **peppermint oil** (see p. 103); **mint oil** (see p. 103); **camphor** (see p. 45); **sage leaf** (see p. 114); **chamomile flower** (see p. 47); **aniseed oil** (see p. 34).

– *Dosage and administration*
  • *Dried sage leaf:* Pour 250 mL of boiling water onto 1 heaped teaspoon of the herb, then cover and steep for 10 minutes. A mixture (equal parts) of sage leaves and chamomile flowers can be used instead.
  • **Tea *Rx*:** Matricariae flos 30.0, Salviae folium 20.0, Thymi herba 10.0. Pour 250 mL of boiling water onto 2 heaped teaspoons of the herbs, then cover and steep for 5 minutes.
  • Use the recommended infusions to gargle or rinse the mouth several times each day.

– *Clinical value:* When treatment is initiated early and the restrictions on use are heeded, these remedies can prevent complications of acute grippal infections and they are very well tolerated.

To Strengthen Immune Defenses of Infection-prone Children

➤ **Purple echinacea**; **pale-flowered echinacea** (see p. 56).

– *Dosage and administration:* Depending on age, 20 to 50 drops of the tincture are taken several times a day. Lozenges, tablets and capsules made from purple echinacea extract can be used instead. Unless otherwise directed, they should be taken 3 times a day for a period of 2 weeks. There is a lack of data supporting the use of the herbal remedy for longer periods.

– *Clinical value:* Comparable synthetic and/or chemical medications do not exist. Patients should seek the advice of a health care practitioner before purchasing these herbal remedies (see Self Care Management, p. 226).

Clinical Considerations

➤ **General comments**
  – A throat infection is generally a sign of a cold. In children, these symptoms are frequently, but not always, accompanied by a high fever.
  – The tonsils should always be inspected.
    • Tonsillitis due to adenovirus infection is likely to be present if the tonsils are red and swollen but otherwise normal, and there is difficulty in swallowing, fever and, in some cases, swollen lymph nodes at the angle of the mandible.
  – If the mucous membranes are coated and other changes are detected, infection with beta-hemolytic streptococci (group A), staphylococci, coxsackievirus, herpesvirus, or Epstein–Barr virus may be present.
  – Inflammations of the mouth can be caused by viral and bacterial pathogens and by various dental problems. Allergies and poisoning are other occasional causes.

➤ **Herbal treatment measures**
  – Tannin-bearing and aromatic herbs are used to treat inflammations of the respiratory passages. Tannins seal the capillaries and inhibit inflammation. The bonds that form between mucosal proteins and tannins are irreversible.
  – Calendula flower has antimicrobial and immunomodulatory effects.
  – Sage flower has antibacterial properties.
  – Chamomile flower is an aromatic herb that inhibits inflammation, protects the mucosae, and promotes epithelialization.

➤ **Clinical value of herbal medicine**
  – If in doubt, the patient should consult a health care practitioner before initiating self- treatment. This is especially important in the case of high fever, unusual changes in the tonsils, and unclassifiable changes in the oral mucosa.
  – Herbal remedies are used for symptomatic treatment of mouth and throat disorders. The available data on their in vitro antibacterial and immunomodulatory effects does not suffice for an assessment of their efficacy.

Recommended Herbal Remedies and Range of Applications

➤ **Tannin-bearing herbs: Silverweed herb** (Potentillae anserinae herba, see p. 117); **bilberry** (Myrtilli fructus); **calendula flower** (Calendulae flos, see p. 90); **sage leaf** (Salviae trilobae folium, see p. 114).

➤ **Aromatic herbs: Chamomile flower** (Matricariae flos, see p. 47).
  – *Action:* The local anti-inflammatory effects help to counteract mouth and throat inflammation.
  – *Contraindications:* For chamomile, see p. 48.
  – *Dosage and administration*
    • *Silverweed:* Steep 4 g of the finely chopped herb in 500 mL of hot water for 15 minutes.
    • *Dried bilberry:* Boil 2 to 3 tablespoons of the herb in 500 mL of water for 30 minutes.
    • *Chamomile flower:* Pour 250 mL of boiling water onto 2 teaspoons of the herb, then cover and steep for 5 minutes.

- *Calendula flower:* Steep 2 teaspoons of the herb in 150 mL of boiling water for 10 minutes.
- *Ribwort plantain:* Preparations should be made using the freshly collected herb (see details regarding catarrhal disorders of the respiratory tract, p. 158).
- *Dried sage leaf:* Pour 250 mL of boiling water onto 1 teaspoon of the herb, then cover and steep for 10 minutes. A mixture of sage leaves and chamomile flowers (equal parts of each) can also be used.
- **Tea *Rx*:** Matricariae flos 30.0, Salviae folium 20.0, Thymi herba 10.0. Pour 250 mL of boiling water onto 2 teaspoons of the herbs, then cover and steep for 5 minutes.
- The preferred infusion or decoction should be used for gargling several times a day.
- Commercial preparations should be used as recommended by the manufacturer.

– *Side effects:* None known.
– *Clinical value*
  - All of the above gargles are safe enough to use long-term, even without medical supervision. Since synthetic drugs have a high potential for side effects, herbal remedies should preferably be administered to pediatric patients whenever feasible (see information on causes of potential complications and general comments on p. 247).
  - Clinical study data and empirical reports are available only for chamomile.

Clinical Considerations

➤ **General comments**
   – Respiratory tract diseases, usually accompanied by fever, are especially common in children.
   – A cold can affect the entire organism, especially in infants and small children without a fully developed immune system.
   – Patients with rhinitis tend to breathe through the mouth, making it more difficult for infants to swallow fluids. Vomiting and diarrhea can also develop owing to the swallowing of infected mucus. If an adequate intake of fluids is not maintained, dehydration, a potentially life-threatening complication, can develop.
   – Narrow air passages are prone to congestion with mucus, which can result in ear infection, sinusitis, or bronchitis.

➤ **Herbal treatment measures**
   – Herbal teas, juices, tinctures and inhalants are recommended.
   – Linden flower tea can be administered to children for prophylactic treatment during the cold season.
   – For details on the action of demulcents (marshmallow root, ribwort plantain herb, and Iceland moss) and saponin-containing herbs (ivy leaf and primula root), see Respiratory Diseases.
   – For information on the treatment of concomitant disorders of the upper respiratory tract, see Colds and Flu, and Mouth and Throat Inflammation.

➤ **Clinical value of herbal medicine**
   – Herbal demulcents and expectorants are generally sufficient for most simple and harmless catarrhal disorders.
   – Children often develop paroxysmal coughs, which respond well to medicinal herbs such as thyme, ribwort plantain, ivy, and sundew. The efficacy of these herbs in whooping cough is questionable, however.
   – ⊙ *Note:* An experienced health care practitioner should be consulted if any of the above-mentioned complications should occur since the herbal remedies are used only as an adjunct to other therapeutic measures.

Recommended Herbal Remedies (Overview)

Demulcents

➤ **Marshmallow root** (Althaeae radix, see p. 91); **ribwort plantain herb** (Plantaginis lanceolatae herba, see p. 60); **Iceland moss** (Lichen islandicus, see p. 79).
➤ For details, see Respiratory Diseases, p. 154.

Expectorants

➤ **Cowslip root** (Primulae radix, see p. 105).
➤ For details, see Respiratory Diseases, p. 155.

Bronchospasmolytics

➤ **Thyme herb** (Thymi herba, see p. 120); **sundew herb** (Droserae herba, see p. 118); **ivy leaf** (Hederae helicis folium, see p. 58).
➤ For details, see Respiratory Diseases, p. 155.

3

➤ **Dosage and administration**
- Commercial products should be used. Administer as recommended by the manufacturer.
- If teas are preferred, the patient should drink 3 to 5 cups daily.

➤ **Other teas and treatments for older children:** See *Respiratory Diseases*, p. 156 ff.

Range of Applications

Catarrhal Disorders of the Upper Respiratory Tract

➤ **Aniseed oil; marshmallow root; thyme herb; spruce needle oil; sundew herb**.
- *Dosage and administration*
  - *Inhalation:* Add 3 drops of aniseed oil to hot water and inhale several times daily, or add 1 g of spruce needle oil to hot water and inhale 3 to 5 times daily.
  - **Expectorant tea *Rx*:** Primulae radix 20.0; Anisi fructus, Foeniculi fructus ad 50.0. Steep 1 teaspoonful in 1 cup of hot water.
  - *For paroxysmal cough:* Use either: thyme syrup, 1 teaspoon, five times daily; or marshmallow root, pour 150 mL of cold water onto 1 teaspoon of the herb and steep for 1 to 2 hours, stirring frequently. Warm slightly before use.
  - *Sundew tincture (1 : 10):* Take 5 drops, 3 times a day.
- *Clinical value*: Herbal remedies are the treatment of choice for catarrhal disorders in children because of the virtual absence of side effects.

Catarrhal Disorders of the Respiratory Tract and Inflammations of the Mouth and Throat

➤ **Ribwort plantain herb** (see p. 60).
- *Dosage and administration:* Immediately after collection of these plants, the aerial parts of ribwort plantain are chopped and the plant juice is extracted. The raw juice is then mixed with equal parts of honey and boiled for 20 minutes. The syrup can be kept refrigerated in a closed container for several days.
  - *Daily dose:* 3 – 6 g of the fresh herb.
- *Clinical value:* An effective treatment with very few side effects.

Paroxysmal Cough and Dry Cough

➤ **Sundew herb** (see p. 118).
- *Dosage and administration*
  - *Sundew tincture (1 : 10):* 5 drops, 3 times a day.
- *Clinical value:* Effective herbal remedy with very few side effects.

Clinical Considerations _____

➤ **General comments**
  – Overeating often causes stomach aches, gas, nausea, and diarrhea in children.
  – Unspecific gastritis and gastritis due to *Helicobacter pylori* infection and peptic ulcers are common, especially in boys over 10 years of age.
  – So-called umbilical colic is characterized by functional and usually psychovegetative, recurrent abdominal pain that persists for at least 3 months. This problem is often associated with a loss of appetite.
  – Dyspepsia and acute unspecific diarrhea are common problems in infants and small children. These conditions are dangerous since they can quickly result in dehydration. The possibility of appendicitis should always be considered, especially if the problems do not clear up within 24 hours or if other symptoms such as lassitude or fever develop.
  – Meteorism of unspecific origin is extremely common in pediatric patients. The possibility of food intolerance (e. g., lactose intolerance) should always be considered.
➤ **General and herbal treatment measures**
  – The underlying cause of habitual constipation (e. g., unhealthy eating habits, diet low in roughage, psychosomatic factors) should first be determined before starting treatment with herbs.
  – Chamomile flower, balm leaf, peppermint leaf, and fennel seed are useful in treating dyspeptic complaints.
  – Because peppermint leaf can irritate the mucous membranes (causing heartburn), it is more suitable for older children and adolescents.
  – Bitter orange peel, angelica, and centaury can be used to stimulate the appetite.
  – Caraway oil can be administered for flatulence.
  – Diarrhea is an indication for dried bilberry, blackberry root, and uzara root (the last is not available in North America). Linseed, psyllium (short-term treatment), and buckthorn fruit are helpful in constipation.
➤ **Clinical value of herbal medicine:** Considering their excellent tolerability and very low rate of side effects, herbal remedies are of very high clinical value in functional disorders of the gastrointestinal tract.

Recommended Herbal Remedies (Overview) _____

Antiphlogistics

➤ **Chamomile flower** (Matricariae flos, see p. 47).
➤ For details, see p. 170.

Spasmolytics

➤ **Balm leaf** (Melissae folium, see p. 84); **peppermint leaf** (Menthae piperitae folium, see p. 102); **chamomile flower** (Matricariae flos, see p. 47).
➤ For details, see p. 170.

Carminatives

➤ **Caraway oil** (Oleum carvi, see p. 45); **fennel seed** (Foeniculi fructus, see p. 65); **peppermint leaf** (Menthae piperitae folium, see p. 102).
➤ For details, see Dyspepsia, p. 174.

13.5 Gastrointestinal Diseases

Bitters

➤ **Centaury** (Centaurii herba, see p. 84); **bitter orange peel** (Aurantii pericarpium, see p. 39); **angelica root** (Angelicae radix, see p. 33).

➤ For details, see Anorexia, p. 165.

Antidiarrheal Agents

➤ **Bilberry fruit** (Myrtilli fructus); **blackberry root** (Rubi fructicosi radix); **raspberry leaf tea** is also used.

➤ For details, see Acute and Chronic Diarrhea, p. 190.

Laxatives

➤ **Linseed** (Lini semen, see p. 66); **psyllium** (Psyllii semen, see p. 106); **buckthorn fruit** (Rhamni cathartici fructus, see p. 42).

➤ For details, see Diseases of the Colon and Rectum, p. 186, and Constipation, p. 196.

– *Dosage and administration:* Unless otherwise instructed, the child should slowly sip a cup of the warm tea as needed. If the symptoms persist, younger children should take 3 cups daily, and older children 5 cups daily. Commercial products should be used as recommended by the manufacturer.

Range of Applications in Acute Diseases

Stomach Complaints

➤ **Chamomile flower** (see p. 47); **caraway seed** (see p. 46); **fennel seed** (see p. 102); **peppermint leaf** (see p. 84); **balm leaf**.

– *Dosage and administration*
  • *Chamomile flower:* Pour 150 mL of boiling water onto 2 heaped teaspoons of the herb, then cover and steep for 5 minutes.
  • **Tea *Rx* 1:** Matricariae flos 10.0, Carvi fructus (chopped) 10.0. Pour 1 cup of boiling water onto 2 heaping teaspoons of the herb, then cover and steep for 5 minutes.
  • **Tea *Rx* 2:** Foeniculi fructus (chopped), Menthae piperitae folium (chopped), Melissae folium (chopped) aa 20.0. Steep 1 teaspoon in 150 mL of boiling water for 10 minutes.

– *Clinical value:* These remedies are all effective. The one the child likes best should be used.

Flatulence, Dyspepsia, or Diarrhea in Infants

➤ **Fennel seed** (see p. 65).

– *Dosage and administration:* Steep 2 teaspoons of the coarsely cut herb (cut using a coffee grinder or blender) in 150 mL of boiling water for 5 minutes.
– *Clinical value:* Its effectiveness has been demonstrated in long years of experience.

Spastic Epigastric Pain due to Functional Problems
(only in older children)

➤ **Peppermint leaf** (see p. 102).

– *Dosage and administration:* Pour 150 mL of boiling water onto 1 teaspoon of the herb, then cover and steep for 5 minutes. Drink while still hot.

- *Side effects:* Heartburn.
- *Clinical value:* Its effectiveness has been demonstrated in long years of experience.

Unspecific Acute Diarrhea

➤ **Bilberry fruit**, **blackberry root**, or **apple sauce** made with the peel and a little honey.
- *Dosage and administration:* Boil 3 tablespoons of dried bilberries in 500 mL of water for 10 minutes. Heat and drink 1 glassful, several times a day, or spoon the cooked berries by the tablespoonful into cream of wheat or yogurt.
- *Clinical value:* Bilberry fruit has proven to be a safe and effective herbal remedy.

Acute Constipation

➤ **Buckthorn berry** (see p. 42); **psyllium** (see p. 106); **linseed** (see p. 66).
- *Dosage and administration*
  - *Buckthorn berry:* Steep 2 teaspoons of the herb in 1 cup of boiling water for 10 minutes. Drink 1 to 2 cups in the evening. Commercial products can be used (see p. 352).
- ◉ *Note:* Buckthorn berries should not be used for more than 1 to 2 weeks without the supervision of a qualified health care practitioner.
➤ **Flaxseed, psyllium:** See p. 66.
- *Contraindications*
  - *Flaxseed:* Imminent or existing bowel obstruction, esophageal stenosis.
  - *Psyllium:* Imminent or existing bowel obstruction, esophageal stenosis, known allergy to psyllium.
  - *Buckthorn berries:* Bowel obstruction, acute inflammatory bowel disease.
- ◉ *Note:*
  - Bulk laxatives (psyllium, linseed) should not be used concomitantly with antidiarrheal agents that inhibit intestinal motility. Linseed can reduce the absorption of other drugs.
  - Taking psyllium without an adequate supply of fluids can result in difficulty of swallowing or in choking. Drink at least 150 ml of liquid.
- *Clinical value:* When used as directed, these herbal remedies are very useful remedies with few side effects and contraindications.

Range of Applications in Chronic Diseases

Anorexia

➤ **Bitter orange peel** (see p. 39); **centaury herb** (see p. 84); **yarrow herb** (see p. 131); **peppermint leaf** (see p. 102).
- *Dosage and administration*
  - Steep 2 g bitter orange peel in 1 cup of boiling water for 5 minutes. Drink one cup before meals.
  - **Tea *Rx*:** Centaurii herba, Millefolii herba, Menthae piperitae folium aa 20.0. Steep 1 teaspoon in 150 mL of hot water. Drink, cold or lukewarm, before meals.
- *Clinical value:* Mild therapeutic action. Alternation of applications is recommended.

3

13.5 Gastrointestinal Diseases

Chronic Meteorism

➤ **Aniseed** (see p. 34); **fennel seed** (see p. 65); **caraway seed** (see p. 46).
  – *Dosage and administration*
    • **Tea *Rx*:** Anisi fructus (chopped), Foeniculi fructus (chopped), Carvi fructus (chopped) aa 20.0. Steep 1 teaspoon in 1 cup of boiling water for 20 minutes. Drink a cup of the warm tea after each meal.
    • **Tincture *Rx*:** Oleum carvi 1.0, Oleum olivarum ad 10.0. Gently massage in a clockwise fashion onto the stomach, especially the region around the navel, up to 3 times daily.

Habitual Constipation

➤ **Flaxseed** (see p. 66); **psyllium** (see p. 106).
  – *Dosage and administration:* Flaxseed is recommended for younger children, whereas psyllium is more effective in adolescents and children over 12 years of age. Flaxseed and psyllium products should always be taken with adequate quantities of fluids, as specified by the manufacturer.
  ◉ *Note:* Taking psyllium without an adequate supply of fluids can result in difficulty swallowing or in choking.
  – *Clinical value:* When used as directed, these herbs are very useful remedies with few side effects and contraindications (see Habitual Constipation, p. 196, and Acute Constipation, p. 196).

Clinical Considerations _____

➤ For introductory information and details regarding urinary tract infections and kidney and ureteral stones, see Diseases of the Urogenital Tract, p. 200. Nighttime bedwetting (nocturnal enuresis) is a common childhood problem that often responds to herbal remedies.

◉ *Important:* Large volumes of so-called kidney teas must be taken. If possible, the tea should not be sweetened at all. If a sweetener is needed, honey should be used instead of refined sugar.

➤ **General comments:** Secondary nocturnal enuresis is characterized by episodic nocturnal bedwetting after long periods of continence. Like irritable bladder, this usually is not an organic disease but a neurotic functional disorder caused by emotional and social problems.

➤ **General and herbal treatment measures:** The recommended herbal remedies are taken by the oral route. They work either through suggestive mechanisms in the sense of a placebo effect (extremely bitter taste of amarogentin and gentiopicroside, which are constituents in gentian root) or through sedative (California poppy) or antidepressant effects (St. John's wort). Controlled clinical studies on the efficacy of herbal remedies in primary nocturnal enuresis have not been conducted.

➤ **Clinical value of herbal medicine:** The herbal remedies recommended as an adjunct to psychotherapy are very safe. Gentle-acting chemical medications for this indication do not exist.

Recommended Herbal Remedies and Range of Applications _____

➤ **Bitters: Gentian root** (Gentianae radix).
➤ **Antidepressants: St. John's wort** (Hyperici herba, see p. 115).
➤ **Sedatives: California poppy herb** and **root** (Eschscholtziae herba et radix).
  – *Contraindications:* Patients with gastrointestinal ulcers should not use gentian root. Patients taking antirejection, antiretroviral, or other life-saving drugs should use St. John's wort cautiously and with the advice of a professional health care provider.
  – *Dosage and administration*
    • **Tea *Rx*:** Hyperici herba 30.0, Chamomillae flos 20.0, Melissae folium 20.0. Steep 2 teaspoons in 250 mL boiling water for 10 minutes. Take 1 to 2 cups each morning and evening for a period of 4 to 6 weeks.
    • Standardized St. John's wort extract, e.g., capsules, tablets. Administer as recommended by the manufacturer.
    • **Gentian Tincture *Rx*:** Tinctura Gentianae 20.0. Take 10 to 20 drops in a little water at noontime and in the evening.
  – *Side effects:* High-dose administration of St. John's wort can lead to photosensitization in fair-skinned individuals.
  – *Clinical value:* Considering the absence of conventional drug treatment alternatives and the positive reports on the effects of herbal remedies, the above-mentioned herbal remedies are certainly worth trying.

13.7 Psychogenic Disorders

Clinical Considerations

➤ **General comments**

- Children suffer from psychogenic disorders such as sleep disorders, psycho-somatic disorders, anxiety disorders and depression more often than is generally assumed. The possibility of organic disease, including cerebral disorders, should always be considered.
- Acute sleep disorders are usually caused by emotional and social stress. Symptoms of certain diseases can also disturb sleep: for example, the pain of an ear infection, the itching of atopic dermatitis (neurodermatitis), or cramplike abdominal pain caused by flatulence. Depression, drug side effects, and diseases that impair the sleep–wake rhythm (anxiety dreams) should be considered if chronic sleep disorders occur in children.
- Recurrent, changing, and multiple physical complaints that usually begin in school age without any discernable physiological cause may indicate a psychosomatic disorder. These problems are more common in girls than in boys. Their foundation is constitutional, but many cases are triggered by psychosocial stress.
- When dealing with anxiety disorders, a distinction should be made between panic disorders and phobias. They are characterized by an excessive intensity of fear, restriction of normal social activities, or unreasonable and unrealistic responses to certain subjects or objects (phobia).

➤ **Herbal treatment measures**

- All of the recommended herbal remedies are taken by the oral route.
- Balm leaf is recommended when difficulty in falling asleep is due to nervous heart or stomach disorders. The herb contains substances with sedative, spasmolytic, and antiflatulent effects.
- Passion flower herb is recommended for restlessness, nervousness, and psychosomatic disorders. In older children, it can be combined with valerian root.
- Lavender oil baths and California poppy are useful with difficulty in falling asleep.
- For anxiety disorders in older children and adolescents, we recommend trying kava root extract or, if depression plays a significant role, St. John's wort.

➤ **Clinical value of herbal medicine**

- Synthetic psychoactive drugs tend to have a lot of side effects and should not be used in pediatric patients unless absolutely necessary. They should preferably be prescribed only by a child psychiatrist.
- Considering their very low rate of side effects, herbal remedies are a highly recommended alternative to synthetic drugs for treatment of childhood psychogenic disorders. They are a useful supplement to psychological counseling.
- Herbal remedies can be used as an adjunct to specific treatment of the primary disease (if applicable) and other measures such as sleep hygiene, autogenous training, physical exercise, elimination of psychosocial stresses, and adequate psychotherapy.

Recommended Herbal Remedies (Overview)

➤ **Dosage and Administration:** All the herbal remedies recommended except for lavender oil (see Herbal Hydrotherapy, p. 285) are administered by the oral route. Commercial products should be administered as recommended by the manufacturer.

Sleep Aids

➤ **Balm leaf** (Melissae folium, see p. 84); **lavender flower** (Lavandulae flos, see p. 59).
➤ For details, see Sleep Disorders, p. 209, and Nervous Anxiety, Tension, and Unease, p. 211.

Daytime Sedatives

➤ **Passion flower herb** (Passiflorae herba, see p. 101); **valerian root** (Valerianae radix, see p. 125); **California poppy** (Eschscholtzia californica).
➤ For details, see Sleep Disorders, p. 209, and Nervous Anxiety, Tension, and Unease, p. 211.

Anxiolytics

➤ **Kava root** (Piperis methystici rhizoma, see p. 82)
➤ For details, see Nervous Anxiety, Tension, and Unease, p. 211.
   – *Contraindications:* Should not be used by children under 12 years of age owing to the lack of adequate study data.

Antidepressants

➤ **St. John's wort** (Hyperici herba, see p. 115).
➤ For details, see Psychovegetative Syndrome, p. 214.

Herbal Remedy Combinations

➤ Valerian root + balm leaf: See Sleep Disorders, p. 209.
➤ Valerian root + balm leaf + passion flower herb: See Sleep Disorders, p. 209.
➤ Passion flower herb + valerian root extract.
➤ Valerian root + balm leaf + orange peel.
➤ St. John's wort extract + valerian root.
➤ Kava root extract + St. John's wort.

Range of Applications

Difficulty in Falling Asleep (Dyskoimesis)

➤ **California poppy.**
   – *Dosage and administration:* Commercial products should be used. Administer as recommended by the manufacturer.
   – *Clinical value:* Clinical studies have not been conducted.

Dyskoimesis with Anxiety-related Heart Consciousness
or Stomach Complaints

➤ **Lemon balm leaf**.
- *Dosage and administration:* Steep 1 to 2 teaspoons of lemon balm leaf (with or without peppermint leaf) in 150 mL of boiling water for 15 minutes. Drink while still warm, directly before retiring. Sweeten with honey if desired.
- *Clinical value:* See Sleep Disorders, p. 209.

Nervous Restlessness in Small Children

➤ **Passion flower herb**.
- *Dosage and administration:* Commercial products should be used. Administer as recommended by the manufacturer.
- *Clinical value:* See Sleep Disorders, p. 209.

Nervous Restlessness, Nervousness, and Psychosomatic Disorders
in Older Children

➤ **Passion flower herb** (see p. 101); **St. John's wort extract** (see p. 115); **valerian root** (see p. 125).
- *Dosage and administration:* Commercial products should be used. Administer as recommended by the manufacturer.
- *Clinical value:* See Sleep Disorders, p. 209.

Anxiety Disorders (in older children and adolescents)

➤ **Kava root** (see p. 82).
- *Dosage and administration:* Commercial products should be used. Administer as recommended by the manufacturer.
- *Clinical value:* See Sleep Disorders, p. 209.

Anxiety Disorders with Depression (in older children and adolescents)

➤ **St. John's wort** (see p. 115); **kava root** (see p. 82).
- *Dosage and administration:* Commercial products should be used. Administer as recommended by the manufacturer.
- *Clinical value:* See Sleep Disorders, p. 209.

Clinical Considerations _____

➤ **General comments**
- *Milk crust (seborrheic dermatitis)*
  - Milk crust is an eczematoid disease of unknown etiology that can occur within in the first 3 months of life.
  - It is characterized by the development of greasy scaling and yellowish crusted patches on the scalp that may spread to the eyebrows, ears, and nose. Yellowish to reddish nonpruritic scales can also develop in the diaper region. Secondary yeast infections (see p. 269) and bacterial infections (see below) can also occur.
  - The symptoms generally disappear within the first year of life. Complications include candidal dermatitis (see p. 269) and bacterial dermatitis (see below).
- *Diaper rash (diaper dermatitis)*
  - Diaper rash is a type of dermatitis of unknown etiology. It is triggered by prolonged contact with irritants in the urine and feces and is more likely to occur when soiled diapers are not changed quickly enough or when waterproof diaper covers are used.
  - Diaper rash is characterized by reddening of the skin in the diaper region. In more severe cases, blistering and erosion of the skin can also occur.
  - Diarrhea, antibiotics, and certain foods and fruit juices promote the development of diaper rash. Secondary bacterial or yeast infections commonly occur.
- *Atopic dermatitis (neurodermatitis):* See p. 267.
- *Herpes labialis*
  - Herpes infections above the waistline are caused by herpes simplex virus type 1 (HSV1). The virus is transmitted through direct contact and remains present in the body as a latent infection.
  - Outbreaks are precipitated by stress, UV irradiation, fever, immunosuppression, and other triggers. The lesions appear as raised areas of skin that conglomerate to form blisters around the mouth (herpes labialis).
- *Bacterial infection:* Inflammation of the skin due to smear infection with or without pus development. *Staphylococcus aureus*, streptococci, and *Haemophilus influenzae* are the main pathogens involved. Dermal bacterial infections are divided into different types as follows:
  - *Impetigo contagiosa:* Superficial pus-filled blisters that rapidly rupture and form a yellowish crust.
  - *Phlegmons:* Suppurative undermining lesions that extend into the subcutaneous tissues.
  - *Erysipelas:* Sharply circumscribed, bright red areas of swelling with chills and fever.
  - *Folliculitis:* Purulent inflammation of the hair follicles, sometimes affecting the surrounding area.
- *Contusions, sprains and injuries:* See Blunt Traumas and Iatrogenic Wounds, p. 278.

➤ **General and herbal treatment measures**
- *Milk crust (seborrheic dermatitis):*
  - The standard scalp medications are oils containing 3% salicylic acid or lotions containing 0.5–1% hydrocortisone.

- The herbal treatment alternatives include oat straw baths (see Herbal Hydrotherapy, p. 288) and heartsease compresses.
- *Diaper rash (diaper dermatitis)*
  - Diaper rash is generally treated with a steroid-free topical zinc fluid, paste or ointment, such as zinc oxide. The parents are also advised to avoid the above-mentioned trigger factors and to apply a diaper rash ointment frequently.
  - Ointments containing chamomile or calendula flower extract can be used as herbal alternatives.
  - *Chamomile extract* is usually recommended. It should be applied at the first signs of diaper rash as well as in the healing phase.
  - *Oily calendula extracts* are more effective in severe cases.
  - *Nystatin* or other antifungals can also be prescribed where there is secondary yeast infection.
- *Atopic dermatitis (neurodermatitis)*
  - Prevention is the main pillar of treatment. If the family has a known history of atopic dermatitis, the infant should be breast fed or given a hypoallergenic milk formula.
  - Skin care includes bathing the infant in a slightly acidic solution and applying an oily ointment after the bath. The regular use of oily bath additives without or without antipruritic agents is also recommended. The infant's clothing should be made of cotton materials.
  - For details on herbal treatment measures, see p. 267.
- *Herpes labialis*
  - Topical aciclovir ointment is the standard treatment.
  - External application of a cream containing a standardized lemon balm leaf extract is a useful herbal alternative when administered at the first signs of an outbreak.
- *Psoriasis (psoriasis vulgaris):* See Psoriasis, p. 263.
- *Bacterial infection of the skin*
  - See Diaper Rash, p. 259 ff.
  - See Herbal Hydrotherapy, p. 288.
➤ **Clinical value of phytotherapy:** The clinical value of phytotherapy is described in the Range of Applications for each clinical picture below.

Recommended Herbal Remedies (Overview)

➤ **Details:** See Dermatological Diseases, p. 262 ff.

Antiphlogistics

➤ **Heartsease herb** (wild pansy) (Violae tricoloris herba, see p. 75); **calendula flower** (Calendulae flos, see p. 90); **chamomile flower** (Matricariae flos, see p. 47); **St. John's wort oil** (Hyperici oleum, see p. 115); **bittersweet stems** (Dulcamarae stipites, see p. 40); **witch hazel leaf and bark** (Hamamelidis folium/cortex, see p. 128); **lemon balm leaf** (Melissae folium, see p. 84).
  - *Action:* See pp. 266, 268.

Immunostimulants with Antimicrobial Effects

➤ **Calendula flower** (Calendulae flos, see p. 90).
  - *Action:* See p. 276.

Antipruritics

➤ **Witch hazel leaf/bark** (Hamamelidis folium/cortex, see p. 128).
  – *Action:* See p. 273.

Virustatics

➤ **Balm leaf** (Melissae folium, see pp. 84, 262).

Antiallergics

➤ **Bittersweet stems** (Dulcamarae stipites, see p. 40).

Range of Applications _____

Milk Crust, Seborrheic Dermatitis

➤ **Antimicrobial immunostimulants: Calendula flower** (see p. 90).
➤ **Anti-inflammatories: Heartsease** (see p. 95); **chamomile flower** (see p. 47); **St. John's wort** (see p. 115); **calendula flower** (see p. 90).
➤ For details, see Eczema, p. 265, and Acne, p. 269.
  – *Dosage and administration*
    • For instructions, see standard treatments for pansy, p. 320.
    • Apply to the affected areas of the skin several times a day.
  – *Clinical value:* Safe alternative to hydrocortisone that is worth trying. Clinical studies have not been conducted.

Diaper Rash

➤ **Anti-inflammatories: Calendula flower** (see p. 90); **chamomile flower** (see p. 47).
➤ **Antimicrobial immunostimulants: Calendula flower**.
  – *Dosage and administration*: A suitable topical preparation should be applied as directed on the product label.
  – *Clinical value:* Useful alternative to standard diaper rash preparations. The parent should seek medical advice if there is no improvement or worsening of symptoms.

Atopic Dermatitis (Neurodermatitis)

➤ **Anti-inflammatory and antipruritic agents: Bittersweet stems**; **balloon-vine herb** (Cardiospermi herba); **witch hazel leaf and bark**.
➤ **Antiallergics: Bittersweet stems**.
  – *Dosage and administration:* A suitable topical preparation should be applied to the affected areas of the skin several times a day, as directed on the product label.
  – *Clinical value:* The recommended herbs are well-tolerated medications with proven effects. They are safe for short or long-term use. The beneficial effects of ointments made from bittersweet, balloonvine, and witch hazel have been demonstrated in clinical studies. A qualified health care provider should supervise treatment.

13.8 Dermatological Diseases

Herpes Labialis

➤ **Virustatic: Lemon balm leaf.**
  – *Dosage and administration:* Commercial products that are applied locally should be used. Administer as recommended by the manufacturer.
  – *Clinical value:* A useful alternative to aciclovir. If treatment is started at the first signs of an outbreak, there is a better chance of success. The most severe types of herpes simplex infection (generalized) do not respond to herbal therapy.

Psoriasis

➤ See Dermatological Diseases: Psoriasis, p. 263.

Bacterial Infection

➤ **Anti-inflammatories: Heartsease herb** (wild pansy); **calendula flower, chamomile flower**.
➤ **Anti-irritants**: **Heartsease herb** (wild pansy); **chamomile flower**.
➤ **Antimicrobial immunostimulants: Calendula flower**.
  – *Dosage and administration*
  – For special formulations for calendula, chamomile, and heartsease extracts see standard treatments on pp. 300, 315, 320.
  – Commercial products should be used. They should be applied locally, as recommended by the manufacturer.
  – *Clinical value:* Herbal ointments and baths alone generally suffice for treatment of mild conditions. If the condition is more severe, the patient should consult a general practitioner and use the herbal remedies for adjunctive treatment only. Clinical study data on chamomile preparations are available.

Contusions, injuries, sprains

➤ See p. 276 ff.

Clinical Considerations

General comments

– Psoriasis is a cornification disorder occurring in intermittent attacks. The disease is characterized by the development of reddish plaques covered by grossly lamellar scales.

– Psoriatic attacks are provoked by certain medications, alcohol, stress, and other skin-damaging factors.

– Different types of psoriasis can be distinguished. Apart from the skin, the nails and especially the joints of the hands and feet can also be affected.

– Psoriasis affects a substantial portion of the Western European population (1–3 %), with about 7 million sufferers of psoriasis in the United States alone. The disease is congenital but the cause is unknown.

General and herbal treatment measures

– Several treatment strategies are available: Topical preparations containing salicylic acid, cignolin, retinoids, glucocorticoids and tar can be used as well as selective ultraviolet radiation in combination with psoralen. More severe cases may warrant systemic therapy with retinoids, cyclosporin A and/or methotrexate.

– Intensive phytotherapy and regular physical measures are important when joint regions are affected.

Clinical value of herbal medicine

– Smaller-scale clinical studies have demonstrated that psoriasis improves with aloe vera and Oregon grape bark.

– These herbs should only be used in mild psoriasis. No data are available on their use in more severe cases.

– *Sarsaparilla* was formerly used for psoriasis in folk medicine, but the Commission E negative monograph states that prolonged use can damage the kidney. Therefore, we do not recommend it.

Recommended Herbal Remedies and Range of Applications

Aloe vera juice (Aloe barbadensis succus); **Oregon grape root/bark** (Mahoniae cortex, see p. 100).

– *Action*
  • Aloe vera gel is the condensed juice of *Aloe barbadensis* leaves. The gel contains enzymes, minerals, vitamins, and saponins and has anti-inflammatory and antibacterial effects. It is commonly added to cosmetics for its moisturizing, regenerative, and elasticity-promoting properties.
  • *Oregon grape root/bark:* Clinical studies have shown that extracts from trunk and root bark of Oregon grape root inhibit cell division in cell cultures and inhibit protein biosynthesis (berberine). Inhibition of T-lymphocyte activity and anti-inflammatory effects have also been reported. The extract is useful in mild to moderate cases of plaque-forming psoriasis.

– *Contraindications:* Oregon grape root should not be used during pregnancy and lactation.

– *Dosage and administration*
  • *Aloe vera gel:* Apply sparingly to affected area of the skin three times a day.
  • Commercial products should be used as directed by the manufacturer.

- *Side effects:* Aloe vera was found to cause allergic and toxic contact eczem in rare cases.
- *Clinical value:* These preparations appear to be effective remedies for mil psoriasis. Further clinical study is required for a final assessment.

Clinical Considerations

▶ **General comments**

– Eczema is a noncontagious type of dermatitis that is usually triggered by hypersensitivity to certain substances.

– Acute attacks are characterized by skin reddening and swelling with papule and blister formation. Crusting and scaling develop after the blisters burst open. Additional skin damage often occurs due to itching and scratching, which is often leads to purulent secondary bacterial infections.

– Chronic eczema is common and can lead to leathery hypertrophy of the skin, or *lichenification*.

– Different types of eczema are distinguished:

  • Allergic contact eczema is precipitated by contact with allergens such as nickel, chromium, preservatives, perfumes, ointment bases, and plant extracts (e. g., arnica).

  • Toxic contact eczema is caused by direct skin damage due to ultraviolet radiation exposure (e. g., sunburn and so-called sun rash).

  • Chronic contact eczema occurs due to constant contact with water and soap, acids, lyes and/or solvents (often job-related).

▶ **General and herbal treatment measures**

– Avoidance of trigger substances is the first and foremost pillar of treatment.

– Standard treatment of acute contact eczema consists of the application of cool, wet compresses with or without short-term cortisone or hydrocortisone treatment as needed. Greasy ointments may also be necessary if skin thinning occurs due to chronic inflammation.

– All of the herbal remedies are applied topically.

▶ **Clinical value of herbal medicine**

– Chamomile flower, witch hazel leaf and bark, balloonvine herb, and oak bark have proven benefits in weeping and, in some cases, bacterially infected, purulent eczema.

– Chamomile flower extract is indicated in mild eczema with or without bacterial infection. Recent studies have shown that chamomile extract is superior to ointment base alone and to 0.5 % hydrocortisone in the treatment of toxic eczema.

– Witch hazel leaf and bark preparations are weaker than 1 % hydrocortisone products and are therefore more suitable for treatment of mild symptoms.

– Balloonvine herb has antipruritic and anti-eczematous effects.

– Oak bark is indicated in acute weeping eczema and is also helpful in secondary bacterial superinfection.

– Bittersweet has not been tested for effectiveness in eczema, but a beneficial effect of the herb seems probable. Bittersweet has a very low rate of side effects and is suitable for long-term use.

Recommended Herbal Remedies and Range of Applications

▶ **Chamomile flower** (Matricariae flos, see p. 47); **bittersweet stems** (Dulcamarae stipites, see p. 40); **witch hazel leaf** and **bark** (Hamamelidis folium/cortex, see p. 128); **oak bark** (Quercus cortex, see p. 99).

14.2 Eczema

- *Action*
  - Chamomile extract contains anti-inflammatory compounds (chamazulene and bisabolol) as well as mucilaginous substances that counteract irritation.
  - Witch hazel contains hamamelitannins that reduce skin redness by decreasing the blood flow to the skin and flavones that inhibit histamine release. Bacteriostatic action has also been reported.
  - Oak bark has a high content of tannins that react with proteins in the superficial layer of the skin and mucous membranes to prevent the penetration of harmful organisms.
  - Bittersweet stems contain tannins as well as steroid alkaloid glycosides with anti-inflammatory, antipruritic, and antiallergic effects.
- *Contraindications:* Oak bark should not be used if there is extensive skin damage. Treatment should be limited to a total of 2 to 3 weeks.
- *Dosage and administration*
  - *Cold wet compresses* made with chamomile flower extract or oak bark decoction are applied to the affected areas of the skin 3 times daily for periods of 1 to 2 hours each (see standard treatment section, Section 4).
  - Exchange the compress for a fresh cold one as soon as it becomes warm and dry. After treatment, place a wet compress over the affected skin and wrap loosely. Do not cover the compress with airtight material.
  - *Oak bark decoction:* Boil 2 tablespoons (10 g) of the herb in 500 mL of water for 15 minutes, then strain. Allow to cool before use. Prepare fresh each day.
  - If commercial products are preferred, they should be used as directed by the manufacturer.
- *Side effects*
  - *Bittersweet stem:* Ointment preparations contain small quantities of alcohol that may cause burning on broken skin.
  - *Chamomile flower:* Although rare, chamomile flower may induce contact eczema. This is usually attributable to adulteration with other plants.
- *Clinical value:* The above herbal treatments are well-tolerated remedies. The efficacy of some has been scientifically proven. They are safe for long-term use. The efficacy of bittersweet, balloonvine, and witch hazel in mild to moderate eczema has been confirmed in clinical studies.

Clinical Considerations

▶ See also section on atopic dermatitis (neurodermatitis) in childhood, p. 259.
▶ **General comments**
– Atopic dermatitis (neurodermatitis) is a familial disorder characterized by intermittent attacks of severely pruritic inflammatory skin changes (eczema) that start, in some cases, as early as the third month of life. Data suggest that longer periods of breast feeding may prevent the disorder.
– Attacks are often provoked by mental or physical stress, infection, skin irritation, or the consumption of certain foods.
– Atopic dermatitis is the most common childhood skin disease. It is characterized by a weeping, patchy skin rash with raised papules, scratching and crusting. The elbows, knee flexures, tops of the feet and hands, and neck are typically involved. The skin is pale, dry, and scaled, especially on the hands. The skin has an abnormal fat composition, often showing a deficiency of unsaturated fatty acids.
– The condition may be complicated by staphylococcus, streptococcus or herpes virus superinfections. It generally is not possible to predict the course of the disease in any given case. The symptoms often disappear during puberty.

▶ **General and herbal treatment measures**
– Skin care measures should include the use of oleaginous ointments and oil baths. Additional skin irritation should be avoided, and cotton underwear is recommended.
– Vacations should be taken in areas with low allergen concentrations, since the current data suggest that allergens (e.g., pollen) are transported through the air to the skin, where they can worsen allergy symptoms.
– When a food allergy is suspected, the food in question should be avoided. Dietary fats such as ones containing the essential fatty acids linoleic and linolenic acids, or eicosapentaenoic acid (EPA) or docosahexaenoic acid (DHA) should preferably be supplied and supplemented by unsaturated fatty acids such as flaxseed oil or fish oils.
– Psychological counseling is helpful.
– If tolerated, ultraviolet radiation can be recommended.
– Nonsteroidal antiphlogistics can be useful in mild cases. Cortisone cremes should only be used in acute attacks.
– Tar preparations are especially useful in cases with chronic itching.
– Superinfection or other aggravated symptoms may require additional treatment with oral antihistamines with or without glucocorticoids.
– Topical herbal remedies prepared from witch hazel bark, bittersweet stems, and balloonvine herb are suitable for adjunctive treatment.
– All of the recommended herbal remedies are applied locally to the affected areas of the skin.

▶ **Clinical value of herbal medicine:** See below. These cases tend to be extremely difficult to manage.

Recommended Herbal Remedies and Range of Applications

▶ **Bittersweet stems** (Dulcamarae stipites); **balloonvine herb** (Cardiospermi herba); **witch hazel leaf** and **bark** (Hamamelidis folium et cortex, see p. 128).

- *Action*
  - Witch hazel bark contain tannins with antipruritic and anti-inflammatory effects.
  - Bittersweet stems contain steroid alkaloid glycosides with anti-inflammatory, antipruritic, and antiallergic effects. The tannins have sealant effects that prevent toxins and pathogens from penetrating the skin.
  - Balloonvine contains halicaric acid, saponins, tannins, sterols, and flavonoids. Anti-inflammatory and antipruritic effects have been reported.
- *Contraindications:* See Eczema, p. 266.
- *Dosage and administration:* Commercial products should be used according to the manufacturer's recommendations.
- *Side effects:* See eczema, p. 266.
  - Bittersweet stems ointments contain small quantities of alcohol and may initially cause burning on broken skin.
- *Clinical value:* The recommended herbs are safe and effective remedies suitable for short-term or long-term use. Clinical studies have demonstrated some beneficial effects, but further research is necessary to evaluate all uses.

Clinical Considerations

▶ **General comments**
- *Acne vulgaris*
  - Acne is a cornification disorder of the hair follicles in which the contents are retained and can become inflamed (pustule formation).
  - Hormonal, hereditary, and external factors (various medications, vitamins B_1, B_6 and B_{12}) play a role.
  - Different types are distinguished. It is not possible to predict the course of the disease, which can persist for several years. Almost every case of acne can be treated with good cosmetic results, provided that treatment is continued until the acne activity spontaneously ceases.
- *Seborrheic dermatitis:* Characterized by the formation of reddish scales in areas of the skin where surface fat is plentiful, e. g., the scalp, eyebrows, and outer part of the auditory canal. Infestation with cutaneous yeast fungi may play an inducing role.

▶ **General and herbal treatment measures**
- Washing the skin regularly with medicated soap several times a day is helpful.
- Acne is generally treated with a combination of topical and oral medications. The topical agents often contain retinoids and antibiotics, systemic therapy uses antibiotics, hormones, and retinoids. Oregon grape can be used as an herbal alternative.
- In seborrheic dermatitis, fungicidal or selenium disulfide-containing shampoos are used to treat the scalp, and ultraviolet radiation, mild glucocorticoids, and fungicidal cremes are used to treat the face. Heartsease (wild pansy) is used for herbal treatment.

▶ **Clinical value of herbal medicine**
- Oregon grape bark is the only herbal remedy available for acne.
- Clinical studies on this use have not been conducted.
- Heartsease is recommended for mild seborrheic dermatitis; clinical study data are not available.

Recommended Herbal Remedies and Range of Applications

▶ **Oregon grape bark** (Mahoniae cortex, see p. 100); **heartsease** (wild pansy) (Violae tricoloris herba, see p. 75).
- *Action*
  - *Oregon grape bark:* Clinical studies have shown that extracts from trunk and root bark of Oregon grape inhibit cell division in cell cultures and inhibit protein biosynthesis (berberine). Inhibition of T-lymphocyte activity and anti-inflammatory effects have also been reported.
  - Heartsease (wild pansy) contains flavonoids with antioxidant and anti-inflammatory effects.
- *Contraindications:* Oregon grape root bark should not be used during pregnancy or lactation.
- *Dosage and administration*
  - *Heartsease (wild pansy):* Steep 1 teaspoon of the finely chopped herb in 1 cup of hot water for 5 minutes, then strain. Use the infusion to prepare wet compresses. Apply 2 to 3 times daily.
  - Commercial tea preparations can be purchased at pharmacies.

3

- *Clinical value:* The herbal preparations are probably effective only in mild cases. Clinical studies have not been conducted.

Clinical Considerations

▶ **General comments**
- Furuncles (boils) are caused by *Staphylococcus* infection of the hair follicles. They most commonly occur on the neck, face, axillary, back, and groin regions.
- The lesions start as coarse red nodules that soon become painful and pustular within a few days. They often heal with scarring. Recurrent furunculosis may be a sign of immune suppression or diabetes.
- ◉ *Important:* Furuncles situated above the upper lip can cause life-threatening complications. The patient should seek medical attention immediately. Furunculosis can affect the eyes and result in the spread of infection to the cerebral veins (thrombosis of venous sinus).

▶ **General and herbal treatment measures**
- Intensive heat application (flaxseed or grass flowers, see p. 308) can accelerate the maturation of the furuncle.
- Hot compresses prepared with oak bark decoction can also be helpful.

▶ **Clinical value of herbal medicine**
- Standard treatment is with oral penicillin or erythromycin for 7 to 10 days. When the central portion of the furuncle softens, it can be opened and drained by a physician.
- Herbal remedies are administered as supplementary treatment measures.

Recommended Herbal Remedies and Range of Applications

▶ **Flaxseed** (Lini semen, see p. 66); **fenugreek seed** (Foenugraeci semen); **oak bark** (Quercus cortex, see p. 99).
- *Action*
  - Linseed contains mucilage and fatty oil. Grass flowers contain a coumarin glycoside that boosts the circulation.
  - Fenugreek contains fatty oils, 20–30 % mucilage, trigonelline, bitter substances, and saponins and has a softening effect.
  - Hot oak bark compresses are especially helpful in recurrent furunculosis. The herbal remedy contains tannins that change the outer layer of the skin, making it more difficult for new infections to occur.
- *Contraindications:* Oak bark should not be used if large areas of the skin are damaged.
- *Dosage and administration*
  - *Flaxseed compresses:* A small linen bag is filled one-third full with flaxseed, sewn together, then boiled briefly. Once the seeds swell, the bag is gently squeezed and applied to the affected site while as hot as tolerable.
  - *Fenugreek poultices:* Mix 50 g fenugreek seed with 1 liter of warm water and apply to the affected area of the skin.
  - *Oak bark compresses:* Place 2 tablespoons of the finely chopped herb in 3 cups of water, bring to a boil and allow to steep for 5 minutes. Apply a hot compress to the affected region several times a day.
  - *Side effects:* Repeated topical application of fenugreek can induce hypersensitivity reactions.
  - *Clinical value:* These measures accelerate the maturation of furuncles. Clinical studies have not been conducted.

14.6 Hair Loss (Effluvium)

Clinical Considerations

➤ **General comments**
  – Hair loss has many causes. Male hormones usually play a role (also in women) but do not have any true pathogenetic significance.
  – Other common causes are hormone disorders, discontinuation of contraceptives, extreme stress, severe infections, systemic diseases, certain heavy metals, certain medications, and fasting. When one of these factors is the cause, hair growth generally normalizes spontaneously within 6 months.
  – Heavy menstruation can provoke hair loss in vegetarian women, as a consequence of low serum iron concentrations.
  – Baldness is hereditary and occurs intermittently. The episodes become less frequent with age.
  – Treatment should be managed by a dermatologist.

➤ **General and herbal treatment measures**
  – Standard treatment of hair loss consists of a number of measures. In addition to treating the causative factors, the patient is generally instructed to shampoo frequently with a mild shampoo, avoid hair-processing chemicals and hair sprays that can cause scalp inflammation, and avoid pulling the hair or wearing long braids or buns, etc.
  – The patient should eat a balanced diet rich in proteins and low in fats. Fasting should be avoided.
  – Alcoholic extracts of stinging nettle are used for herbal therapy.

➤ **Clinical value of herbal medicine:** The use of herbal remedies is most effective when hair loss is associated with depleted states with fatigue.

Recommended Herbal Remedies and Range of Applications

➤ **Stinging nettle herb** (Urticae herba, see p. 97).
  – *Action:* When applied topically, stinging nettle gently increases the local blood flow.
  – *Dosage and administration*
    • **Hair tonic *Rx*:** Tinctura urticae herba 10.0. Spiritus rosmarini ad 100.0 Massage vigorously into the scalp 2 to 3 times daily.
  – *Clinical value:* The herbal remedy appears to be useful in the above indication. Clinical studies have not been conducted.

Clinical Considerations

▶ **General comments**
  – Itching is an unpleasant sensation on the skin surface that leads to scratching. Pruritus can also cause sleep disturbance.
  – Many diseases can lead to itching. Hence, the health care practitioner should always try to identify the underlying cause.
  – Certain tissue hormones (e. g., substance P) are released within the skin, thereby activating receptors that trigger itching sensations.

▶ **General and herbal treatment measures**
  – The main effort should be concentrated on treating the underlying cause of pruritus. Herbal remedies can be used if UVB radiation therapy cannot be performed.
  – Capsaicin gel is a standard medication.
  – Oleaginous ointments containing uric acid are used to treat dry skin.
  – Oat straw baths can also be recommended (see Herbal Hydrotherapy, p. 289).

▶ **Clinical value of herbal medicine:** See below.

Recommended Herbal Remedies and Range of Applications

▶ **Heartsease** (wild pansy) (Violae tricoloris herba, see p. 75); **cayenne** (Capsici fructus, see p. 46); **Spanish paprika** (Capsici fructus); **peppermint leaf** (Menthae piperitae folium, see p. 102).
  – *Action*
    • Cayenne and Spanish paprika contain pungent capsaicinoids. Capsaicin, the active principle in these herbs, stimulates free nerve endings on the skin surface. This produces skin reddening and a hot, burning sensation for around 20 minutes, presumably due to the release of substance p. The intensity of the reaction gradually decreases after repeated use.
    • Menthol, the monoterpene active principle in peppermint oil, also has an antipruritic effect. It cools the skin and raises the sensory threshold for skin irritations.
    • Heartsease (wild pansy) contains flavonoids, saponins, and methylsalicylates that are presumed to have antioxidant and anti-inflammatory effects.
  – *Contraindications*
    • *Capsaicin:* Skin diseases, dermatitis, skin damage. Should not come in contact with the mucous membranes. Should not be used by children under 12 years of age.
    • *Peppermint oil and mint oil* should not be applied to the face of infants and small children.
  – *Dosage and administration*
    • *Heartsease (wild pansy):* Steep 1 teaspoon of the finely chopped herb in 1 cup of hot water for 5 minutes, then strain. Use the liquid to make wet compresses.
    • *Capsicum tincture (1 : 10):* Massage a few drops onto the affected area of the skin several times a day. When treating generalized pruritus, try treating only one particular region of the body.
    • *Mint oil, peppermint oil:* Apply topically, 2 to 3 times daily.
    • *Heartsease herb (tea):* Apply a compress of heartsease herb tea.

14.7 Itching (Pruritus)

> ◉ *Note:* The topical mint oils and heartsease compress should not be use
> together.
- • **Oat straw baths:** See Herbal Hydrotherapy, p. 289.
- – *Side effects:* When used for prolonged periods, capsaicin can cause skin in
  flammation with blistering or ulceration. Therefore, preparations contain
  ing capsaicin should not be used for more than 3 days without medical su
  pervision.
- – *Clinical value*
  - • The effects of the individual herbal preparations vary greatly, and it
    not possible to predict the results of long-term treatment.
  - • Menthol-containing preparations and heartsease (wild pansy) are suit
    able for long-term use. Controlled clinical studies have not been con
    ducted.

Clinical Considerations

➤ **General comments**
– A number of factors can lead to excessive perspiration (hyperhidrosis): for example, diffuse disorders of temperature regulation, psychological problems (perspiration mainly in the palms of the hands, armpits, groin, and soles of the feet), stress, and recovery from illness. Hyperhidrosis can also be a sign of an underlying disease, such as hyperthyroidism, in menopause, and diabetes.
– The problem can cause considerable distress, both objectively measurable and subjective.

➤ **General and herbal treatment measures**
– Aluminum chloride hexahydrate is used in standard therapy.
– Sage leaves are used in herbal medicine.

➤ **Clinical value of herbal medicine**
– Sage is used because of the pharmacological properties of its active constituents. Clinical studies have not been conducted.

Recommended Herbal Remedies and Range of Applications

➤ **Sage leaf** (Salviae folium, see p. 114).
– *Action:* Sage leaves contain tannic acid, an anti-inflammatory compound, and an essential oil with antibacterial and anti-inflammatory effects attributable to the compounds thujone, 1,8-cineole, camphor, and carnosol.
– *Contraindications:* Pregnant women should not use alcohol-based sage extracts or pure sage oil.
– *Dosage and administration*
  • Sage preparations are administered internally in the form of tea or commercial medicinal products, and externally as liniments or bath additives. Liniments are prepared by diluting the tincture or fluid extract in water.
  • *Tea:* Steep 1–2 g sage leaves in 150 mL of hot water and allow to cool. Drink 30 minutes before meals.
  • *Tincture (1 : 5):* Dilute ½ teaspoon in a small amount of water and take twice daily before meals.
  • *Daily dose for internal use:* 4–6 g (tea).
  ◉ *Important:* Sage tea should not be used for extended periods or during pregnancy or nursing owing to the thujone content (see Sage, p. 114).
– *Side effects:* Epileptiform convulsions have been observed after prolonged use of alcoholic sage extracts and pure sage oil.
– *Clinical value:* Empirical observations from various sources indicate that sage is an effective alternative to the standard drugs. Clinical study data are not available.

Clinical Considerations

➤ **General comments**
  – Every injury produces a wound, that is, a tissue defect that the body must seal off by fibrous tissue scarring and skin regeneration.
  – In primary wound healing, the wound heals with a minimal amount of scar formation within a few days. This requires secure wound coverage, cleanliness, and a good blood supply to the wound.
  – In secondary wound healing, the healing process is slower and more complicated. Bacterial invasion is usually involved. Wounds that do not begin to heal within 8 weeks are called chronic wounds, e. g., leg ulcers, diabetic foot ulcers, bed sores (decubitus ulcers), and surgical wounds.

➤ **Herbal treatment measures**
  – All of the recommended herbal remedies are applied locally as watery extracts or ointments. Wet compresses are the preferred vehicle for cleaning wounds and stimulating the healing process. Once the wound starts to heal, the patient can switch to ointments, which are sparingly applied to the edges of the wound.
  – Chamomile flower extracts are beneficial in all phases of wound healing.
  – An oily calendula flower extract should preferably be used if there is more severe involvement.
  – Small, circumscribed wounds heal quickly when treated with St. John's wort oil.
  – Compresses soaked in arnica tincture are recommended for wounds with a slimy and adhesive coating, poor granulation, and first signs of lymphangitis. It contains helenalin, a compound known to cause contact allergies, with increased inflammation in susceptible individuals. Spanish *Arnica montana* varieties contain only small quantities of the compound and should be used wherever possible and available. Before using arnica, the potential risk should be carefully weighed against the expected benefits of treatment, and the duration of use should be limited. Study data supporting this use are still lacking.
  – Fresh plant juice extracted from purple echinacea has immunomodulatory constituents. Echinacea stimulates granulation for new tissue.

➤ **Clinical value of herbal medicine:** Every attempt should be made to treat the underlying disease. The recommended herbal preparations are safe adjunctive treatment measures to accelerate wound healing.

Recommended Herbal Remedies and Range of Applications

➤ **Calendula flower** (Calendulae flos, see p. 90); **chamomile flower** (Matricariae flos, see p. 47); **arnica flower** (Arnicae flos, see p. 35); **St. John's wort oil** (Hyperici oleum see p. 115); **purple echinacea** (Echinaceae purpureae herba, see p. 56).
  – *Action*
    • *Anti-inflammatory:* Calendula flower, chamomile flower, arnica flower, St. John's wort oil. The essential oil in chamomile flowers contains the anti-inflammatory compounds chamazulene and bisabolol in addition to soothing mucilages.
    • *Antimicrobial and immunostimulant:* Calendula flower, arnica flower. Their most important constituents are bitter principles with potent

anti-inflammatory and antimicrobial (antibacterial and antifungal) effects. The essential oil, which contains thymol and thymol ether, is also antimicrobial. These herbs boost the circulation and alleviate pain. Their polysaccharide constituents stimulate the immune system. Researchers also found that calendula flower contains some carotinoids that are known to promote wound healing.

- *Immunostimulant:* Calendula stimulates the immune system through macrophages and granulocytes, promotes the formation of new tissue, and prevents the spread of infection.

⊙ *Note:* The active principles in chamomile flowers are present in active form only in alcoholic extracts and corresponding essences.

- *Contraindications:* Arnica, calendula, and chamomile should not be used by individuals with a known allergy to arnica and other composite plants. Arnica should not be used by children under 12 years of age.
- *Dosage and administration*
  - *Compresses:* Wet with a mixture of calendula tincture and Ringer's solution (1 : 10).
  - *Small wounds:* Apply *Hypericum* oil directly to the wound three times a day. The *Hypericum* oil should be of a rich red color to be effective.
  - The above formulations or commercial products are applied locally, several times a day. Compresses soaked with the plant extract are applied for 1 to 2 hours, 3 times daily. Each compress should be left on for only around 15 to 20 minutes (until it becomes warm and dry), then replaced by a fresh one. Commercial products should be used as directed by the manufacturer.

⊙ *Warning:* Arnica should not be allowed to come in contact with the eye or applied to the eye region. Arnica-containing ointments should not be applied to mucous membranes or open wounds. The hands should be washed after using arnica products.

- *Side effects*
  - *Chamomile flower:* Although rare, contact allergies can occur. This is, in most cases, attributable to adulteration with corn chamomile.
  - *Arnica flower:* Prolonged use of the herb or tincture on damaged skin can lead to edematous inflammation with blistering or eczema. Concentrated helenalin-containing extracts can provoke contact eczema. Hence, undiluted arnica tincture should never be used or applied to an open wound. Arnica tincture has a greater potential for sensitization than arnica ointment.
  - *Clinical value:* The above herbal measures are used to promote the healing process, especially in chronic wounds or those with secondary healing. Clinical studies have been conducted on chamomile flower extract and echinacea. Calendula flower extract is reputed to greatly accelerate granulation.

15.2 Blunt Traumas and Iatrogenic Wounds

Clinical Considerations

➤ **General comments:** Blunt trauma is common after impact due to sports injuries and accidents. The tearing of lymph and blood vessels leads to the seepage of lymph and blood into the surrounding tissues. Nerves, muscles and tendons can also be damaged. Pain, swelling, and a restricted range of movement are the unpleasant consequences. Comparable symptoms sometimes occur after surgery and bone fractures.

➤ **Herbal treatment measures**

– Wet compresses soaked with diluted arnica tincture accelerate blood and lymph absorption and alleviate pain. Compresses are especially effective for contusions. Since helenalin can trigger contact eczema, arnica extracts usually are not applied to open wounds (see Wounds, p. 276). The herb is however, very useful for treating insect bites. Arnica ointment is also useful in the initial stages, but its effects are not as strong as those of the extract.

– Comfrey compresses can be helpful after the acute symptoms have subsided. The herb should only be used externally, and not on open wounds, because it contains hepatotoxic substances (pyrrolizidine alkaloids).

– In folk medicine, poultices made from onion pulp are applied at this stage They ease pain and reduce swelling.

– In the further course of healing or in conditions attributable to bone fractures, sprains and surgery, we recommend liniments made of juniper, calamus or angelica spirits. The liniment should be applied directly after an application of heat. Empirical reports on these uses are available.

➤ **Clinical value of herbal medicine:** Immobilization and cold wet compresses especially arnica compresses, are recommended for acute contusions and sprains. The compresses have cooling effects and reduce inflammation. Once the acute symptoms have subsided, comfrey compresses and liniments containing essential oils can usefully supplement conventional measures such as hot air treatment and active exercise.

Recommended Herbal Remedies and Range of Applications

➤ **Arnica flower** (Arnicae flos, see p. 35); **comfrey root** (Symphyti radix); **onion bulb** (Cepae bulbus); **calamus root** (Calami rhizoma, see p. 44); **juniper berry** (Juniperi fructus, see p. 80); **angelica root** (Angelicae radix, see p. 33).

– *Action*

• *Arnica flower* (see p. 35): Contains sesquiterpene lactones (e. g., dihydrohelenalin), which are potent anti-inflammatories. Prevents the cell membranes from releasing arachidonic acid, a substance required for the biosynthesis of inflammation-promoting chemicals.

• *Comfrey root:* Contains allantoin, mucilages, and tannins. Like uric acid allantoin plays an active role in osmosis and stimulates the local blood flow, as well as promoting wound-healing and reducing sclerosis. Preparations made from comfrey root have analgesic and anti-inflammatory effects and reduce swelling.

• *Juniper:* The essential oil extracted from the berries of juniper contains alpha and beta pinenes which are known to act as skin irritants and increase the local blood supply.

- *Calamus root:* The essential oil extracted from the calamus rhizome contains camphor and is thus spasmolytic and increases the local blood supply.
- *Contraindications:* Arnica should not be used by individuals with eczema and known hypersensitivity to arnica or other composite plants. Calamus oil contains a variable percentage of beta-asarone, depending on where the raw herb was grown. Since the compound can damage the genetic material, calamus should not be used during pregnancy or lactation or by children. Comfrey root preparations should not be applied to open wounds or damaged skin and should not be allowed to come in contact with the eyes or mucous membranes.
- *Dosage and administration*
  - *Compresses:* Acute injuries are treated with linen compresses soaked in one of the above plant extracts. The compresses are applied locally to the affected area for 1 to 2 hours, 3 times daily (see Wounds, p. 276). They should not be covered with airtight material. Commercial products should be used as directed by the manufacturer.
  - *Acute injuries:* Dilute 1 tablespoon of arnica tincture in 500 mL of cold water. Wet a compress with the solution and apply to the affected area. Repeat frequently.
  - **Liniments:** Apply three times daily. Liniments are especially effective when warmed prior to use.
  - **Liniment *Rx* 1:** Oleum Juniperi 2.0, Spiritus Calami ad 100.0.
  - **Liniment *Rx* 2:** Oleum Calami 2.0, Spiritus Angelicae Compos. ad 100.0.
  - *Onion poultices:* Stir finely chopped onion, water, and a little salt to a pulp and apply to affected area.
- ◉ *Note:* Comfrey root should not be used for more than 4 to 6 weeks a year. The maximum daily dose of pyrrolizidine alkaloids is 100 (g. The herbal remedy should not be used during pregnancy unless the expected benefits clearly outweigh the risks.
- *Side effects:* Although rare, comfrey root can lead to hypersensitivity reactions at the application site, leading to reddening and nodule or blister formation, usually in conjunction with itching. Treatment should be discontinued if such effects are observed.
- *Clinical value:* If the limitations and contraindications are heeded, these herbal remedies represent cheap and effective treatment alternatives. However, comparative clinical studies have yet to be conducted.

15.3 Leg Ulceration

Clinical Considerations

➤ **General comments:** Leg ulceration is due either to impaired venous flow or—more rarely—impaired arterial flow. Venous stasis is usually the result of deep leg vein thrombosis that occurred many years previously or represents the final stage of chronic venous insufficiency. Hence, both arterial and venous leg ulcers can be attributed to local oxygen and nutrient deficiencies.

➤ **Herbal treatment measures**
 – Most of the treatment recommendations apply to venous leg ulcers. However, arterial ulceration is difficult to diagnose and was probably treated along with venous ulceration in the past.
 – Regarding the aqueous extract of red wine leaves, a recent postmarketing surveillance study demonstrated that the preparation has a favorable effect on simple venous ulcers. The preparation was used in combination with esculin, a coumarin derivative obtained from the leaves and bark of the horse chestnut tree.
 – In light of its allantoin content, local therapy with preparations made from comfrey root should promote granulation. Aloe gel also contains allantoin and is often recommended as an external application.
 – Ointments containing coneflower extract can strengthen local immune defenses, thereby inhibiting wound infection.
 – If acute dermatitis develops around an old ulcer, we recommend the application of wet compresses soaked in oak bark decoction or soaking the affected region of the skin in the decoction. The use of arnica extract, a popular remedy, is not to be recommended in this situation since it rather frequently induces massive contact allergies.
 – Calendula is recommended for initial treatment of secondary leg ulcer infections (see Wounds, p. 276).

➤ **Clinical value of herbal medicine:** The above herbal remedies are recommended as adjunctive treatment measures. The primary goal of treatment is to improve the circulation. Arterial and venous ulcers are treated differently. If the underlying cause cannot be eliminated, which is usually the case, new ulcers can be expected during the course of treatment. It is therefore imperative that the patient faithfully follows the instructions of the supervising health care provider, especially in the periods where no ulcers are present. It is equally important that the patient consults the health care provider immediately after a new ulcer has developed. Attempts of self-treatment are usually futile and they could worsen the overall condition. Recent findings on wound care (see p. 276) should naturally be considered.

Recommended Herbal Remedies and Range of Applications

➤ **Comfrey root** (Symphyti radix); **purple echinacea herb** (Echinacea purpureae herba, see p. 56); **red wine leaf** (Vitis viniferae folium); **calendula flower** (Calendulae flos, see p. 90); **oak bark** (Quercus cortex, see p. 99).
 – *Action:* See Herbal treatment measures.
 – *Contraindications:* Comfrey root should not be applied to open wounds or damaged skin and should not be allowed to come in contact with the eyes or mucous membranes. See p. 278 for restrictions on use.

- *Dosage and administration*
  - All of the recommended herbal remedies except red wine leaf are applied locally. Ointments are applied to the edges of the ulcer.
- *Compresses soaked in oak bark extract:* Apply fresh compresses for 1 to 2 hours, 3 times daily. A fresh compress is applied as soon as the previous one has become warm and dry. Between treatments, a wet compress should be applied to the wound and loosely wrapped. The compresses should not be covered with airtight material. Commercial products should be used as directed by the manufacturer.
- *Oak bark decoction:* Boil 2 tablespoons of oak bark in 500 mL of water for 15 minutes, then strain. Allow to cool and use the undiluted decoction to prepare wet compresses. The decoction should be prepared fresh each day.
- *Side effects:* For those associated with comfrey root, see p. 278.
- *Clinical value:* If the limitations and contraindications are heeded, these remedies represent cheap and well-tolerated adjunctive treatment measures. Further research on their clinical efficacy should be conducted.

16.1 Fundamentals of Hydrotherapy

Physiological Effects of Medicinal Baths

➤ **Action:** The therapeutic action of medicinal baths is a result of the physiological effects of water temperature (36–38 °C) and water pressure.
  – Warm baths dilate blood vessels in the skin, thus improving the circulation.
  – Full-submersion baths exert considerable pressure on the body. Therapeutic baths should therefore be limited to a duration of 10 to 20 minutes, followed by a resting period of at least 30 minutes.

➤ **Contraindications**
  – Patients with high blood pressure or heart failure should not take full baths unless directed by a physician. Individuals with mild varicose leg veins can take warm baths, but should spray cold water onto the legs at the end of the bath. When making baths for elderly patients, the tub should be filled only three-fourths full. This is compensated for by slightly raising the water temperature.
  – *Contraindications for full baths:* Acute or extensive skin disease, large areas of damaged skin, severe febrile or infectious disease, WHO stage III hypertension (organ damage), NYHA stage III/IV heart failure, and deep vein thrombosis. Partial-submersion baths can be used to treat problems limited to a specific area of the body.

Specific Effects of Herb Baths

➤ **Action and effects of herbal extracts**
  – The effects of herbal bath additives are transmitted by stimulation of receptors on the skin and/or by reflex mechanisms.
  – Essential oils are inhaled with vapors from the bathwater. The oils travel to the respiratory tract and olfactory nerve, thereby exerting direct effects on the limbic system and stimulating the senses (aromatherapy).

➤ **Emulsifying agents**
  – *Pure essential oils* require the addition of an emulsifying agent to improve their dispersion in water. This prevents high local concentrations of the oil and related skin irritation.
  – *Fatty oils* (soybean oil, evening primrose oil) used for supportive treatment of dry skin diseases do not require an emulsifying agent. The oil should form a protective film on the skin surface after leaving the bathtub.

Range of Uses

➤ **Typical indications for herbal baths**
  – Colds and flu
  – To improve the circulation
  – Nervousness and sleep disorders
  – Rheumatic complaints
  – Inflammatory skin diseases

Clinical Considerations

➤ **General considerations:** See Section 5.2, Colds and Flu, p. 150.
  - Herbal baths effectively stimulate the circulation. Since the blood flow to the extremities can be impaired during the early stages of catarrhal disorders, hydrotherapy can play an important role in their treatment. When a cold develops, local nonspecific immune defense mechanisms are weakened, and the blood supply to the mucous membranes of the mouth, nose and throat decreases also, owing to a reflex mechanism.

➤ **Hydrotherapy measures**
  - The deep-heating effect is a key therapeutic element of baths for cold and flu. The warm water dilates the peripheral vessels and, by way of reflex transmission, increases the blood flow to the mucous membranes of the mouth, nose, and throat.
  - Spruce and pine needle oil as well as eucalyptus and thyme oil enhance the peripheral blood flow when absorbed transdermally. The oil particles inhaled in steam from the bathwater take direct action in the respiratory passages, where they effectively decrease nasal congestion, liquefy viscous bronchial secretions, and improve expectoration.

➤ **Clinical value of hydrotherapy**
  - Herbal cold and flu baths are recommended for supportive treatment of acute or chronic catarrhal disorders.

Herbal Remedies and Range of Uses

Aromatic Herbs

➤ **Drugs used: Thyme oil** (Thymi aetheroleum, see p. 120); **eucalyptus oil** (Eucalypti aetheroleum, see p. 61); **pine needle oil** (Pini aetheroleum, see p. 104); **spruce needle oil** (Piceae aetheroleum).
➤ **Action:** Bacteriostatic, bactericidal, virustatic, expectorant, bronchospasmolytic, hyperemic.
➤ **Contraindications:** The above contraindications for full baths apply. Herbal cold and flu baths are not recommended for infants or small children under 3 years of age.
➤ **Administration:** Full baths are administered in the early stages of cold development.
➤ **Clinical value:** The recommended baths are safe and effective adjunctive treatment measures, provided no contraindications apply.
➤ Cf. Section 5.2, Colds and Flu, p. 150 ff.

16.3 Circulatory Disorders

Clinical Considerations

➤ **General considerations**
  - *Constitutional hypotension* is a relatively common disorder associated with a variety of circulatory problems, the most common of which are hypoperfusion of the hands and feet and general vegetative dysregulation. The etiology is unknown.
  - *Nervous heart* without an identifiable organic cause is also common.
➤ **Hydrotherapy measures:** Full baths supplemented with the herbal additives listed below, provided no contraindications apply.
➤ **Clinical value of hydrotherapy:** Herbal baths can be recommended as a supplement to physical therapy measures for constitutional hypotension and nervous heart, especially since standard drug therapies for the disorders do not exist.

Herbal Remedies and Range of Uses

➤ **Drugs used: Balm leaf** (Melissae folium, see p. 84); **lavender flower** (Lavandulae flos, see p. 59); **rosemary leaf** (Rosmarini folium, see p. 112).
➤ **Action:** Balm oil, a calming and relaxing herb, is recommended for nervous heart. Recent data indicate that one of its constituents, rosmarinic acid, may also block thyrotropin (TSH), a thyroid-stimulating hormone. Lavender oil has a generalized relaxing and stabilizing effect on the autonomic nervous system (ANS). Lavender baths are therefore recommended for ANS and menopausal disorders. Rosemary leaf oil stimulates the circulation. Applied topically, its counterirritant and circulation-stimulating effects make it a useful remedy for general lassitude, fatigue, and symptomatic hypotension.
➤ **Contraindications:** See p. 282.
➤ **Administration**
  - *Rosemary bath:* Steep 50 g of rosemary leaves in 1 liter of hot water for 30 minutes, well covered. Strain and add to the bathwater.
  - *Balm bath:* Steep 10 g of balm leaves in 2 liters of hot water for 5 minutes, well covered. Strain and add to the bathwater.
  - *Administration:* Balm and lavender baths should preferably be administered in the evening, whereas rosemary baths should be taken in the morning. A resting period is recommended after all of these herbal baths.
➤ **Clinical value:** The above herbal baths are safe and effective adjunctive treatment measures, provided no contraindications apply.

Clinical Considerations

▶ **General considerations:** See Disorders and Diseases of the Nervous System, p. 209 ff.

▶ **Hydrotherapy measures:** Relaxing warm baths supplemented with lavender, balm or valerian extract are recommended. The drop in body temperature after a warm bath is very conducive to sleep. Hence, the baths are best taken at night.

▶ **Clinical value of hydrotherapy:** Herbal baths are an excellent supplement to general sleep hygiene measures and oral medications.

Herbal Remedies and Range of Uses

▶ **Herbs used: Balm leaf** (Melissae folium, see p. 84); **lavender flower** (Lavandulae flos, see p. 59); **valerian root** (Valerianae radix, see p. 125); **hop flowers** (Lupuli flos, see p. 75).

▶ **Action: Balm oil** and **citronella oil** (Indian balm) are recommended for nervous heart due to their calming and relaxing effects. Recent data indicate that one of the constituents, rosmarinic acid, may also block thyrotropin (TSH), a thyroid-stimulating hormone. Lavender baths are recommended for autonomic nervous system (ANS) disorders, nervous agitation, and menopausal complaints because of the generalized relaxing and stabilizing effects of lavender oil on the ANS. The central depressant and antispasmodic properties of valerian root oil promote relaxation and sleep induction. Hop baths have a relatively mild sedative effect, so a series of baths must be taken before the effects are felt.

▶ **Administration**
  – *Balm bath:* Steep 10 g of balm leaves in 2 liters of hot water for 5 minutes, well covered. Strain and add to the bathwater.
  – See p. 284 for additional instructions.
  – These baths should be taken in the evening.
  ⊙ *Important:* Valerian baths can have rather potent effects on some people, so someone should always be on hand to monitor the bathing patient.

▶ **Clinical value:** The recommended baths are safe and effective adjunctive treatment measures, provided no contraindications apply.

16.5 Rheumatic Pain

Clinical Considerations

➤ **General considerations**
- The term "rheumatism" is often used to refer to all degenerative or chronic diseases associated with joint or soft-tissue inflammation.
- Degenerative types of rheumatism (usually nonactivated arthrosis) are typically associated with pain after exercise due to irritating and inflamed lesions in the synovial membrane resulting from erosion of cartilage particles. When the pain is more severe, the surrounding muscles tighten, leading to postural compensation and additional erosion.
- In inflammatory rheumatism, the pain is not associated with exercise but occurs mainly at night. The joints are red, tender, and swollen.

➤ **Hydrotherapy measures**
- Herbal baths are used for deep heat therapy. They warm the joints, enhance synovial secretion, produce vasodilatation, facilitate the elimination of metabolites responsible for pain production, and relax the muscles. A bathwater temperature of over 36 °C is recommended for patients with rheumatoid diseases.

➤ **Drugs used: Eucalyptus leaf** (cineole); **menthol**; **juniper oil** (alpha- and betapinenes); **rosemary leaf** (camphor, cineole); and **pine needles** (essential oils and tannins).

➤ **Clinical value of hydrotherapy:** Heat therapy measures such as herbal baths, Kneipp hydrotherapy, and grass flower pillow application can reduce the pain of nonactivated arthrosis.

Herbal Remedies and Range of Uses

➤ **Drugs used: Spruce needle oil** (Pini aetheroleum); **rosemary leaf** (Rosmarini folium, see p. 112); **grass flowers** (Graminis flos); **eucalyptus oil** (Eucalypti aetheroleum, see p. 61); **juniper berry** (Juniperi fructus, see p. 80).

➤ **Action:** These herbal bath additives have a general vasodilative effect due to the essential oils. Grass flowers have high concentrations of essential oils and coumarins that increase the blood flow locally and in the internal organs.

➤ **Contraindications**
- *Spruce needle oil:* Hypersensitivity to turpentine, extensive skin damage, acute skin injuries of unknown origin, febrile and infectious diseases.
- *Eucalyptus oil:* Extensive skin damage, acute skin injuries of unknown origin, and febrile and infectious diseases.
- ◉ *Note:* Warming baths are recommended only for non-inflammatory processes. The general contraindications for herbal baths (see p. 282) should be heeded.

➤ **Administration**
- *Grass flower pillow:* Heat to 42 °C and apply to the affected area for 40 minutes (see Standard Treatments, p. 308).
- *Grass flower bath:* Add 500 g grass flowers to 4 to 5 liters of water and bring to a boil. Strain and add to the bathwater.
- *Rosemary bath:* Steep 50 g of rosemary leaves in 1 liter of hot water for 30 minutes, well covered. Strain and add to the bathwater. The patient should bathe for 15 to 20 minutes, 2 to 3 times a week.
- Juniper oil: Refer to commercially available products.

➤ **Side effects:** Spruce needle oil can cause cutaneous hypersensitivity reactions in rare cases. Soaps should not be used with spruce needle oil as they diminish its therapeutic effects.

➤ **Clinical value:** These herbal remedies are useful supplements to other pain-relieving measures, especially because of their relaxing effect.

16.6 Inflammatory Skin Diseases

Clinical Considerations

➤ **General considerations:** See Eczema, p. 265 ff.
➤ **Hydrotherapy measures**
  – Tannin-containing astringents such as oak bark and oatstraw extract are useful remedies for itching and weeping eczema.
  – Chamomile oil or extract, yarrow extract, or horsetail extract are used to prepare herbal baths for inflammatory skin problems.
  – Peppermint oil, lavender oil, and thyme oil are useful bath additives when itching is a problem.
  – Oil baths for dry skin should be rich in moisturizers and contain no emulsifying agents.
➤ **Clinical value of hydrotherapy:** Herbal baths can be recommended for supportive treatment of skin diseases, such as eczema, inflammatory skin lesions, and pruritus.

Herbal Remedies and Range of Uses

➤ **Drugs used: Oak bark** (Quercus cortex, see p. 99); **horsetail** (Equiseti herba, see p. 78); **yarrow** (Millefolii herba, see p. 131); **thyme** (Thymi herba, see p. 47); **chamomile flowers** (Matricariae flos, see p. 102); **oatstraw** (Avenae stramentum); **wheat bran**; **peppermint leaves** (Menthae piperitae folium, see p. 102).
➤ **Action**
  – *Tannin-containing astringents:* Oak bark contains anti-inflammatory flavonols. Oatstraw extract contains silicic acid and steroid saponins presumed to be responsible for the drug's therapeutic action.
  – *Chamomile oil and extract:* The volatile oil has anti-inflammatory and wound-healing properties. α-Bisabolol inhibits bacterial and fungal growth.
  – *Yarrow:* The volatile oil kills bacteria and reduces inflammation.
  – *Horsetail* contains flavonoids and more than 10% mineral compounds, especially silicic acid.
  – *Menthol* stimulates cold receptors, resulting in local anesthesia and cooling.
  – *Thyme oil* has antiseptic properties.
  – *Wheat bran* reduces itching and inflammation.
➤ **Contraindications**
  – *Yarrow:* Hypersensitivity to composite plants.
  – *Oak bark:* Extensive skin damage.
➤ **Administration**
  – *Full- and partial-submersion baths:* 1 to 2 times a week, in accordance with the type and severity of the complaints.
  – *Oak bark bath:* Add 5 g of the drug to 1 liter of water, bring to a boil and steep for 15 to 20 minutes. Strain and add to the bathwater (full bath).
  – *Yarrow bath:* Add 100 g drug to 20 liters of bathwater.
  – *Thyme bath:* Add 1 g drug to 1 liter of bathwater.
  – *Chamomile bath:* Add 50 g drug to 10 liters of bathwater.
  – *Horsetail bath:* For each 10 liters of bathwater 100 g herb. are needed. First boil the drug for 5 to 10 minutes in a smaller quantity of water, then steep for another 15 minutes. Strain and add to the bathwater (final dilution: 100 g/10 liters).

- *Oatstraw bath:* Pour 4 liters of boiling water onto 100 g of the drug and allow to cool to room temperature. Strain and add to the bathwater.

▶ **Clinical value:** The recommended baths are safe and effective adjunctive treatment measures, provided no contraindications apply.

17.1 Arnica Wrap for Heart Ailments

General Considerations

➤ See **Arnica** (*Arnica montana* L.), p. 35.
➤ **Indications**
  - Angina (angina pectoris).
  - To reduce the strain on the heart in febrile elderly patients.
➤ **Contraindications:** Allergy to arnica.
➤ **Action**
  - The effects of the drugs are transmitted by nerves and reflexes across Head's zones, resulting in an increased blood supply and reduction of the cardiac load.
  - Clinical practice has shown that arnica compresses are effective in relieving anginal symptoms. Patients report a sensation of heat spreading from the inside out, and an increased perception of the feet. The aromatherapy effect also plays an important role.
➤ **Materials**
  - 1 cup of water, heated to body temperature
  - 1 tablespoon of 70 % arnica tincture (arnica blossoms and ethanol 70 % v/v 1 : 10)
  - Bowl and tablespoon
  - Compress (folded cotton cloth, ca. 15 × 20 cm)
  - Flannel or wool sheet somewhat larger than the compress

Procedure

➤ **Preparation:** Fill the bowl with 1 cup (150 mL) of water heated to body temperature (ca. 35 °C). Add 1 tablespoon of 70 % arnica tincture (final concentration of the wrap should be 7 % tincture). Dip the compress in the bowl until thoroughly soaked with arnica water.
➤ **Application**
  - Place bowl with soaked compress by the patient's bedside.
  - Allow the patient to inhale the vapors from the arnica water. Squeeze excess water out of the compress and place on chest over the heart region. Wrap flannel or wool sheet around chest. Dress the patient in a nightshirt or pajamas. Loosely cover the shoulders and arms with a blanket.
  - ◉ *Warning:* Do not use a hot water bottle!
➤ Duration of treatment: 15 to 30 minutes.
➤ **Tips**
  - Lower doses or ointment-type compresses are recommended for patients with circulatory instability.
  - Lower concentrations of arnica solution should be used in patients with sensitive skin by using more water.
  - Acute anginal pain may require repeated treatment. The compresses do not alter the regulation of body temperature.
  - Comment: In angina, the arnica wrap is a purely adjunctive measure. Adequate diagnosis and treatment should not be missed.

General Considerations

➤ See **Rosemary** (*Rosmarinus officinalis* L.), p. 112.
➤ **Indications**
  – Hypotension
  – Venous insufficiency
  – Chronic debility and convalescence
  – For patients with perceptual disorders and basal stimulation
➤ **Contraindications:** Allergy to rosemary, pregnancy.
➤ **Action:** Invigorating. Conveys a sense of bodily boundaries to patients with perceptual disorders.

Procedure

➤ **Preparation**
  – *Method 1*
    • Pour warm water (28 – 32 °C) into a washbowl.
    • Mix 5 drops of rosemary essential oil with $^1/_2$ cup of milk and add to water.
  – *Method 2*
    • Steep 3 tablespoons of dried rosemary leaf in 1 liter of water for 15 minutes, allow to cool to 28–32 °C, then pour into the washbowl.
➤ **Application:** The treatment is performed like a standard whole-body wash. Start with the upper body, applying the rosemary water against the direction of hair growth. It is helpful to place the hands and feet of the patient directly into the washbowl. The patient is also dried by rubbing a towel counter to the direction of hair growth.
➤ **Frequency of treatment:** 1 to 2 times daily, as needed.

18.1 Flaxseed Poultice for Sinusitis

General Considerations

- ➤ See **Flaxseed** (*Linum usitatissimum* L.), p. 66.
- ➤ **Indications:** Sinusitis, i. e., inflammation of nasal and/or frontal sinuses.
- ➤ **Contraindications:** Circulatory instability, coagulopathy.
- ➤ **Action:** Reduces mucosal inflammation, relieves pain, and improves the discharge of pus and mucus.
- ➤ **Materials**
  - 300 g flaxseed (whole)
  - Saucepan, spoon, and water
  - 6 to 8 small linen cloths, wool cloth, 2 hot water bottles

Procedure

- ➤ **Preparation:** Place flaxseed in pot of water (ratio of 1 : 2, i. e., 300 g linseed in 600 mL water). Bring to a boil and allow to simmer until the mixture reaches the proper consistency for gruel. Add more water if too thick, or add more linseed if too thin. Wrap 1 to 2 tablespoons of the gruel in a linen cloth and place between 2 hot water bottles filled with hot water (Fig. **4**). Repeat to make a total of 6 to 8 poultices.
- ➤ **Application:** Apply the poultices to the regions of the nasal and frontal sinuses, as hot as the patient can stand them (Fig. **4**). Cover with a small towel or wool cloth. Apply a fresh poultice every 4 to 5 minutes or so, since they are effective only when hot.
- ➤ **Duration of treatment:** 20 to 30 minutes.
- ➤ Frequency of treatment: 1 to 3 times daily.
- ◉ *Note:* Chamomile steam baths (p. 48), horseradish poultices (p. 293), and mustard footbaths (p. 312) are also helpful for sinusitis.

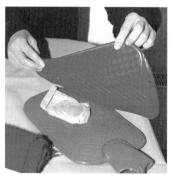
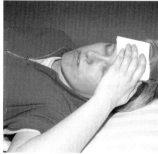

Fig. 4 Linseed poultices. **a** Preparation. **b** Application. Reproduced with permission from A. Sonn, *Wickel und Auflagen*, Thieme, Stuttgart, 1998.

General Considerations

➤ **Horseradish root** (Armoraciae radix).
➤ **Indications**
  – Sinusitis, i. e., inflammation of the nasal and/or frontal sinuses
  – Headaches
➤ **Contraindications:** Allergy to horseradish; broken skin or inflammation in the affected area.
➤ **Action:** Increases the blood flow and dissolves mucus.
➤ **Materials**
  – 2 tablespoons grated horseradish root, either freshly prepared or commercially processed without chemical additives, at room temperature
  – Compress (gauze or small linen cloth), washcloth
  – Olive oil

Procedure

➤ **Preparation:** Spread a 1–2 cm thick layer of grated horseradish onto compress and fold over the edges securely.
➤ **Application:** Apply the horseradish poultice to the upper neck region and cover with the washcloth.
➤ **Duration of treatment:** 2 to 5 minutes, or as long as tolerated by the patient. The duration can be extended to a maximum of 10 to 12 minutes in later treatments.
➤ **Aftercare**
  – The poultice will usually cause the skin to redden. After removing it, do not wash the skin with water, but wipe sparingly with olive oil. This preserves the heat and moisturizes the skin.
  – Instruct the patient to keep the feet warm (wool socks, blanket, etc.).
➤ **Frequency of treatment:** 1 to 2 times daily. Inspect the skin before the next poultice application. If redness or irritation from the previous application is still detected, treatment should be interrupted for a day. Long-term treatment is recommended in chronic disease.
◉ *Warning:* Horseradish poultices can cause skin burns if left on for too long. Check the skin for redness or irritation during poultice application. Observe the patient's reaction and remove the poultices if they cause undue burning or discomfort. Stay with the patient during first-time treatment. Carefully monitor individuals with sensitive skin, elderly individuals, and patients who are not mentally alert.
  ◉ *Note:* Horseradish poultices are also helpful in patients with cystitis (especially when chronic), indwelling catheters, and irritable bladder. In the latter case, the poultice is applied to the bladder region.

18.3 Thyme Oil Compress

General Considerations

➤ See **Thyme** (*Thymus vulgaris* L.), p. 120.

◉ *Note:* Commercial high-quality thyme oil should be used for this indication. Linalool/geraniol type thyme oil is recommended for use in children, though it might prove difficult to obtain, and the thujanol type is recommended for adults.

➤ **Indications**
  – Colds, bronchitis
  – Asthma, whooping cough
  – To dissolve viscous mucus in ventilated patients
  – To promote secretolysis after extubation
  – Chronic obstructive respiratory tract disease

➤ **Contraindications:** Allergy to thyme, pregnancy, epilepsy, aversion to the smell of thyme.

➤ **Action**
  – Antispasmodic, antiseptic, expectorant, secretomotor.
  – Clinical practice has shown that thyme oil relieves cough, dissolves viscous mucus, boosts the immune system of patients with infectious diseases, and is a potent disinfectant. It is especially effective in fighting staphylococcal infections.

➤ **Materials**
  – 1 tablespoon 10 % thyme oil*
  – Compress (gauze or linen cloth), 20 × 30 cm
  – Small plastic bag
  – Hot water bottle
  – Washcloth, wool cloth
  – Flannel sheet

Procedure

➤ **Preparation:** Open the plastic bag, place the gauze or linen compress inside and add 1 tablespoon of the 10 % thyme oil. Close the bag and squeeze compress until saturated with oil but not dripping. Fill the hot water bottle with water (60–70 °C). Place the plastic bag with compress as well as the washcloth and wool cloth onto the hot water bottle to warm.

➤ **Application:** Check the feet. If cold, warm by placing a hot water bottle directly underneath them or over the stomach. Keep the shoulders warm. After taking it out of the plastic bag, place the heated compress over the upper sternal region and cover with heated washcloth or wool cloth. Dress the patient in a nightshirt or pajama top. Wrap flannel sheet around the chest if desired. Wakeful patients should be instructed to place one hand over the compress for enhanced perception of its mild warming effect. If the patient is unable to respond to instructions, the therapist should lay the patient's hand over the compress.

◉ *Note:* Heat is relaxing.

---

* A bulk quantity of 10 % thyme oil can be made by mixing 45 mL of sunflower oil with 5 mL of 100 % thyme oil. This is filled into a dark bottle and labeled with name and date (shelf life 3 months). A single dose is prepared by mixing 1 tablespoon of cold-pressed sunflower or olive oil with 5 drops of 100 % thyme oil.

➤ **Duration of treatment:** 30 minutes. The compress can be left on longer, even overnight if the patient falls asleep during an evening treatment.
➤ **Aftercare:** Return the compress to the plastic bag, close securely, and save for next treatment (repeat above procedure). Each compress can be used for up to 1 week before discarding.

18.4 Thyme Chest Wrap

General Considerations

➤ See **Thyme** (*Thymus vulgaris* L.), p. 120.
➤ Indications
   – Coughing (bronchitis, convulsive cough, whooping cough)
   – Asthma
   – **Contraindications:** Allergy to thyme, circulatory instability
   – **Action**
      • Antispasmodic, anti-inflammatory, immunostimulant, antibacterial.
      • Clinical practice has shown that thyme chest wraps are very effective in alleviating severe dry cough. Wet heat is relaxing and promotes sleep.
➤ **Materials**
   – 1 tablespoon thyme leaf, $1/2$ liter boiling water
   – Measuring cup, tea strainer, saucepan
   – Compress (e. g., diaper cloth) with or without cover cloth
   – Dishcloth
   – Terrycloth towel
   – Flannel sheet (wrap)
   – Hot water bottle

Procedure

➤ **Preparation**
   – *Patient:* If the patient's feet are cold, place a hot water bottle (ca. 60 °C) underneath them. Measure peak flow value and respiration rate if indicated. Spread the flannel sheet onto the bed.
   – *Wrap:* Take $1/2$ liter of boiling water (measuring cup) and add 1 tablespoon of thyme leaf. Steep for 5 minutes, then strain into a saucepan and keep warm. Wrap the compress in the dishcloth, dip into the hot thyme infusion until fully soaked, then wring out excess liquid.
➤ **Application:** Have the patient sit up in bed. Take the hot compress out of the dishcloth and check for heat tolerance by touching the compress to the underside of forearm. Place the compress, as hot as the patient feels comfortable with, over the patient's chest, either directly or wrapped in a cover cloth. Cover the compress with the towel and wrap the chest in the flannel sheet.
   ◉ *Note:* The wrap should be applied neatly and securely. Speed is required to finish before the compress cools. When completed, place a half-filled hot water bottle over the chest.
➤ **Duration of treatment:** 20 to 30 minutes, i. e., until the wrap has cooled.
➤ **Aftercare:** Treatment should be followed by a 30-minute resting period. Peak flow and respiration rate values should be measured if necessary.

➤ For more information on mustard, see **White mustard** (*Sinapis alba* L.), p. 127.

➤ **Indications**
  – Acute pneumonia, pleuritis
  – Bronchitis, asthma
  – For prevention of pneumonia
  – To improve breathing difficulties
  – ◉ *Warning:* It is imperative to watch for signs of respiratory distress and the need for intubation.
  – **Contraindications:** Allergy to mustard, broken skin on affected area.

➤ **Action**
  – Activates the local metabolism and relieves inflammation in the respiratory passages. Helps the patient breathe more deeply, thereby saturating the blood with more oxygen. In febrile conditions, the wrap helps to eliminate excess body heat.
  – Clinical practice has shown that mustard wraps induce productive cough within 30 to 60 minutes after application. Deep and restful sleep occurs 4 to 6 hours after treatment.

➤ **Materials** (Fig. **5**)
  – 4 tablespoons powdered black mustard seed (Sinapis nigrae semen)
  – Absorbent cloth (e. g., diaper cloth or dishcloth)
  – Multi-ply paper toweling (3 sheets) and adhesive tape
  – Small bowl of lukewarm water (ca. 35–40 °C)
  – Small towel, flannel sheet (wrap) (see p. 296)
  – Olive oil
  – Timer (optional)

Procedure

➤ **Patient preparation:** Same as for thyme chest wrap (see p. 296). Document oxygen saturation and respiration rate if the patients is on a ventilator.

➤ **Wrap preparation:** Lay the diaper cloth on the countertop and place a paper towel on top. Spread 4 tablespoons of mustard powder onto the center of the paper towel to form a small square. Fold over the edges of the paper towel, then of the diaper cloth, to produce a closed packet. Secure with adhesive tape. Roll the finished poultice and soak in a small bowl of warm water (ca. 35–40 °C) for 2 to 3 minutes.

➤ **Application**
  – Have the patient sit up in bed. Remove the poultice from the bowl and squeeze out excess water. Apply to the lower chest region and cover with a towel. Have the patient lie down on the flannel sheet and wrap the sheet snugly around the patient.
  – Stay with the patient during treatment and encourage the patient to breathe deeply. Set the timer for 2 minutes.

➤ **Duration of treatment**
  – 1st wrap: 2 to 3 minutes.
  – 2nd wrap: 3 to 4 minutes.
  – The duration of treatment for all subsequent wraps can be increased by 2 to 3 minutes. Check the skin after 2 minutes of treatment. Remove the wrap if slight reddening occurs. If the skin does not react, the wrap can be left on 1 to 2 minutes longer.

18.5 Mustard Wrap

- ◉ *Note:* The patient response and skin reaction determine how long the wrap should be left on. The maximum application time for mustard wraps is 12 minutes.
- ◉ *Warning:* Mustard wraps can cause severe skin reddening and blistering (skin burns) if left on too long. Never leave the patient unattended once the mustard wrap has been applied.

▶ **Aftercare:** Remove the wrap and use a towel to remove any traces of mustard powder. Apply olive oil to the application site. Then re-wrap the patient in flannel cloth and have the patient rest for 30 minutes. Measure and record peak flow value or, in ventilated patients, oxygen saturation and pulse rate.

▶ **Frequency of treatment**
- *Once daily.* For proper adaptation to the physiological regulation of body temperature, mustard wraps are best applied in the afternoon.
- Mustard wraps can be used for a therapeutic course of treatment. We generally recommend 5 days of treatment followed by a 2-day break. Treatment should be interrupted for a day if signs of redness are observed at the application site on the day after treatment.
- Mustard wraps also help to reduce fever.

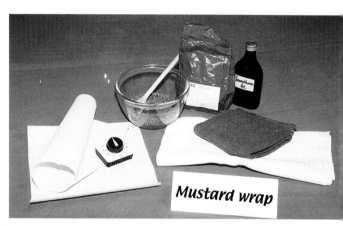

Fig. 5 Materials required for a mustard wrap. Reproduced with permission from A. Sonn, *Wickel und Auflagen*, Thieme, Stuttgart, 1998.

General Considerations

➤ See Section 6.3, Reflux, Gastritis, Gastroduodenal Ulcers, Dyspepsia, p. 170 ff.

➤ **Indications:** Gastroenteritis, gastroduodenitis (with or without vomiting), Crohn's disease and colitis, flatulence and tenesmus, irritable bowel syndrome, constipation, scar pain after major stomach surgery, stress and nervousness, menstrual cramps, stomach ache in children.

➤ **Contraindications:** Acute abdominal pain of unclear origin, febrile gastritis, appendicitis, severe heart failure, coagulopathies, thrombocytopenia, circulatory instability, tetraplegia and other forms of paralysis, acute renal or biliary colic with fever.

➤ **Action**
   – Depending on the clinical picture, stomach wraps are used to reduce gastrointestinal spasms and peristalsis. The effects of the wrap are transmitted across the solar plexus and throughout the body.
   – Clinical practice has shown that hot stomach compresses are relaxing, calming, analgesic, and antispasmodic. Moreover, they significantly boost the well-being of the patient.

➤ **Materials**
   – Small bowl with ca. 400 mL of hot water (80 °C)
   – 2 compresses (diaper cloth), 1 dishtowel, 1 small towel, 1 flannel sheet (wrap)
   – 2 hot water bottles

Procedure

➤ **Preparation:** Fill the bowl with hot water. Fold the compress to an appropriate width and place inside the dishcloth. Dip both in the bowl of water until fully saturated. Hold the ends of the dishcloth and wring out excess water.
   ◉ *Note:* The drier the compress, the better, as far as heat tolerance is concerned.

➤ **Application:** Remove the compress from the dishcloth and test for heat tolerance by lightly touching a few times on the stomach. Apply while as hot as the skin can stand without burning. Cover with a towel to prevent leakage and wrap securely in a flannel sheet. Place a warm water bottle on the right and another on the left side of the stomach to preserve the heat.

➤ **Duration of treatment:** 20 to 30 minutes, or until the wrap becomes too cool.

➤ **Aftercare**
   – Remove the wrap after 20 to 30 minutes; dry off the patient with a towel. Again wrap in the flannel sheet and apply hot water bottles.
   – Allow the patient to rest for 30 to 60 minutes.
   – Record treatment (patient's opinion of effects).
   ◉ *Note:* Slight redness of the skin after wrap removal is normal. Prevent skin burns by checking for heat tolerance before wrap application.

19.2 Hot Chamomile Wrap

➤ See **Chamomile** (*Chamomilla recutita* L. Rauschert), p. 47.
➤ **Indications:** Abdominal or intestinal cramps, flatulence, constipation, stomach tension, menstrual cramps, painful uterine involution and postpartum pain, scar pain after stomach surgery, sleep disorders, nervous disorders, stress, cold feet.
➤ **Contraindication:** Allergy to chamomile, circulatory instability, acute abdominal pain of unknown origin.
➤ **Action**
  – Antispasmodic, relaxing, warming, analgesic.
  – Clinical practice has shown that the hot wet compresses ease inner tension. Some patients even fall asleep during the treatment.
➤ **Materials**
  – 1 tablespoon dried chamomile flower, $1/2$ liter boiling water
  – Measuring cup, tea strainer, saucepan
  – 1 compress (diaper cloth or round pad), 1 kitchen towel, 1 small towel, 1 flannel sheet
  – 1 hot water bottle

Procedure

➤ **Preparation:** Place 1 tablespoon chamomile flower in the measuring cup and add $1/2$ liter of boiling water. Steep for 5 minutes, then strain into saucepan and keep warm. Wrap compress in dishcloth, dip into hot chamomile infusion until fully soaked, then wring out excess liquid.
➤ **Application:** Have the patient sit up in bed. Take the hot compress out of the dishcloth and check for heat tolerance by touching the compress to the underside of patient's forearm. Place the compress, as hot as the patient feels comfortable with, over the patient's stomach, either directly or wrapped in cover cloth. Cover the compress with the towel and wrap the abdominal region in flannel sheet. Speed is required to finish before the compress cools. The wrap should fit snugly. When completed, place a half-filled hot water bottle over the stomach.
➤ **Duration of treatment:** 20 to 30 minutes, i. e., until the wrap has cooled.
➤ **Aftercare:** Treatment should be followed by a 30-minute resting period.

General Considerations

➤ See **Fennel** (*Foeniculum vulgare*), p. 65.
➤ **Indications:** Digestive problems, flatulence, cramps, hiccups, nausea and vomiting.
➤ **Contraindications:** Allergy to fennel, epilepsy, aversion to smell of fennel.
➤ **Action**
  – Warming, antispasmodic, induces menstruation (emmenagogue), promotes the flow of milk in nursing mothers (galactagogue).
  – Clinical experience has shown that these compresses are very effective in relieving cramps and stomach trouble, even after stomach surgery.
➤ **Materials**
  – 1 tablespoon 10% fennel oil *or*
    1 tablespoon olive oil + 5 drops 100% fennel oil
  – Compress (linen cloth, 20 × 30 cm, or gauze compress, 20 × 30 cm)
  – Small plastic bag, hot water bottle
  – Wash cloth, wool cloth, flannel sheet.

Procedure

➤ **Preparation:** Open the plastic bag, place the gauze or linen compress inside and add oil. Close the bag and squeeze the compress until saturated with oil but not dripping. Fill the hot water bottle with hot water (60 °C). Place the plastic bag with compress as well as washcloth and wool cloth onto the hot water bottle to warm.
➤ **Application:** Remove the heated compress from the bag and check for heat tolerance by touching onto the forearm. Place over the stomach in the region where the pain is worst. Cover with the heated washcloth and wrap the patient in the flannel sheet. Place a half-filled hot water bottle onto the stomach, additionally onto the feet if cold.
➤ **Duration of treatment:** Leave the compress on for 30 minutes, then remove it. The compress can be left on longer, even overnight if the patient falls asleep during an evening treatment.
➤ **Aftercare:** Return the compress to the plastic bag, close the bag securely, and save for the next treatment (repeat the above procedure). Each compress can be used for up to 1 week before discarding.

19.4 Hot Yarrow Wrap

General Considerations

➤ See **Yarrow** (*Achillea millefolium*), p. 131.
➤ **Indications:** Liver diseases, metabolic disorders, to stimulate liver activity, to promote digestion after heavy meals, constipation, depression, atopic dermatitis.
➤ **Contraindications:** Allergy to yarrow, circulatory instability.
➤ **Action**
   – Antispasmodic, relaxing, promotes digestion, stimulates liver metabolism and regeneration.
   – Clinical experience has shown that hot yarrow wraps alleviate the pain and tension of disorders associated with increased epigastric pressure (e. g., liver metastases).
➤ **Materials**
   – 3 to 4 tablespoons yarrow herb, $1/2$ liter boiling water.
   – See Hot Chamomile Wrap, p. 300.

Procedure

➤ **Preparation:** Place 1 tablespoon yarrow herb in measuring cup and add $1/2$ liter of boiling water. Steep for 5 minutes, then strain into saucepan and keep warm. Wrap compress in dishcloth, dip into hot yarrow infusion until fully soaked, then wring out excess liquid.
➤ **Application:** See Hot Chamomile Wrap, p. 300.
➤ **Duration of treatment:** 20 to 30 minutes, i. e., until the wrap has cooled.
➤ **Aftercare:** Treatment should be followed by a 30-minute resting period.

General Considerations

➤ See **Eucalyptus Oil** (*Eucalyptus globulus* L. B.), p. 61
➤ See Chapter 7, Diseases of the Urogenital Tract, p. 200 ff.
➤ **Indications:** Cystitis, retention of urine.
➤ **Contraindications:** Allergy to eucalyptus, aversion to smell of eucalyptus.
➤ **Action**
  – Antiseptic and antispasmodic.
  – Clinical experience has shown that eucalyptus oil compresses are effective in treating retention of urine and cystitis. Around 70 % of patients are able to pass urine spontaneously up to 2 hours after treatment. The compresses also achieve good effects in patients with urinary retention following coronary angiography. Many patients with cystitis reported that the pain on urination disappeared after 2 to 3 days of treatment. Urine cultures have shown that oil compresses alone are not sufficient, but are an excellent adjunct to pharmaceutical treatment.
➤ **Materials**
  – 1 tablespoon 10 % eucalyptus oil (pharmaceutical quality) *or* 1 tablespoon sunflower or olive oil + 5 drops of 100 % eucalyptus oil
  – 1 compress (folded linen or gauze material, 20 × 30 cm)
  – Small plastic bag, hot water bottle
  – Washcloth, wool cloth, flannel sheet

Procedure

➤ **Preparation:** Open the plastic bag, place the gauze or linen compress inside, and add eucalyptus oil. Close the bag and squeeze the compress until saturated with oil but not dripping. Fill the hot water bottle with water (60 – 70 °C). Place the plastic bag with the compress as well as the washcloth and the wool cloth onto the hot water bottle to warm.
➤ **Application:** Apply the heated compress to the stomach region and cover with the heated washcloth or wool cloth. Dress the patient in underpants and nightshirt or pajamas to cover. Place the half-filled hot water bottle over the lower stomach region.
➤ **Duration of treatment:** 30 minutes, or until the wrap becomes too cool. If the feet are cold, have the patient put on wool socks and/or place a second hot water bottle under the feet.
➤ **Frequency of treatment:** Twice daily.
➤ **Aftercare:** Treatment should be followed by a 30-minute resting period.
  ◉ *Note:* Instruct the patient to drink plenty of fluids, especially a suitable herbal bladder tea.

20.2 Horseradish Poultice

General Considerations

➤ **Horseradish root** (Armoraciae radix)
➤ See Section 7.1, Urinary Tract Infection, p. 200 ff.
➤ **Indications:** Cystitis.
➤ **Contraindications:** Allergy to horseradish, broken skin, eczema.
➤ **Action:** Increases cutaneous blood flow, induces a reflex increase in blood flow to the bladder, stimulates the metabolism and promotes the healing of inflammatory processes.
➤ **Materials**
  – 4 tablespoons grated horseradish root, either freshly prepared or commercially processed without chemical additives, at room temperature
  – Compress (gauze or linen material) and adhesive tape
  – Olive oil
  – Towel, flannel sheet, hot water bottle (as needed)

Procedure

➤ **Preparation:** Spread a 1–2 cm thick layer of grated horseradish onto compress, fold over edges and secure with tape.
➤ **Application:** Allow the patient to void before starting treatment. Apply the horseradish poultice to the stomach in such a way that there is only one layer of cloth between the compress and the skin. Place the towel over the compress and wrap the stomach region in the flannel sheet. If the patient's feet are cold, place a hot water bottle under them.
➤ **Duration of treatment:** No more than 4 to 5 minutes, while checking for skin irritation.
➤ **Aftercare:** Wipe the skin with olive oil and allow the patient to rest for 30 minutes.
➤ **Frequency of treatment:** Check the skin for irritation on the second day of treatment before reapplication. Take a day's break in treatment if there are signs of reddening or irritation.

➤ See Chapter 8, Disorders and Diseases of the Nervous System, p. 209 ff.

➤ **Indications:** Stress, exhaustion, and fatigue, reactive depression (e. g., after cancer diagnosis).

➤ **Contraindications:** Allergy to plants used for treatment; pregnancy. The treatment can increase the effects of alcohol. The patient should abstain from alcohol around treatment.

➤ **Action**
  – Mood-enhancing, relaxing, promotes feeling of well-being.
  – Actions according to essential oil used
    • *Benzoin:* Balancing, calming, helpful in stress and depression.
    • *Jasmine:* Lifts the spirits, e. g., in depression and anxiety.
    • *Clary sage:* Enhances the mood, stabilizes the emotional state, has stimulating effects in fatigue and low-energy anxiety.

➤ **Materials**
  – 2 tablespoons sea salt
  – 5 to 10 drops 100 % clary sage
  – 5 to 10 drops 100 % benzoin
  – 1 to 3 drops 100 % jasmine oil
  – ca. 300 mL boiling water
  – Compress (several thicknesses of diaper cloth), dish towel, towel, flannel sheet
  – Hot water bottle

Procedure

➤ **Preparation:** Put the sea salt in a bowl and add boiling water. Stir for a few minutes until the salt is completely dissolved. Add the essential oils to the hot salt water. Dip the compress into the salt water and oil solution, then wrap in the dish towel and wring out.

➤ **Application:** Spread the flannel sheet on the bed and have the patient lie down on it. Check the compress for heat tolerance by touching it lightly on the underside of the forearm. Place the compress over the upper abdominal region (solar plexus) and cover with the towel. Wrap the stomach region in the flannel sheet. If the feet are cold, place the hot water bottle under the feet or over the stomach.

➤ **Duration of treatment:** 20 to 30 minutes, or until the wrap has become too cool.

➤ **Aftercare:** Remove the compress after 30 minutes and re-wrap patient in the flannel sheet. Allow the patient to rest for 30 minutes.

◉ *Note:* Because of its mood-enhancing effect, this treatment should be performed in the morning. In crisis situations, it can also be performed at other times of the day or at nighttime.

21.2 Lavender Oil Chest Compress

General Considerations

➤ See **Lavender** (*Lavandula angustifolia* Mill.), see p. 59
➤ See Chapter 8, Disorders and Diseases of the Nervous System, p. 209 ff.
➤ **Indications:** Nervousness, anxiety, difficulty in falling asleep or sleeping though the night, coughing, bronchitis.
➤ **Contraindications:** Allergy to lavender, aversion to the smell of lavender.
➤ **Action**
   – Calming, balancing, antispasmodic, secretolytic, expectorant, antiseptic, inhibits growth of *E. coli*, *Candida albicans*, and *Staphylococcus aureus* in vitro.
   – Clinical experience has shown that lavender oil chest compresses are very effective calming treatments for stressed patients. It improves the patient's ability to fall asleep or sleep through the night, provided the patient is not a habitual sleeping aid user. The compresses give family members a chance to get involved in treatment, especially in long-stay, seriously ill, or dying patients. The family members should be encouraged to apply the compress, placing one hand on the compress and caressing the patient with the other. These compresses are also a good choice for children with problems in falling asleep.
➤ **Materials**
   – 1 tablespoon 10 % lavender oil *or*
     1 tablespoon cold-pressed sunflower or olive oil + 5 drops 100 % lavender oil.
   – Compress (linen cloth, 20 × 30 cm, or gauze compress, 20 × 30 cm)
   – Small plastic bag, hot water bottle
   – Wash cloth, wool cloth, flannel sheet

Procedure

➤ **Preparation:** Open the plastic bag, place the gauze or linen compress inside, and add the oil. Close the bag and squeeze the compress until saturated with oil but not dripping. Fill the hot water bottle with hot water (60 °C). Place the plastic bag with the compress as well as the washcloth and the wool cloth onto the hot water bottle to warm.
➤ **Application:** Check the feet. If cold, warm by placing a hot water bottle directly underneath them or over the stomach. Keep the shoulders warm. Place the heated compress over the upper sternal region and cover with the heated washcloth or wool cloth. Dress the patient in a nightshirt or pajama top. Wrap the flannel sheet around the chest if desired. Wakeful patients should be instructed to place one hand over the compress for enhanced perception of its mild warming effect. If the patient is unable to respond to instructions, the therapist should lay the patient's hand over the compress.
➤ **Duration of treatment:** Leave the compress on for 30 minutes, then remove it. The compress can be left on longer, even overnight if the patient falls asleep during an evening treatment.
➤ **Aftercare:** Return the compress to the plastic bag, close securely, and save for next treatment (repeat the above procedure). Each compress can be used for up to 1 week before discarding.

General Considerations

➤ See **Lavender** (*Lavandula angustifolia* Mill.), p. 59.
➤ **Indications:** Restless anxiety, pain-related restlessness, difficulty in falling asleep, stress, anxiety related to the diagnosis of cancer or a scheduled surgery, hypertension, hyperthyroidism, postinfarction debility, terminal illness.
➤ **Contraindications:** Severe depression, akinesia.
➤ **Materials**
  - 5 drops of lavender oil in $1/2$ cup of milk *or*
    1 liter lavender infusion (3 tbsp. lavender flower in 1 liter boiling water for 5 minutes)
  - 3 to 4 liters of warm water
  - Washpan, soft sponge, washcloth, towel

Procedure

➤ **Preparation:** Mix lavender oil and milk, then add to wash water heated to 40 °C. As the water cools during the washing procedure, the evaporation on the patient's skin still induces a pleasant feeling of warmness.
➤ **Application:** See p. 32

22.1 Grass Flower Pillow

General Considerations

➤ **Indications:** Rheumatoid diseases, muscle tension, arthrosis. Also used in menstrual cramping, chronic liver disease and vegetative dystonia.
➤ **Contraindications:** Allergy to grass flowers, acute neuralgia (ice therapy is better), circulatory instability. Can be safely used in patients on warfarin (Phenprocoumon).
➤ **Action:** Reduces pain, increases the local blood flow, thereby enhancing tissue metabolism, reduces increased muscle tone, increases the elasticity of the connective tissues, is calming and relaxing.
➤ **Materials**
  – Grass flowers, linen or cotton bag, safety pins *or* commercial grass flower pillow
  – Towel, flannel sheet, or large bath towel
  – Wide pot and colander that fits on top, pressure cooker with colander element or hospital pressure heater

Procedure

➤ **Preparation:** Fill the cloth bag with the hay flowers until half full, leaving plenty of room for expansion after wetting. Close the bag securely with safety pins. Pour water into the wide pot and heat to boiling, then place the colander on top. Place the grass flower pillow on the colander or leaf steamer and steam-heat for approximately 30 minutes.
➤ **Application:** Carefully place the hot pillow over the troubled area, as hot as the patient can stand it. Cover with a towel to prevent leakage, and wrap snugly in the flannel sheet.
➤ **Duration of treatment:** 20 to 40 minutes, or until the pillow has become too cool.
➤ **Aftercare:** Remove the grass flower pillow and re-wrap the treated area in the flannel sheet. Allow the patient to rest for 30 minutes. Each grass flower pillow can be used 4 to 5 times before discarding. Use only on the same patient. Hang to air-dry after each use.
➤ **Frequency of treatment:** 1 to 2 times daily.

General Considerations

➤ See **Ginger** (*Zingiber officinale* Roscoe), p. 70
➤ **Indications:** Chronic joint disease, rheumatism, gout, back pain, muscle tension, shoulder pain, acute shoulder-arm syndrome, psoriasis with joint involvement, to promote excretion, chronic bronchitis.
➤ **Contraindications:** Arterial hypertension, schizophrenia.
➤ **Action:** Warms the entire body, enhances simultaneous breathing exercises (stressed inhalation), dissolves mucus, stimulates urine excretion, improves joint mobility, reduces pain.
➤ **Materials**
  – 3 tablespoons freshly grated ginger root (rhizome) *or*
    2 tablespoons powdered dry ginger root
  – Four layers of smooth cotton cloth, folded to the size of the treatment area
  – Dish towel, towel, and flannel sheet
  – Hot water bottle
  – Neutral vegetable oil (e. g., olive oil)

Procedure

➤ **Preparation:** Place the ginger root (freshly grated or powdered) in a small plastic bowl. Add approximately 500 mL of hot water (80 °C) and steep for 3 to 5 minutes. Dip the cotton cloth in the ginger water until completely soaked. Wrap in the dish towel and wring out excess liquid.
➤ **Application:** Place the hot, wet cloth over the lumbar spine. Cover with the towel and wrap using the flannel sheet. Tuck the patient snugly in bed, ensuring that the shoulders are well covered. Check the feet; if cold, place hot water bottle underneath and tuck in under the bedcovers. Darken the room and ensure absolute peace and quiet.
  ◉ *Note:* Good wrapping technique is essential. An additional sheet may be needed to eliminate air holes in wraps for patients with pronounced spinal curvature.
➤ Duration of treatment: 20 to 40 minutes.
➤ **Aftercare:** Remove the compress and apply neutral oil to the treated area. Then re-wrap the patient in the flannel sheet and instruct the patient to rest for another 30 minutes.
➤ **Frequency of treatment:** Once daily. To respect the normal rules of body temperature regulation, this treatment should be performed in the morning. Ginger wraps can be used for a therapeutic course of treatment, especially in chronic illnesses. In such a case, we generally recommend 5 days of treatment followed by a 2-day break, then another 5 days of treatment. The number of treatments is determined by the type and severity of disease.

22.3 Arnica Joint Wrap

General Considerations

➤ See **Arnica** (*Arnica montana* L.), p. 35 ff.
➤ **Indications:** Joint pain, rheumatic joint complaints, infectious arthritis, contusions, sprains, bruises, torn ligaments, fracture-related edema.
➤ **Contraindications:** Allergy to arnica.
➤ **Action**
  – Alleviates pain, reduces swelling, anti-inflammatory, stabilizes the blood vessels.
  – Clinical experience has shown that it is better to treat hot joints with cold compresses, arthritis with lukewarm compresses, and cold joints with hot compresses.
➤ **Materials**
  – 1 tablespoon 70 % arnica tincture (arnica blossoms and 70 % ethanol v/v 1 : 10)
  – Several thicknesses of linen cloth or compress
  – Elastic bandage
  – Waterproof sheet

Procedure

➤ **Preparation:** Fill a small bowl with 300 mL of water heated to the appropriate temperature (see Action above). Add arnica essence and mix. Dip the cloth (compress) into the arnica solution.
➤ **Application:** Allow the patient to inhale the vapors from the arnica solution. Wring out the cloth (compress) and place on the affected area. Wrap with elastic bandage and spread waterproof sheet underneath.
➤ **Duration of treatment:** 30 minutes to 2 hours, depending on the severity of inflammation. Treatment can be repeated liberally. If the bandage dries, wet with more arnica solution. For chronic joint problems, the wrap is best applied for 30 minutes in the morning and evening.

General Considerations

➤ See **Arnica** (*Arnica montana* L.), p. 35 ff.
➤ **Indications:** Rising fever (see below), cold hands and/or feet, centralization of blood flow, narrowing of peripheral vessels.
➤ **Contraindications:** Allergy to arnica.
➤ **Action**
  – Widens the peripheral arteries.
  – Clinical experience has shown that pulse wraps widen the peripheral arteries in patients with a rising temperature. A bout of sweating can sometimes stop the increase of temperature. As the peripheral vessels widen, the body becomes warmer from head to toe. This is the right time to apply a cooling calf wrap or give the patient a cooling wash (see p. 314).
➤ **Materials**
  – 10 mL of 60 % arnica essence (arnica blossoms and 70 % ethanol v/v 1 : 10).
  – 4 cotton or silk wrap cloths, 10 × 25 cm each
  – 4 narrow flannel cloths, 12 × 26 cm each
  – 1 dish towel
  – 200 mL of hot water (80 °C)

Procedure

➤ **Preparation:** Pour hot water and arnica essence into a small bowl. Wrap one pulse wrap cloth in the dish towel and dip into the hot arnica water.
➤ **Application:** Apply the wrap, after wringing out excess liquid by squeezing the dish towel, as hot as the patient can stand it, to the pulse site and wrap the flannel cloth around it. Discard used arnica water. Replace the used pulse wrap with a fresh one, prepared with fresh arnica solution, every 10 minutes. Repeat for a total of 3 wrap applications. The wraps can be left in place longer, even over night, if the patient falls asleep during treatment.
➤ **Duration of treatment:** 30 minutes.

23.2 Mustard Powder Footbath

General Considerations

➤ For more information on mustard, see **White mustard** (*Sinapis alba* L.) p. 127.
➤ **Indications:** Budding colds, sinusitis, tonsillitis, headaches.
➤ **Action:** Topical application of mustard powder can reduce congestion. Mustard increases the blood flow to the skin through local irritation.
➤ **Materials**
  – *Either*
    • 2 tablespoons black mustard powder
    • Small foot tub (water up to ankle)
  – *or*
    • 4 tablespoons black mustard powder
    • High foot tub (water up to knee or calf)
  – Measuring cup, towel , oily skin care product, wool socks
  ◉ *Note:* Use pharmaceutical quality powdered black mustard seed (Sinapis nigrae semen).

Procedure

➤ **Preparation:** Fill foot tub ²/₃ full with water heated to 37 °C. Add mustard powder and mix.
➤ **Application:** Have the patient place their feet in the water. Ensure that the water temperature remains constant by adding more hot water after ca. 5 minutes. After 10 minutes of treatment, rinse the feet with clear, lukewarm water, paying careful attention to the ankles and areas between toes. Dry feet well.
➤ **Duration of treatment:** 10 minutes; can be extended to a total of 20 minutes, depending on the individual skin tolerance, e. g., occurrence of skin reddening and the severity of disease.
➤ **Aftercare:** Apply hypericum oil or another high-quality vegetable oil (e.g., olive oil) to feet. Have the patient put on the wool socks and rest for 30 minutes. If the footbath is administered at night, this should be done immediately before retiring.
  ◉ *Note:* Mustard seed causes the skin to redden, usually immediately, but sometimes only after several baths. If the redness persists until the next day, discontinue treatment for a day.

General Considerations

➤ **Indications:** Budding throat inflammation with difficulty in swallowing, chronic throat inflammation.
➤ **Contraindications:** Allergy to lemon, inflammation of the skin in the affected area, aversion to the smell of lemon.
➤ **Action:** Astringent, antiseptic, antibacterial.
➤ **Materials**
  – 1 lemon, preferably without chemical additives
  – 500 mL of hot water
  – 2 diaper cloths, 1 dish towel, 1 wool or silk scarf

Procedure

➤ **Preparation:** Wash the lemon and cut it in two. Pour boiling water into a bowl and add the lemon, cut surface facing downwards. use a fork to hold the lemon under the water. Use a knife to scratch the surface and flesh of the lemon under the water. Use a drinking glass to press the juice and essential oil out of the lemon. Fold a diaper cloth to width of patient's neck, then wrap in the dish towel and dip in the hot lemon water until completely soaked.
➤ **Application:** Wring out the cloth and apply, as hot as the patient can stand it, to the front and sides of the neck, leaving the cervical spine uncovered (Fig. **6**). Cover with the dry piece of diaper cloth and wrap with wool or silk scarf.
➤ **Duration of treatment:** The wrap should be left on until it becomes too cool.
  ◉ *Note:* Cold water should be used if the patient has severely painful dysphagia. In that case, the wrap should be left on until it becomes too warm and has lost its cooling effects.
➤ **Aftercare:** Keep the neck warm by wrapping in a scarf or cloth.

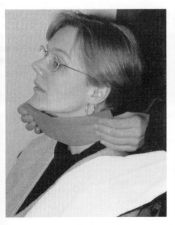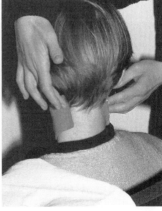

b

Fig. **6** Application of lemon neck wrap. Reproduced with permission from A. Sonn, *Wickel und Auflagen*, Thieme, Stuttgart, 1998.

23.4 Fever-Reducing Whole-Body Peppermint Wash ▰▰

General Considerations

➤ See **Peppermint** (*Mentha piperita* L), p. 102.
➤ Indications: Temperature over 39 °C (102 °F).
➤ **Contraindications:** Use with caution in allergy patients.
   ◉ *Note:* The body has to be completely warm, including the hands and feet. The treatment should not be performed if blood flow is centralized.
➤ **Action:** The menthol contained in peppermint leaves has a cooling effect on the skin.
➤ **Materials**
   – 3 tablespoons peppermint leaf
   – 3 to 5 drops of peppermint essential oil
   – 1 liter of boiling water
   – Wash cloth, towel

Procedure

➤ **Preparation:** See instructions for whole-body wash (p. 32). The water temperature should be 1–2 °C less than the patient's body temperature. Pour 1 liter of boiling water onto 3 tablespoons of peppermint leaf and steep for 5 minutes. Strain and add 3 to 5 drops of peppermint oil, then add the infusion to 3 to 4 liters of wash water.
➤ **Application:** Dip the washcloth in the warm peppermint water, wring out and start by washing the arms and legs. When finished, do not towel dry, but gently dab off excess water. The evaporation of the liquid on the skin has an additional cooling effect.
➤ **Frequency of treatment:** Repeat any time the temperature rises above 39 °C, provided the blood flow is not centralized.

General Considerations

➤ See **Calendula** (*Calendula officinalis* L.), p. 90.
➤ **Indications:** Poor wound healing, dirty wounds, leg ulceration, radiation ulcers, decubitus ulcers grade II/III, complex wound healing disorders (e. g., in diabetes), poor healing of amputation stumps, surgical wounds.
➤ **Contraindications:** Allergy to composite plants.
➤ **Action:** Disinfectant, anti-inflammatory, promotes the development of granulation tissue, stimulates the lymph system. Ringer's solution contains potassium. Wet dressings soaked in Ringer's solution provide the calcium needed for granulation tissue development and maintain the moist wound environment needed for wound cleanliness for more than 12 hours.
➤ **Materials**
  – 70 % calendula tincture
  – Ringer's solution
  – Wet dressings
  – Sterilized and unsterilized gloves
  – Sterile syringes, cannulas (select size according to wound type and size)
  – Sterile gauze compresses, sterile pledgets
  – Dressing materials (gauze and adhesive tape)
  – Anatomic/surgical forceps
  ◉ *Note:* If patient is allergic to adhesive tape, use hydrocolloid dressings instead.

Procedure

➤ **Preparation:** Prepare a mixture of 10 % Ringer's solution and calendula tincture (see Table **3** for mixing ratio). Draw into an ear syringe bulb, apply to Tender-Wet compresses, and allow to soak for 3 minutes.
➤ **Application**
  – Wash hands with disinfectant and put on unsterilized gloves.
  – Take off the old dressing and inspect the wound, noting the color of the exudate, the presence or absence of necrosis and the extent, smell, color, and temperature of the wound.
  – Wash the hands again and put on sterile gloves.
  – Use forceps to clean the wound with pledgets and compresses soaked with Ringer–calendula solution.
  – Fill the wound with soaked wet dressings, making sure the entire wound surface is covered. Cover with 1 to 2 layers of sterile compresses, secure with tape.
➤ **Frequency of treatment:** The dressings should be changed every 12 hours according to recommendation of the manufacturer. Some wet dressings only have to be changed every 24 hours. This is useful when the wound is relatively clean.

24.1 Ringer–Calendula Mixture for Wet Dressings

Table 3 Dosage and mixing ratio for 10 % Ringer-calendula solution to be applied to wet dressings according to dressing size

Dressing Size	Total Volume	Mixing Ratio
10 × 10 cm	60 mL	51 mL Ringer's solution + 9 mL calendula tincture
7.5 × 7.5 cm	30 mL	25.5 mL Ringer's solution + 4.5 mL calendula tincture
5.5 × 5.5 cm	15 mL	12.5 mL Ringer's solution + 1.5 mL calendula tincture
4 × 4 cm	10 mL	8.5 mL Ringer's solution + 1.5 mL calendula tincture

General Considerations

➤ See **Calendula** (*Calendula officinalis* L.), p. 90.
➤ **Indications:** Deep decubitus ulcers stage III/IV, wounds with frayed edges and deep pockets, wounds due to tumors, weeping deep wounds, proctological wounds, deep radiation ulcers, bite and stab wounds.
➤ **Contraindications:** Allergy to calendula, dry wounds.
➤ **Action**
  – See Ringer–Calendula Mixture for Wet Dressings, p. 316.
  – Sorbalgon is a loose, non-woven dressing made of high-quality calcium alginate fibers. It has an excellent gel-forming capacity. Sorbalgon dressings have a high absorption capacity: they absorb wound exudate at a rate of approx. 10 mL per gram of dressing. Germs and detritus are taken up into the fibers and kept inside the gel upon transformation. This ensures effective wound cleansing and significant germ reduction.
  – Cutinova foam is a hydrophilic dressing that stimulates natural wound cleansing and regulates moisture and heat regulation without sticking to the wound.
➤ **Materials**
  – Ringer's solution, 70 % calendula tincture
  – Sorbalgon dressing, either 5 × 5 cm or 10 × 10 cm, depending on the size of the wound
  – Cutinova foam dressing (available in sizes 5 × 6 cm, 10 × 10 cm, and 15 × 20 cm) or similar product
  – Disinfectant hand cleaner, 2 pairs of sterile gloves
  – 2 sterile 10-mL syringes, cannula
  – Forceps, pledgets, tape

Procedure

➤ **Preparation:** See instructions on p. 315. Use 8.5 mL of Ringer's solution and 1.5 mL of 70 % calendula tincture.
➤ **Application:** Irrigate the wound with Ringer's solution and dab with pledgets if necessary (change gloves). Use the forceps to insert the Sorbalgon dressing into the wound and wet with Ringer–calendula solution. Cover the wound with Cutinova foam dressing or similar product. The hydroactive dressing is applied with the sticky side facing the cleansed wound surface. The dressing should extend at least 2 – 3 cm beyond the edges of the wound to ensure secure adhesion on the dry surrounding skin. Secure edges with tape.
➤ **Frequency of treatment:** The dressings should be changed every 24 hours or whenever the exudate from the wound seeps through the dressing.

24.3 Rhatany Tincture for Wound Treatment

General Considerations

➤ See **Rhatany** (*Krameria trianda* Ruiz et Par.), p. 111.
➤ **Indications:** Abrasions, bleeding through spontaneous skin fissures during cortisone treatment, ureteral bleeding due to indwelling catheters, fever blisters/herpes zoster, efflorescences, oozing hemorrhages in hemophiliacs, nosebleeds.
➤ **Contraindications:** Allergy to rhatany.
➤ **Action:** Disinfectant, astringent, hemostyptic, antibacterial.
➤ **Materials:** Used in combination with conventional dressing materials.

Procedure

➤ **Severe nosebleeds:** Soak a tampon or small sterile cotton ball with rhatany tincture and insert in the nostril.
➤ **Wound disinfection:** Clean the wound with the undiluted tincture. Dressings are generally not necessary.
➤ **Frequency of treatment:** Can be applied several times a day as needed.

General Considerations _____

➤ See **Arnica** (*Arnica montana* L.), p. 35.
➤ **Indications:** Hematoma, inflammation due to insect bites, superficial phlebitis, phlegmons, furunculosis, erysipelas.
➤ **Contraindications:** Allergy to arnica.
➤ **Action**
  – Analgesic, detumescent, anti-inflammatory, vessel-stabilizing.
  – Clinical experience has shown that arnica wraps are effective in treating extensive hematomas as well as acute inflammation and severe swelling around insect bites.
➤ **Materials**
  – 1 tablespoon 70% arnica tincture (arnica blossoms and 70% ethanol v/v 1 : 10)
  – 300 mL cold water
  – Several layers of folded linen cloth
  – Roll of gauze
  – Waterproof sheet

Procedure _____

➤ **Preparation:** Mix the arnica tincture and water in a bowl. Dip the linen cloth into the arnica water.
➤ **Application:** Allow the patient to inhale the vapors from the arnica water. Cover bedding with the waterproof sheet. Wring out the linen cloth and apply to the affected area. Secure with gauze if necessary.
➤ **Duration of treatment:** $1/2$ to 2 hours, depending on the severity of inflammation. If the dressing becomes dry, it can be re-wetted with more of the arnica water.

24.5 Whole-Body Wash with Heartsease Infusion ▮▮▮

General Considerations ───────────────

➤ See **heartsease** (*Viola tricolor* L.). p. 75
➤ **Indications:** Allergy, eczema-related itching old age related itching, itching associated with liver or kidney diseases.
➤ **Contraindications:** Allergy to heartsease.
➤ **Action:** Antipruritic and calming. The effects of topical heartsease preparations can be enhanced by drinking heartsease tea (prepared as specified below, 1 cup, 3 times daily).
➤ **Materials**
  – 3 tablespoons heartsease, 1 liter boiling water
  – 3 to 4 liters of cold water
  – Washcloth and towel

Procedure ───────────────

➤ **Preparation:** Steep 3 tablespoons heartsease in 1 liter of boiling water for 5 minutes. Add 3 to 4 liters of boiling water to yield a water temperature of 30–35 °C.
➤ **Application:** Use for a calming wash, see p. 32.
➤ **Frequency of treatment:** 1 to 3 times daily, depending on the severity of symptoms.

General Considerations

▶ **Indications:** Blister-forming and pustule-forming skin diseases, acne, impetigo, erysipelas, phlegmons, gangrene, abscess, infected wounds, felons, urticaria, acute atopic dermatitis, insect bites, bite wounds, burns (cooling, calming), herpes zoster (apply the juice), mastitis, lymph congestion, thrombophlebitis, leg ulceration (apply poultice or leaves), gout, rheumatoid arthritis, suppurative arthritis.

▶ **Action:** Reduces inflammation and swelling and has softening, cooling and calming effects.

▶ **Materials**
- Fresh head of white cabbage
- Knife, cutting board, empty water bottle, cotton cloth or compress, wool cloth
- Fixation materials such as elastic bandage or flannel sheet, depending on the size and position of the affected area

Procedure

▶ **Preparation:** Use a sharp knife to remove the individual leaves of the cabbage. Wash carefully and pat dry.

▶ **Application**
- Place the prepared cabbage leaves so that they overlap over the affected area. Cover the cabbage leaves with the cotton cloth, compress or diaper cloth. To treat hot joints, crush the leaves and apply at room temperature. If the joints are cold, place the crushed leaves in a plastic bag and warm on a hot water bottle before applying. When finished, wrap the flannel sheet or elastic bandage around the cabbage leaves and cover cloth.
- *Dressing for open wounds, e.g., leg ulcers:* Cover wound edges with calendula creme. Pack the wound with pureed cabbage leaves or with thinly sliced (1–2 mm) cabbage leaves, ensuring that the cabbage leaves do not extend over the edges of the wound. Cover the cabbage puree with several layers of gauze to absorb any secretions. If profuse amounts of exudate are secreted from the wound, it should be cleaned with Ringer's solution and the dressing should be changed frequently.

▶ **Duration of treatment:** 1 to 12 hours. It is helpful to leave the poultice on overnight if there is joint pain. In wound treatment, the frequency of dressing changes is determined by the amount of exudate secreted from the wound.

▶ **Aftercare:** After removing the old dressing, wash the skin with lukewarm water. Sparingly apply olive oil to sensitive skin.

▶ **Effects of cabbage poultices on wound healing**
- Soften and dissolve areas of necrosis, liquefy hardened secretions, and promote the discharge of stinking, whitish-brown fluid.
- Demarcate the wound from the surroundings, and promote granulation and epithelialization.
- Promote clean scar formation.
- ◉ *Note:* Radiating pain can develop after treatment of previously painless wounds (e.g., heel ulcers). The pain goes away, to be replaced by the well-known "itch of healing."

General Considerations

➤ **Indications:** Damaged hair, hair damage due to chemical treatments, hair loss, dandruff, seborrheic scalp eczema, hair loss in long-standing patients due to stress, fever, or antibiotics.
➤ **Action:** Egg yolk and oils smooth the hair; rosemary oil improves the blood flow to the scalp; and eucalyptus oil disinfects and reduces itching and dandruff.
➤ **Materials**
  – 1 egg yolk for short hair or 2 for long hair
  – 3 tablespoons of vegetable oil for short hair or 6 for long hair (e.g., sunflower, safflower, or olive oil)
  – Dash of lemon juice
  – 5 drops of 100% rosemary oil
  – 5 drops of 100% eucalyptus oil

Procedure

➤ **Preparation:** Mix egg yolk and oil at room temperature to mayonnaise consistency. Mix in lemon juice and essential oils.
➤ **Application:** Apply mixture to dry hair and briefly massage the head. Cover hair with a plastic bag and wrap in a pre-warmed towel.
➤ **Duration of treatment:** Leave on for 30 minutes.
➤ **Aftercare:** Rinse the scalp and hair thoroughly with lukewarm water. Wash with a mild shampoo. The hair should now be shiny and easy to comb through.
➤ **Frequency of treatment:** For severe hair loss or dandruff, apply the hair mask once a week until the condition improves.

General Considerations

➤ **Indications:** See Egg Yolk Hair Mask, p. 322.
➤ **Action:** Egg yolk and oils smooth the hair; cedar oil revitalizes the hair and detoxifies the scalp; bayberry oil stimulates hair growth.
➤ **Materials**
  – 1 egg yolk for short hair or 2 for long hair
  – 3 tablespoon jojoba oil for short hair, 6 for long hair
  – Dash of lemon juice
  – 5 drops of 100 % cedar oil
  – 5 drops of 100 % bayberry oil

Procedure

➤ See Egg Yolk Hair Mask, p. 322.

25 Herbal Oils for Musculoskeletal Diseases

Table 4 Herbal oils for musculoskeletal diseases

Mud and lavender oil	Rheumatism, meteorosensitivity, spinal syndrome, neuralgia, chronic pain, metastasis-related pain
Aconite oil (nervine oil)*	Rheumatic joint disease, neuralgia, neuritis
Arnica oil (5%)	Myogelosis, subacute and chronic joint disease, pain after muscular exertion, hematoma, blunt trauma, strained muscles, contusions
Rosemary oil (10%)	Rheumatic diseases with tendency to generalized cold sensations
Birch oil	Painful, traumatic, inflammatory or rheumatic muscle and joint diseases
Birch–arnica oil	Same as birch oil, but more potent
Hypericum oil (5%)	Backache, root irritation syndrome, muscular rheumatism
Camphor oil (5%)	Painful rheumatic conditions, neuralgia, peripheral circulation disorders
Horsetail oil (10%)	Chronic inflammatory, degenerative diseases of the joints and nerves

* Commercial products only

Latin Plant Name	Common Plant Name	Parts Used
Achillea millefolium	Yarrow	Flowering aerial parts
Acorus calamus	Calamus (sweetflag)	Rhizome
Actaea racemosa	Black cohosh	Rhizome
Adonis vernalis	Adonis	Aerial parts
Aesculus hippocastanum	Horse chestnut	Seeds/bark/leaves
Alcea rosea	Hollyhock	Flowers
Alchemilla xanthochlora (A. vulgaris)	Lady's mantle	Aerial parts
Allium cepa	Onion	Bulb
Allium sativum	Garlic	Bulb
Allium ursinum	Bear paw garlic, ramson	Aerial parts
Aloe ferox	Aloe vera (Cape aloe)	Leaves
Aloe vera (Aloe barbadensis)	Aloe vera (Barbados aloe)	Leaves
Alpinia officinarum	Lesser galangal	Rhizome
Althaea officinalis	Marshmallow	Leaves/root
Ammi visnaga	Khella	Fruit
Ananas comosus	Pineapple	Raw bromelain
Angelica archangelica	Angelica	Root
Arctium lappa (A. major)	Great burdock	Root
Arctostaphylos uva-ursi	Uva-ursi (bearberry)	Leaves
Armoracia rusticana	Horseradish	Root
Arnica montana	Arnica	Flowers
Artemisia absinthium	Wormwood	Flowering aerial parts
Atropa belladonna	Belladonna	Leaves/root
Avena sativa	Oats	Oatstraw
Baptisia tinctoria	Wild indigo	Root
Berberis vulgaris	Barberry	Fruit/Root bark
Beta vulgaris	Sugar beet	Root juice (betanin)
Beta vulgaris var. conditiva	Red beet	Root juice (betanin)
Betula pendula, B. pubescens	Birch	Leaves
Brassica nigra	Black mustard	Seeds
Calendula officinalis	Marigold (calendula)	Flowers
Capsella bursa-pastoris	Shepherd's purse	Aerial parts
Capsicum annuum L. var. annuum	Cayenne	Fruit
Carica papaya	Papaya	Fruit
Carum carvi	Caraway	Fruit (seeds)/essential oil
Centaurium minus (erythraea)	Lesser centaury	Flowering aerial parts
Cephaelis ipecacuanha	Ipecac (ipecacuanha)	Root
Cetraria islandica	Iceland moss	Thallus
Chelidonium majus	Greater celandine	Flowering aerial parts
Cinchona pubescens	Red cinchona	Bark
Cinnamomum camphora	Camphor	Bark (camphor)
Citrus × aurantium)	Bitter orange	Peel
Citrus limon	Lemon	Fruit

26.1 Latin–English Plant Glossary

Latin Plant Name	Common Plant Name	Parts Used
Cnicus benedictus	Blessed thistle	Aerial parts
Coffea arabica	Coffee	Seed, roasted outer parts of seed
Cola nitida	Cola (kola)	Seeds
Colchicum autumnale	Autumn crocus (Meadow saffron)	Seeds, corms, flowers
Commiphora molmol	Myrrh	Oleo-gum-resin
Convallaria majalis	Lily-of-the-valley	Flowering aerial parts
Coriandrum sativum	Coriander	Fruit (seeds)
Crataegus laevigata, C. monogyna	Hawthorn	Leaves and flowers/fruit (berries)
Cucurbita pepo	Pumpkin	Seeds
Curcuma longa	Turmeric	Rhizome
Cynara scolymus	Artichoke	Leaves
Cytisus scoparius	Scotch broom	Flowering aerial parts
Drosera rotundifolia	Sundew	Aerial parts with root fragments
Echinacea pallida	Pale coneflower	Root
Echinacea purpurea	Purple coneflower	Aerial parts
Eleutherococcus senticosus	Eleuthero	Root
Elymus repens	Couch grass	Rhizome
Ephedra spp.	Ephedra	Aerial parts/root
Equisetum arvense	Horsetail	Sterile green stems
Eryngium planum	Plains eryngo	Root
Eschscholtzia californica	California poppy	Aerial parts
Eucalyptus globulus	Eucalyptus	Leaves/eucalyptus oil
Euphrasia stricta	Eyebright	Aerial parts
Filipendula ulmaria	Meadowsweet	Flowers
Foeniculum vulgare	Fennel	Fruit (seeds)
Frangula alnus	Frangula (alder buckthorn)	Bark (frangula bark)
Frangula purshiana	Cascara sagrada	Bark (cascara bark)
Fumaria officinalis	Fumitory	Flowering aerial parts
Galega officinalis	Goat's rue	Aerial parts
Gelsemium sempervirens	Gelsemium (Yellow jasmine)	Rhizome
Gentiana lutea	Gentian	Root
Ginkgo biloba	Ginkgo	Leaves
Glycyrrhiza glabra	Licorice	Root
Graminis flos	Grass flowers, hay flowers	Flower parts and glume
Gratiola officinalis	Hedge hyssop, gratiola	Aerial parts
Hamamelis virginiana	Witch hazel	Bark/leaves
Harpagophytum procumbens	Devil's claw	Root
Hedera helix	English ivy	Leaves
Herniaria glabra	Rupturewort	Aerial parts
Humulus lupulus	Hops	Cones (strobiles)
Hyoscyamus niger	Henbane	Leaves
Hypericum perforatum	St. John's wort	Flowering aerial parts
Ilex paraguariensis	Maté	Leaves

Latin Plant Name	Common Plant Name	Parts Used
Jasminium odoratissimum	True yellow jasmine	Flowers
Juglans regia	English walnut	Leaves
Juniperus communis	Juniper	Fruit (berries)
Krameria lappacea	Rhatany (Peruvian rhatany)	Root
Lamium album	White deadnettle	Flowers
Lavandula angustifolia	English lavender	Flowers
Leonurus cardiaca	Motherwort	Aerial parts
Levisticum officinale	Lovage	Root
Lichen islandicus	See *Cetraria islandica*	
Linum usitatissimum	Flax	Seeds (linseed)
Lycopus europaeus	European bugleweed	Aerial parts
Lycopus virginicus	Bugleweed (Virginian bugleweed)	Aerial parts
Mahonia aquifolium	Oregon grape (mountain grape, holly-leaf barberry)	Root/bark
Malva sylvestris	Mallow	Flowers/leaves
Marrubium vulgare	Horehound	Aerial parts
Marsdenia condurango	Condurango	Bark
Matricaria recutita	Chamomile (German chamomile)	Flowers
Melilotus officinalis	Yellowsweet clover, melilot	Aerial parts
Melissa officinalis	Lemon balm (balm)	Leaves
Mentha piperita	Peppermint	Leaves/essential oil
Menyanthes trifoliata	Bog bean (buckbean)	Leaves
Oenothera biennis	Evening primrose	Seeds (oil)
Olea europaea	Olive	Leaves
Orthosiphon aristatus	Java tea	Leaves
Panax ginseng	Asian ginseng (Chinese ginseng)	Root
Passiflora incarnata	Passion flower	Aerial parts
Paullinia cupana	Guarana	Seeds
Petasites hybridus	Purple butterbur	Rhizome
Petroselinum crispum	Parsley	Aerial parts/root
Peumus boldus	Boldo	Leaves
Phaseolus vulgaris	Common bean	Pods
Pimpinella anisum	Aniseed	Fruit
Pimpinella saxifraga	Burnet saxifrage	Root
Pinus spp.	Pine tree	Needles (pine) needle oil/twigs/turpentine
Piper methysticum	Kava, Kava-kava, pepper plant	Rhizome
Plantago arenaria	Psyllium	Seeds
Plantago lanceolata	English plantain (ribwort)	Aerial parts/leaves
Plantago ovata	Indian plantain (blond psyllium, isphagula)	Husks
Podophyllum peltatum	Mayapple (American mandrake)	Rhizome (resin)

Latin Plant Name	Common Plant Name	Parts Used
Polygonum aviculare	Knotweed	Aerial parts
Polygonum hydropiper	Smartweed (water pepper)	Aerial parts
Populus spp.	Poplar (cottonwood)	Buds
Potentilla anserina	Silverweed (goosewort)	Flowering aerial parts
Potentilla erecta	Cinquefoil (Tormentill)	Rhizome
Primula elatior	Oxlip	Flowers/root
Primula veris	Primula (primrose)	Flowers/root
Quercus robur	Oak	Bark from twigs and shoots
Raphanus sativus	Radish	Root
Rhamnus cathartica	Buckthorn	Fruit (berries)
Rheum palmatum	Chinese rhubarb	Root
Ribes nigrum	Black currant	Fruit (berries)
Rosa canina	Dog rose	Fruit (rose hips)
Rosmarinus officinalis	Rosemary	Leafy shoots with flowers
Rubus fructicosus	Blackberry	Leaves
Rubus idaeus	Raspberry	Leaves
Ruscus aculeatus	Butcher's broom	Rhizome
Salvia officinalis	Sage	Leaves
Sambucus nigra	European elder	Flowers
Saponaria officinalis	Soapwort (bouncing bet)	Root
Secale cornutum	Ergot	Fungus (ergot)
Senna alexandrina	Senna	Leaves/fruit (pods)
Serenoa repens (Sabal serrulata)	Saw palmetto	Fruit (berries)
Silybum marianum	Milk thistle, Marian thistle	Fruit
Sinapis alba	White mustard	Seeds
Solanum dulcamara	Bittersweet, bitter nightshade	Stems
Solidago virgaurea	European goldenrod	Flowering aerial parts
Symphytum officinale	Comfrey	Root
Syzygium aromaticum	Clove	Flower buds
Taraxacum officinale	Dandelion	Root and aerial parts
Thuja occidentalis	Thuja, Arbor vitae, tree of life, Northern white cedar	Twig tips and young shoots
Thymus vulgaris	Thyme	Leaves and flowers
Tilia cordata	Linden (small-leaved lime)	Flowers
Tilia platyphyllos	Linden (large-leaved lime)	Flowers
Trigonella foenum-graecum	Fenugreek	Seed
Tropaeolum majus	Nasturium, Indian cress	Aerial parts including leaves, flowers and seeds
Tussilago farfara	Coltsfoot	Leaves
Urginea maritima	Red squill	Bulb
Urtica dioica L. ssp. dioica	Stinging nettle, common nettle	Aerial parts/root

Latin Plant Name	Common Plant Name	Parts Used
Urtica urens	Dwarf nettle, small nettle	Aerial parts/root
Usnea barbata	Usnea (Old man's beard)	Lichen
Vaccinium myrtillus	Bilberry	Fruit/leaves
Valeriana officinalis	Valerian	Root
Verbascum densiflorum	Mullein	Flowers
Veronica officinalis	Speedwell	Flowering aerial parts
Viola odorata	Sweet violet	Flowers/root
Viola tricolor	Heartsease, wild pansy	Flowering aerial parts
Viscum album	European mistletoe	Young twigs including leaves, flowers, and fruit
Vitex agnus-castus	Chaste tree	Fruit (berries)
Vitis viniferae	Grape	Red leaves
Xysmalobium undulatum	Uzara	Root
Zingiber officinalis	Ginger	Rhizome

26.2 English–Latin Plant Glossary

Common Plant Name	Latin Name	Pharmaceutical Name
Adonis	*Adonis vernalis*	Adonidis herba
Aloe	*Aloe vera* (*Aloe barba-densis*), *A. capensis*	Aloe folium
Angelica	*Angelica archangelica*	Angelicae radix
Aniseed	*Pimpinella anisum*	Anisi fructus
Arbor vitae	See Thuja	
Arnica	*Arnica montana*	Arnicae flos
Artichoke	*Cynara scolymus*	Cynarae folium
Asian ginseng (Chinese ginseng)	*Panax ginseng*	Ginseng radix
Autumn crocus (Meadow saffron)	*Colchicum autumnale*	Colchici semen
Balm	See Lemon balm	
Barberry	*Berberis vulgaris*	Berberidis fructus, Berberidis cortex
Bean	See Common bean, Bog bean	
Bear paw garlic (ramson)	*Allium ursinum*	Allii ursini herba
Bearberry	See Uva-ursi	
Belladonna	*Atropa belladonna*	Belladonnae folium, Belladonnae radix
Bilberry	*Vaccinium myrtillus*	Myrtilli folium, Myrtilli fructus
Birch	*Betula* spp.	Betulae folium
Bitter nightshade	See Bittersweet	
Bitter orange	*Citrus × aurantium*	Aurantii pericarpium
Bittersweet (bitter nightshade)	*Solanum dulcamara*	Dulcamarae stipites
Black cohosh	*Actaea racemosa*	Cimicifugae rhizoma
Black currant	*Ribes nigrum*	Ribis nigri fructus
Black mustard	*Brassica nigra*	Sinapis nigrae semen
Blackberry	*Rubus fruticosus*	Rubi fructicosi folium
Blessed thistle	*Cnicus benedictus*	Cnici benedicti herba
Blond psyllium	See Indian plantain	
Bog bean (buckbean)	*Menyanthes trifoliata*	Menyanthidis folium
Boldo	*Peumus boldus*	Boldo folium
Buckbean	See Bogbean	
Buckthorn	*Rhamnus cathartica*	Rhamni cathartici fructus
Buckthorn, alder	See Frangula	
Bugleweed	See European bugleweed, Virginia bugleweed	
Burdock	See Great burdock	
Burnet saxifrage	*Pimpinella saxifraga*	Pimpinellae radix
Butcher's broom	*Ruscus aculeatus*	Rusci aculeati rhizoma
Butterbur	See Purple butterbur	
Calamus (sweetflag)	*Acorus calamus*	Calami rhizoma
Calendula	See Marigold	
California poppy	*Eschscholtzia californica*	Eschscholtziae herba
Camphor	*Cinnamomum camphora*	Cinnamomi cortex

Common Plant Name	Latin Name	Pharmaceutical Name
Caraway	*Carum carvi*	Carvi fructus, Carvi aetheroleum
Cascara sagrada	*Frangula purshiana*	Rhamni purshiani cortex
Cayenne	*Capsicum annuum* L. var. *annuum*	Capsici fructus
Celandine	See Greater celandine	
Centaury	See Lesser centaury	
Chamomile	*Matricaria recutita*	Matricariae flos
Chaste tree	*Vitex agnus-castus*	Agni casti fructus
Chestnut	See Horse chestnut	
Chinese ginseng	See Asian ginseng	
Chinese rhubarb	*Rheum palmatum*	Rhei radix
Cinchona	See Red cinchona	
Cinquefoil (tormentil)	*Potentilla erecta*	Tormentillae rhizoma
Clove	*Syzygium aromaticum*	Caryophylli flos
Coffee	*Coffea arabica*	Coffea semen, Coffea carbo
Cohosh	See Black cohosh	
Cola tree	*Cola nitida*	Colae semen
Coltsfoot	*Tussilago farfara*	Tussilagi folium
Comfrey	*Symphytum officinale*	Symphyti radix
Common bean	*Phaseolus vulgaris*	Phaseoli pericarpum
Common nettle	See Stinging nettle	
Condurango	*Marsdenia condurango*	Condurango cortex
Coneflower	See White echinacea, Purple echinacea	
Coriander	*Coriandrum sativum*	Coriandri fructus
Cowslip	See Primula	
Crocus	See Autumn crocus	
Dandelion	*Taraxacum officinale*	Taraxaci radix cum herba
Deadnettle	See White deadnettle	
Devil's claw	*Harpagophytum procumbens*	Harpagophyti radix
Dog rose	*Rosa canina*	Cynosbati fructus
Echinacea	See White echinacea, Purple echinacea	
Elder	See European elder	
Eleuthero (Siberian ginseng)	*Eleuterococcus senticosus*	Eleutherococci radix
English ivy	*Hedera helix*	Hederae helicis folium
English lavender	*Lavandula angustifolia*	Lavandulae flos
English plantain (ribwort)	*Plantago lanceolata*	Plantaginis lanceolatae folium, Plantaginis lanceolatae herba
English walnut	*Juglans regia*	Juglandis folium
Ephedra	*Ephedra* spp.	Ephedrae herba, Ephedrae radix
Ergot	*Secale cornutum*	Secale cornutum
Eucalyptus	*Eucalyptus globulus*	Eucalypti folium, Eucalypti aetheroleum

26.2 English–Latin Plant Glossary

Common Plant Name	Latin Name	Pharmaceutical Name
European bugleweed	*Lycopus europaeus*	Lycopi europaei herba
European elder	*Sambucus nigra*	Sambuci flos
European goldenrod	*Solidago virgaurea*	Virgaureae herba
European mistletoe	*Viscum album*	Visci herba
Evening primrose	*Oenothera biennis*	Oenothera biennis aetheroleum
Eyebright	*Euphrasia stricta*	Euphrasiae herba
Fennel	*Foeniculum vulgare*	Foeniculi fructus
Fenugreek	*Trigonella foenum-graecum*	Foenugraeci semen
Flax	*Linum usitatissimum*	Lini semen
Frangula (alder buckthorn)	*Frangula alnus*	Frangulae cortex
Fumitory	*Fumaria officinalis*	Fumariae herba
Galangal	See Lesser galangal	
Garlic	*Allium sativum*	Allii sativi bulbus
Gelsemium (yellow jasmine)	*Gelsemium sempervirens*	Gelsemii rhizoma
Gentian	See Yellow gentian	
Ginger	*Zingiber officinalis*	Zingiberis rhizoma
Ginkgo	*Ginkgo biloba*	Ginkgo bilobae folium
Ginseng	See Asian ginseng, Eleuthero (Siberian ginseng)	
Goat's rue	*Galega officinalis*	Galegae herba
Goldenrod	See European goldenrod	
Goosewort	See Silverweed	
Grape	*Vitis viniferae*	Vitis viniferae folium
Grass flowers	*Graminis flos*	Graminis flos
Gratiola	See Hedge hyssop	
Great burdock	*Arctium lappa*	Bardanae radix
Greater celandine	*Chelidonium majus*	Chelidonii herba
Guarana	*Paullinia cupana*	Paulliniae semen
Hawthorn	*Crataegus laevigata, C. monogyna*	Crataegi folium cum flos, Crataegi fructus
Hay flowers	See Grass flowers	
Heartsease	*Viola tricolor*	Violae tricoloris herba
Hedge hyssop	*Gratiola officinalis*	Gratiolae herba
Henbane	*Hyoscyamus niger*	Hyoscyami folium
High mallow	See Mallow	
Hollyhock	*Alcea rosea*	Malvae arboreae flos
Hops	*Humulus lupulus*	Lupuli strobulus
Horehound	*Marrubium vulgare*	Marrubii herba
Horse chestnut	*Aesculus hippocastanum*	Hippocastani semen, Hippocastani cortex, Hippocastani folium
Horseradish	*Armoracia rusticana*	Armoraciae radix
Horsetail	*Equisetum arvense*	Equiseti herba
Iceland moss	*Cetraria islandica*	Cetrariae lichen
Indian plantain	*Plantago ovata*	Plantaginis ovatae semen

Common Plant Name	Latin Name	Pharmaceutical Name
Indigo	See Wild indigo	
Ipecac, ipecacuanha	*Cephaelis ipecacuanha*	Ipecacuanhae radix
Ivy	See English ivy	
Jasmine, Yellow	See Gelsemium, True yellow jasmine	
Java tea	*Orthosiphon aristatus*	Orthosiphonis folium
Juniper	*Juniperus communis*	Juniperi fructus
Kava	*Piper methysticum*	Piperis methystici rhizoma
Khella	*Ammi visnaga*	Ammeos visnagae fructus
Knotweed	*Polygonum aviculare*	Polygoni avicularis herba
Kola tree	See Cola tree	
Lady's mantle	*Alchemilla xanthochlora* (*A. vulgaris*)	Alchemillae herba
Lavender	See English lavender	
Lemon	*Citrus limon*	Limonii fructus
Lemon balm	*Melissa officinalis*	Melissae folium
Lesser centaury	*Centaurium minus* (*erythraea*)	Centaurii herba
Lesser galangal	*Alpinia officinarum*	Galangae rhizoma
Lichen islandicus	See Iceland moss	
Licorice	*Glycyrrhiza glabra*	Liquiritiae radix
Lily-of-the-valley	*Convallaria majalis*	Convallariae herba
Lime tree	See Linden	
Linden (large-leaved lime)	*Tilia platyphyllos*	Tiliae flos
Linden (small-leaved lime)	*Tilia cordata*	Tiliae flos
Lovage	*Levisticum officinale*	Levistici radix
Mallow	*Malva sylvestris*	Malvae flos, Malvae folium
Mandrake	See Mayapple	
Marian thistle	See Milk thistle	
Marigold (Calendula)	*Calendula officinalis*	Calendulae flos
Marshmallow	*Althaea officinalis*	Althaea folium, Althaea radix
Maté (yerba maté)	*Ilex paraguariensis*	Maté folium
Mayapple (mandrake)	*Podophyllum peltatum*	Podophylli rhizoma
Meadow saffron	See Autumn crocus	
Meadowsweet	*Filipendula ulmaria*	Spireae flos
Melilot	See Yellow sweetclover	
Milk thistle (marian thistle)	*Silybum marianum*	Cardui mariae fructus
Mistletoe	See European mistletoe	
Moss	See Iceland moss	
Motherwort	*Leonurus cardiaca*	Leonuri cardiacae herba
Mountain grape	See Oregon grape	
Mullein	*Verbascum densiflorum*	Verbasci flos
Mustard	See Black mustard, White mustard	
Myrrh	*Commiphora molmol*	oleo-gum-vesin

26.2 English–Latin Plant Glossary

Common Plant Name	Latin Name	Pharmaceutical Name
Nasturtium	*Tropaeolum majus*	Tropaeoli herba
Nettle	See Small nettle, Stinging nettle	
Nightshade	See Bittersweet	
Oak	*Quercus robur*	Quercus cortex
Oats	*Avena sativa*	Avenae herba
Old man's beard	See Usnea	
Olive	*Olea europaea*	Oleae folium
Onion	*Allium cepa*	Allii cepae bulbus
Orange	See Bitter orange	
Oregon grape (mountain grape)	*Mahonia aquifolium*	Mahoniae cortex, Mahoniae radix
Orthosiphon	See Java tea	
Oxlip	*Primula elatior*	Primulae flos, Primulae radix
Papaya	*Carica papaya*	Caricae papayae fructus
Parsley	*Petroselinum crispum*	Petroselini herba, Petroselini radix
Passion flower	*Passiflora incarnata*	Passiflorae herba
Peppermint	*Mentha × piperita*	Menthae piperitae folium
Pine tree	*Pinus* spp.	Pini picea, Pini turiones
Pineapple	*Ananas comosus*	Bromelain
Plaintain	See Indian plaintain, English plantain	
Plains eryngo	*Eryngium planum*	Eryngi radix
Poppy	See California poppy	
Primrose	See Evening primrose, Primula	
Primula	*Primula veris*	Primulae flos cum calycibus, Primulae radix
Psyllium	*Plantago arenaria*	Psyllii semen
Psyllium, blond	See Indian plaintain	
Pumpkin	*Cucurbita pepo*	Cucurbitae semen
Purple butterbur	*Petasites hybridus*	Petasitidis rhizoma
Purple echinacea	*Echinacea purpurea*	Echinaceae purpureae herba
Radish	*Raphanus sativus*	Raphani sativi radix
Ramson	See Bear paw garlic	
Raspberry	*Rubus idaeus*	Rubi foliae
Red Beet	*Beta vulgaris* var. *conditiva*	Betae succus
Red cinchona	*Cinchona pubescens*	Cinchonae cortex
Red squill	*Urginea maritima*	Scillae bulbus
Rhatany	*Krameria lappacea*	Ratanhiae radix
Rhubarb	See Chinese rhubarb	
Ribwort	See English plantain	
Rose	See Dog rose	
Rosemary	*Rosmarinus officinalis*	Rosmarini folium
Round-leaved sundew	*Drosera rotundifolia*	Droserae herba

Common Plant Name	Latin Name	Pharmaceutical Name
Rue	See Goat's rue	
Rupturewort	*Herniaria glabra*	Herniariae herba
Saffron, meadow	See Autum crocus	
Sage	*Salvia officinalis*	Salviae folium
St. John's wort	*Hypericum perforatum*	Hyperici herba
Saw palmetto	*Serenoa repens*	Sabal fructus
Saxifrage	See Burnet saxifrage	
Scotch broom	*Cytisus scoparius*	Scoparii herba
Senna	*Senna alexandrina*	Sennae folium, Sennae fructus
Shepherd's purse	*Capsella bursa-pastoris*	Bursae pastoris herba
Siberian ginseng	See Eleuthero	
Silverweed (goosewort)	*Potentilla anserina*	Anserinae herba
Small nettle	*Urtica urens*	Urticae herba, Urticae radix
Smartweed	*Polygonum hydropiper*	Polygoni hydropiperis herba
Soapwort	*Saponaria officinalis*	Saponariae rubrae radix
Speedwell	*Veronica officinalis*	Veronicae herba
Spring adonis	*Adonis vernalis*	Adonidis herba
Squill	See Red squill	
Stinging nettle	*Urtica dioica* ssp. *dioica*	Urticae herba, Urticae radix
Sugar Beet	*Beta vulgaris*	Betae succus
Sundew	See Round-leaved sundew	
Sweet violet	*Viola odorata*	Violae odoratae flos, Violae odoratae radix
Sweetclover	See Yellow sweetclover	
Sweetflag	See Calamus	
Thistle	See Blessed thistle, Milk thistle	
Thuja	*Thuja occidentalis*	Thujae herba
Thyme	*Thymus vulgaris*	Thymi herba
Tormentil	See Cinquefoil	
True yellow jasmine	*Jasminium odoratissimum*	Jasmini flos
Turmeric	*Curcuma longa*	Curcumae longae rhizoma, Curcumae xanthorrhizae rhizoma
Usnea	*Usnea barbata*	Usnea barbata
Uva-ursi (bearberry)	*Arctostaphylos uva-ursi*	Uvae ursi folium
Uzara	*Xysmalobium undulatum*	Uzarae radix
Valerian	*Valeriana officinalis*	Valerianae radix
Violet	See Sweet violet	
Virginia bugleweed	*Lycopus virginicus*	Lycopi virginici herba
Walnut	See English walnut	
White deadnettle	*Lamium album*	Lamii albi flos
White echinacea	*Echinacea pallida*	Echinaceae pallidae radix
White mustard	*Sinapis alba*	Sinapis albae semen

26.2 English–Latin Plant Glossary

Common Plant Name	Latin Name	Pharmaceutical Name
Wild indigo	*Baptisia tinctoria*	Baptisia tinctoriae radix
Wild pansy	See Heartsease	
Witch hazel	*Hamamelis virginiana*	Hamamelidis cortex, Hamamelidis folium
Wormwood	*Artemisia absinthium*	Absinthii herba
Yarrow	*Achillea millefolium*	Millefolii herba
Yellow gentian	*Gentiana lutea*	Gentianae radix
Yellow jasmine	See Gelsemium, True yellow jasmine	
Yellow sweetclover (melilot)	*Melilotus officinalis*	Meliloti herba
Yerba mate	See Maté	

Table 5 Dosages for herbal remedies commonly recommended in Europe and North America

Disease/Condition	Part of Plant Used in Therapy	Recommended Form	Recommended German Dosage	Recommended US Dosage	Warnings	Notes	See Page
Angelica, *Angelica archangelica*							33
Anorexia and functional upper abdominal complaints	Root	Tea	1 tsp in 1 cup boiled water 1 cup, 3 times/day, before meals	0.5–2 g of the powdered root simmered for 5 minutes; steep for 15 minutes for each cup of water. Drink ½ cup tea before 2 main meals	May cause photosensitization. Do not use during pregnancy		167
		Tincture	20–30 drops in a glass of water	0.5–2 mL in a little water before meals	May cause photosensitization. Do not use during pregnancy		167
Blunt trauma, iatrogenic wounds	Root	Compress	Apply locally to affected area for 1–2 hours. 3 times/day Do not cover with airtight material	Same			279
		Liniment	Apply 3 times/day. Especially effective when warmed prior to use	Same			279

5

Table 5 Continued

Disease/Condition	Part of Plant Used in Therapy	Recommended Form	Recommended German Dosage	Recommended US Dosage	Warnings	Notes	See Page
Aniseed, *Pimpinella anisum*							34
Bloating and meteorism	Fruit	Oil	3 drops on cube of sugar, several times/day	Same	Do not use during pregnancy		176
	Fruit	Tea	Pour 1 cup of boiled water onto 1 tsp crushed seeds, steep for 10 minutes. 1 cup, 3–5 times/day	Pour 1 cup of boiled water onto 1 tsp of whole seeds; steep for 20 minutes. Drink 1 cup after meals			176
Fever, colds and flu. Cough, runny nose, bronchitis. Inflammations of the mouth and throat. Acute pharyngitis	Fruit	Liniment	Every 30–60 minutes (acute) or 1–3 times/day (chronic)	Same			155
		Tea	One cup morning and/or evening	0.5–1.0 g/cup infusion after main meals			156
Dyspeptic complaints. Anorexia	Fruit	Medicament	Infant: 1 tsp/day (in bottle) Adults: 1 tbsp/day Daily dose: 3 g dried seed	Give 1–3 dropperful (1–3 mL) to infant of the mild infusion (as above)			174, 176

Catarrhal disorders of the upper respiratory tract in children	Fruit	Oil	3 drops in hot water, inhale several times/day	Same	Do not use during pregnancy	250

Arnica, *Arnica montana*

Angina tonsillaris, peritonsillar abscess	Flowers	Gargle	1 tsp of tincture (1:10) in a glass of hot water	Same	Do not apply high concentrations and undiluted tinctures	35, 163
Angina (angina pectoris) and to reduce strain on the heart in febrile elderly patients	Flowers	Wrap	1 cup of water heated to body temperature and 1 tbsp 60% arnica essence	Same	Do not apply high concentrations and undiluted tinctures	310, 311
Acute hemorrhoidal inflammation	Flowers	Sitz bath	1–2 tsp of tincture (1:10) in 500 mL water	Same	Do not apply high concentrations and undiluted tinctures	188
Blunt trauma, iatrogenic wounds	Flowers	Compress	1 tbsp tincture (1:10) in 500 mL cold water. Apply to affected area and repeat frequently	Same	Do not apply high concentrations and undiluted tinctures	279

5

Table 5 Continued

Disease/Condition	Part of Plant Used in Therapy	Recommended Form	Recommended German Dosage	Recommended US Dosage	Warnings	Notes	See Page
Arnica, *Arnica montana* (continued)							35
	Flowers	Compress	Dose: See Section 15.1, wounds, p. 276 Apply locally to affected area for 1–2 hours, 3 times/day. Do not cover with airtight material	Same	Do not apply high concentrations and undiluted tinctures		277
		Tincture	Dilute 1 tbsp in 500 mL cold water. Apply as a compress to affected area	Same	Do not apply high concentrations and undiluted tinctures		277
Joint pain, rheumatic joint complaints, infectious arthritis, contusions, sprains, bruises, torn ligaments, fracture-related edema	Flowers	Wrap	1 tbsp 60 % arnica essence. Mix with 300 mL cold/lukewarm/hot water as necessary. Dip compress into solution Compress for 30 minutes to 2 hours, depending on inflammation. Can be repeated as necessary	Same	Do not apply high concentrations and undiluted tinctures		310

Flowers	Wrap	10 mL 60 % arnica essence. 200 mL hot water. Apply wrap to the pulse site and replace every 10 minutes. Repeat for a total of 3 wraps. Duration of treatment 30 minutes	Same	Do not apply high concentrations and undiluted tinctures	311
Flowers	Wrap	Mix 1 tbsp 60 % arnica essence and 300 mL cold water. Apply for ½ to 2 hours, depending on severity of inflammation	Same	Do not apply high concentrations and undiluted tinctures	319
Flowers			Apply also for strains and sprains; do not apply to cuts or where skin is broken; discontinue if allergic reaction with inflammation develops. Apply 1–2 mL, several times daily		
	Ointment	10–20 % tincture in a neutral ointment base		Do not apply high concentrations and undiluted tinctures	The tincture should be made 1 : 10, calculated on a dry-weight basis	279

Increasing body temperature, cold hands and/or feet, centralization of blood flow, narrowing of peripheral vessels

Hematoma, inflammation due to insect bites, superficial phlebitis, phlegmons, furunculosis, erysipelas

Thrombophlebitis. Furunculosis and inflammations resulting from insect bites. Inflammation of the skin. Rheumatic muscle and joint complaints. Contusions

Table 5 Continued

Disease/Condition	Part of Plant Used in Therapy	Recommended Form	Recommended German Dosage	Recommended US Dosage	Warnings	Notes	See Page
Arnica, *Arnica montana* (continued)							
							35
		Tincture	1 : 10 (DAB*)	Dilute 2–3 mL 1 : 10 tincture of flowers (calculated on a dry weight basis) in 6–18 ml of water, rub in well. 2–3 times daily; discontinue if irritation or allergic reaction occurs	Do not apply high concentrations and undiluted tinctures		279
Inflammation of the mouth and throat	Flowers	Fomentation	1–3–10 parts (no exact dose statement)	Dilute 10–20 drops of the 1 : 10 tincture in 18–36 ml of water. Gargle 1–2 tsp several times daily; discontinue if irritation or allergic reaction develops	Do not apply high concentrations and undiluted tinctures		163
		Mouthwash	1 : 10 (no exact dose statement)	Same as above	Do not apply high concentrations and undiluted tinctures		163

* DAB = The Dispensatory of the United States of America

Indication	Part	Preparation	Dose	Administration	Contraindications	Page
Muscle pain and tension, sore muscles, pulled muscles and contusions, massages after sports, connective tissue massages	Flowers	Tincture	Apply up to 4 times/day (no exact dose statement)	Apply 1–2 mL of 1:10 tincture on unbroken skin; discontinue if allergic reaction with inflammation develops		234

Artichoke, *Cynara scolymus*

Indication	Part	Preparation	Dose	Administration	Contraindications	Page
Anorexia. Meteorism. Liver and gall bladder complaints. Hyperlipoproteinemia	Leaves	Fresh and dried leaves, juice and extracts	6 g/day	6–9 g of the dried leaf, simmered in 1 quart of water for 20 minutes; steep for 15 minutes. Drink ½ cup before meals; 2–4 mL of a hydroalcoholic tincture (1:6 on a dry weight basis) in a little water before meals	Do not use in obstructive diseases of biliary system or in cholecystolithiasis	144, 165, 182
Atherosclerosis	Leaves	Extract	320–640 mg, 3 times/day, daily dose 960–1920 mg/day	300–640 mg three times daily of the standardized extract (for instance to 15% chlorogenic acid, 5% cynarin)	Do not use in obstructive diseases of biliary system or in cholecystolithiasis	144

5

Table 5 Continued

Disease/Condition	Part of Plant Used in Therapy	Recommended Form	Recommended German Dosage	Recommended US Dosage	Warnings	Notes	See Page
Asian Ginseng, *Panax ginseng* C.A. May							37
Exhaustion, convalescence. Decreased mental and physical performance and concentration. Fatigue and debility	Root	Tea	3 g dried herb in boiling water, cover and steep for 5–10 mins. One cup 3–4 times/ day. Daily dose, dry extract 1–2 g/day	Simmer 3–6 g of the root slices or pieces for 45 minutes; strain and add enough water to cover well, simmer again for 20 minutes and combine decoctions. Drink 1 cup twice daily as needed	Do not overdose. Use caution concurrently with caffeine-containing preparations or drinks. Not usually indicated for anyone under the age of 30 years	Traditional Chinese medicinal dose is 3–15 g in each prescription; seldom used alone	
Barbados aloe, *Aloe vera* (*Aloe barbadensis*)							263
Psoriasis	Leaves	Gel	Apply sparingly to affected area 3 times/day	Apply liberally to affected area 1–2 times/day			

Belladonna, *Atropa belladonna*

Gastritis, dyspepsia, complaints of the biliary tract	Leaves	Extract	As prescribed	The dry standardized extract should contain 1% total alkaloids (BPC*). The average dose is 15 mg	Do not overdose	171, 185
Gastric colic	Leaves	Tincture	8–10 drops in water, 3 times/day	Standardized belladonna tinctures are also available (1% +/−0.05%). Dose is about 20 drops; do not exceed recommended dose	Do not overdose	172

Bilberry, *Vaccinium myrtillus*

Acute glossitis and aphthous stomatitis	Fruit	Gargle	1–3 tbsp dried berries in 1 L of water. Gargle several times/day	Simmer dried blueberries or huckleberries for 10 minutes, steep for 15 minutes		162
Chronic stomatitis, chronic pharyngitis, smoker's catarrh	Fruit	Astringent mouthwash	1–3 tbsp dried fruit per L of water	Same as above		163

---

* BPC = British Pharmaceutical Codex, Published by the Council of the Pharmaceutical Society of Great Britain, 1911

Table 5 Continued.

Disease/Condition	Part of Plant Used in Therapy	Recommended Form	Recommended German Dosage	Recommended US Dosage	Warnings	Notes	See Page
Bilberry, *Vaccinium myrtillus* (continued)							
Infant dyspepsia (infantile dystrophy)	Fruit	Extract	Suspend herb in water or chamomile tea to yield 5% suspension, then boil. 150–200 g/kg body weight/day	Same		Blend the dried or fresh fruit to create suspension, then simmer for 5 minutes, steep for 15 minutes	192
Acute diarrhea in small children	Fruit	Suspension	Suspend ground and sieved fruit in water or chamomile tea to yield 10–20% suspension; boil; bind with rice flour. 3–5 tsp, 3–5 times/day	Same		Or blend the fruit in a blender with the liquid until smooth	192
Acute diarrhea of any origin	Fruit	Tea	Simmer 3 tbsp in ½ L water. 1 cup, 3–5 times/day. Heat each portion before use	Same		Blend the fruit with the liquid, then filter or consume the fruit with the liquid	191

Unspecific acute diarrhea in children	Fruit	Tea	Boil 3 tbsp dried bilberries in 500 mL water. 1 glass, hot, several times/day, or mix with cream of wheat or yogurt	Same	Same as above	253
Inflammations of the mouth and throat in children	Fruit	Gargle	2–3 tbsp herb in 500 mL water	Same	Blend the fruit with the liquid, then filter	247

Birch, *Betula pendula* Roth

Rheumatic diseases (supportive treatment). Diuretic to flush bacteria out of the lower urinary tract and to flush out renal gravel	Leaves	Tea	1–2 tablespoons in 150 mL hot water. 3–4 cups/day, between meals. Daily dose: 12 g	Same	Do not use for treatment of cardiac or renal edema	Simmer for 10 minutes, steep for 20 minutes, strain and drink	39
Dysuria, irritable bladder, urolithiasis	Leaves	Tea	As above. 1 cup, 3–5 times/day	Same. Daily dose 6–12 g of the dried leaves	Do not use for treatment of cardiac or renal edema		39

5

5

Table 5 Continued

Disease/Condition	Part of Plant Used in Therapy	Recommended Form	Recommended German Dosage	Recommended US Dosage	Warnings	Notes	See Page
Bitter orange, *Citrus aurantium*							
Anorexia. Dyspeptic complaints	Peel	Tea	2 g in 1 cup boiling water. 1 cup before meals. 10–15 mg herb daily	2–4 g, 2–3 times daily before meals. Traditional dose in Chinese medical prescriptions is 3–9 g of the dried herb as a decoction, twice daily		Simmer for a few minutes in a covered pan; turn off heat; steep for 20 minutes	165
Bittersweet (Bitter nightshade), *Solanum dulcamara*							
Eczema, boils, acne. Warts. For supportive treatment of chronic eczema	Stems	Compress	1–2 g herb in 250 mL water. Apply compress several times/day	Same	Do not use during pregnancy and nursing	Simmer for 15 minutes	40
Blackberry, *Rubus fruticosus*							
Acute diarrhea of any origin	Leaves	Powder	Make an infusion from 1 tsp 3–5 times/day	Make an infusion from 4–6 g of the dried leaves. Drink 1 cup several times daily			191

Root	Tea	1 tsp chopped herb in 1 cup boiled water. 1 cup between meals, 3–5 times/day	Make a decoction from 3–7 g of the dried root and rhizomes. Drink 1 cup after meals			
	Powder	1 tsp, 3–5 times/day	Same			

Black cohosh, *Actaea racemosa*

Menopausal complaints. Premenstrual syndrome (PMS). Menstrual cramps	Rhizome	Tincture	10 drops on a cube of sugar, 3 times/day. Daily dose 3 g herb	2–4 mL (1 : 10 tincture BPC*), several times a day	Do not use during pregnancy and nursing	1–3 mL 1 : 5 tincture, several times daily
						41
		Capsules; Tablets	1 twice daily	500 mg to 2 g of the powder in capsules, 2–3 times daily, or as a decoction	Do not use during pregnancy and nursing	Standardized extracts are available, for instance, to 1 mg triterpene glycosides calculated as 27-deoxyactein per tablet; dose, 1 tablet twice daily
						240

---

* BPC = British Pharmaceutical Codex, Published by the Council of the Pharmaceutical Society of Great Britain, 1911

Dosages

Table 5 Continued

Disease/Condition	Part of Plant Used in Therapy	Recommended Form	Recommended German Dosage	Recommended US Dosage	Warnings	Notes	See Page
Black currant, *Ribes nigrum*							
Prevention and treatment of upper respiratory tract infections	Fruit	Juice	Dilute with hot water. 1 glass with meals at noon and in the evening	Same		Commercial juices may contain refined sugar, a known immune suppressant	152
Debility, fatigue, adaptive and functional disorders. Convalescence	Fruit	Juice	Dilute with hot water. 1 glass noon and in the evening	Same		Note above	221
Acute diarrhea of any origin	Fruit	Juice	1 glass, 3–5 times/day	Same		Note above	191
Blessed thistle, *Cnicus benedictus*							
Anorexia; dyspepsia	Aerial parts	Tea	2 tsp in 1 cup boiled water. 2–3 cups/day, before meals	Steep 0.5–3 g of the herb for 30 minutes; strain. Drink ½ cup several times a day just before meals	Do not use during pregnancy	A hot tea is more stimulating and can produce sweating	167

Indication	Plant part	Form	Dosage	Dosage	Contraindications	Notes	Page
Bog Bean (Buck Bean), Menyanthes trifoliata							
Chronic stomatitis; chronic pharyngitis	Leaves	Tincture	10–30 drops in a liqueur glassful of water	2–3 mL (1:6 hydroethanolic tincture) in a little water, several times a day before meals	Do not use during pregnancy		167
	Leaves	Bitter mouthwash	1–2 tsp tea mixture to 1 L of water	Mix 1–2 mL in 4 ounces of water and gargle every 2–3 hours			164
Anorexia; dyspepsia	Leaves	Tincture	20–40 drops in ½ glass of water	1–3 mL in a little water 2–3 times/day before meals	Do not use in diarrhea, dysentery, colitis	Excessive doses can cause GI irritation and nausea	166
Boldo, Peumus boldus							
Gastrointestinal spasms with Gallbladder Dyskinesia	Leaves	Tea	2 tsp ground herb in 1 cup boiled water. 1 cup, 2–3 times/day	1–2 tsp dried leaf infused in 1 cup of boiled water for 20 minutes	Do not overdose		183
Buckthorn, Rhamnus cathartica							
Acute constipation in children beyond 12 years	Fruit	Tea	2 tsp berries in 1 cup boiling water. Drink 1–2 cups in the evening	For North America, the dried fruits of cascara (Rhamnus purshiana) or California coffee berry	Do not use over longer times; during pregnancy or nursing; in obstructive diseases of the	1–2 weeks is the usual period of use for acute constipation; excessive doses can cause	253

Table 5 Continued

Disease/Condition	Part of Plant Used in Therapy	Recommended Form	Recommended German Dosage	Recommended US Dosage	Warnings	Notes	See Page
Buckthorn, _Rhamnus cathartica_ (continued)							
				(_R. californica_) will also serve	bowels; in acute enteritis	intestinal cramps, especially in susceptible individuals	42
Constipation	Fruit	Tea	4 g berries (1 tsp) in 1 cup boiled water. One cup morning and night. Daily dose: 2–5 g	See above	Do not use over longer times; during pregnancy or nursing; in obstructive diseases of the bowels; in acute enteritis		
Butcher's broom, _Ruscus aculeatus_							
Hemorrhoids. Varicose veins	Root	Externally	7–11 mg total ruscogenins/day. Use commercial products as directed	Use commercial products as directed		Commercial creams are available, for instance standardized to 22 % sterolic heterosides	43

	Internally		Tablets or capsules: standardized extract (9 % to 11 % ruscogenin) 100 mg 3 times/day	100–200 mg total ruscogenins/day. Use commercial products as directed			43

Calamus (Sweetflag), *Acorus calmus*

Dyspeptic complaints	Root	Tea	1–1.5 g (2 tsp) herb in 150 mL boiled water. One cup with each meal	Make an infusion from 1–3 g of the dried rhizome. Drink 1 cup after meals	Do not use long-term	Avoid during pregnancy	44
Induce local hyperemia, to treat exhaustion	Root	Bath additive	250–500 g as infusion in bath water	Same			44
Anorexia in severe organic diseases such as cancer	Root	Tincture	20 to drops in a glass of water, 15–30 minutes before meals, 3 times/day	1–3 mL (1 : 5 tincture) in a little water; drink after meals	Do not use long term	North American calamus root (as opposed to Asian or European material) is reported to have little or no β-asarone, a known mutagen	168
Subacute and chronic proctitis	Root	Irrigation	2 tsp in 150 mL water	Same			188

Table 5 Continued

Disease/Condition	Part of Plant Used in Therapy	Recommended Form	Recommended German Dosage	Recommended US Dosage	Warnings	Notes	See Page
Calamus (Sweetflag), *Acorus calmus* (continued)							
Blunt trauma, iatrogenic wounds	Root	Compress	Apply locally to affected area for 1–2 hours, 3 times/day. Do not cover with airtight material	Simmer 3–5 g of the dried rhizome in 1 quart of water for 20 minutes on low heat in a covered pot; soak a washcloth and apply hot			279
		Liniment	Apply 3 times/day. Especially effective when warmed prior to use	Same			
Camphor, *Cinnamomum camphora*							
Cardiac arrhythmias. Coughs and bronchitis. Low blood pressure. Nervous heart disorders. Rheumatic complaints	Bark → camphor	Ointment; liniment	Apply to skin several times/day	Same	Do not use during pregnancy and in infants and children. May cause allergic dermatitis	Commercial products such as Vick's Vap-o-Rub, Tiger Balm, Blistex Medicated Lip Ointment, Chapstick, Ben-Gay, Campho-Phenique, Deep-Down Pain Relief Rub all contain camphor	45

		Spirit	9.5 – 10.5 % Camphor (DAB 10). Apply to skin several times/day	Same	Do not use during pregnancy and in infants and children. May cause allergic dermatitis	See above	45
Acute bronchitis	Bark → camphor	Inhalation	Apply to skin or use for inhalations several times/day	Same	Do not use during pregnancy and in infants and children. May cause allergic dermatitis	See above	157
Muscle pain and tension; sore muscles; pulled muscles and contusions; massages after sports; connective-tissue massages	Bark → camphor	Tincture	Apply up to 4 times/day	Same	Do not use during pregnancy and in infants and children. May cause allergic dermatitis	See above	234

Caraway, *Carum carvi*

Roemheld's complex with poor evacuation of the bowels	Fruit	Tea	1 – 2 tsp in 1 cup of boiling water. 1 cup mornings and evenings	Same		Boil water, turn off head, steep for 15 minutes, strain and drink	178
Dyspeptic complaints	Essential oil	Oil	1 – 2 drops on sugar, 3 – 6 drops/day	Same		Or add 1 – 2 drops to a cup of peppermint tea	176

5

Disease/Condition	Part of Plant Used in Therapy	Recommended Form	Recommended German Dosage	Recommended US Dosage	Warnings	Notes	See Page
Caraway, *Carum carvi* (continued)							
	Fruit	Tea	1–2 tsp (1.5 g) crushed in 150 mL water. Daily dose 1.5–6 g herb	Same			176
Severely distended and painful stomach	Essential oil	Oil	2–3 drops in water at meal times	Same		Use warm water for best results	176
	Fruit	Tea	Pour 1 cup of boiled water onto 1 tsp crushed seeds. 1 cup at or after meals	Same			176
Chronic meteorism in children	Essential oil	Tincture	Massage into stomach region, up to 3 times/day.	Same		Or use a tincture of caraway seeds	176
Cayenne, *Capsicum annuum*							
Muscular tension. Rheumatic diseases	Fruit	Tincture	(1 : 10). Apply to affected area several times/day	Same	Do not overdose		47

Condition	Part	Preparation	Dosage		Page
Itching (pruritus)	Fruit	Tincture	(1:10) Massage a few drops onto affected area several times/day	Same	273
				Cayenne pepper is a common ingredient in tinctures and liniments; may cause burning at first, but this feeling usually subsides after a few days of use	

Chamomile, *Chamomilla recutita*

Condition	Part	Preparation	Dosage		Page
Angina tonsillaris	Flowers	Extract	10 drops in 1 glass water, or apply directly to affected sites. Rinse the mouth and gargle	10 drops of a 1 : 5 tincture in 2 mL of water. Gargle every hour or two	163
Angina tonsillaris	Flowers	Tincture	20–30 drops in 1 glass water. Gargle	Same	163
Acute gastritis and esophagitis (in viral infection); ulcers with nocturnal pain and localized epigastric hunger pain	Flowers	Tea	2–3 cups from 15–30 g of the dried flowers before eating in the morning	Use 15–30 g of the dried flowers as a daily dose	171
		Extract	To be taken before eating in the morning according to the recommendations of the producer	Take 3–4 cups of the strong tea made with up to 30 g of the dried flowers throughout the day	171

Table 5 Continued

Chamomile, *Chamomilla recutita* (continued)

Disease/Condition	Part of Plant Used in Therapy	Recommended Form	Recommended German Dosage	Recommended US Dosage	Warnings	Notes	See Page
Acute hemorrhoidal inflammation	Flowers	Extract	1 tsp in 500 mL water, external use	1 tsp of the 1:5 tincture, or soak a cloth in strong tea made from up to 30 g of the dried flowers/day in 4 ounces of warm water			188
Acute proctitis	Flowers	Irrigation	1 tsp herb in 150 mL water	Same			187
Abnormal bacterial flora	Flowers	Tea	1 cup strong tea, sweetened with 1 to 2 tsp lactose, 3–4 times/day	Same			192
Abdominal or intestinal cramps; flatulence	Flowers	Wrap	1 tbsp dried flower, ½ L boiling water; steep for 5 minutes, strain and keep warm. 20–30 minutes until wrap has cooled	Use 1–3 tbsp for ½ quart of water			300

Stomach complaints in children	Flowers	Tea	Pour 150 ml boiling water onto 2 heaped tsp herb	Same	For infants, make a light infusion and give 1–3 droppersful as needed	252
Colds and fever; coughs and bronchitis; decreased resistance to infections	Flowers	Tea	1 tbsp (3 g) in 1 cup hot water. One cup, freshly prepared, between meals, 3–4 times/day	Steep for 15–20 minutes, strain and drink warm	48
Acute rhinitis	Flowers	Drops or cream	Apply to each nostril, 3–4 times/day	Use cream, or add several drops of chamomile blue oil to an unscented cream base	148
	Flowers	Tea	2–3 tbsp dried flower, 1 tsp extract, or 5 drops of essential oil in boiling water, inhale several times daily	Steam of dried flowers contains very little essential oil; use pure essential oil (chamomile blue) for best results	148
Inflammation of the skin	Flowers	Bath additive	50 g herb in 1 L hot water. Steam bath: Pour hot water onto ca. 6 g herb	Same	48
Inflammations of the mouth and throat	Flowers	Mouthwash and gargle	Rinse with fresh tea several times/day.	Same	48

Dosages

5

Table 5 Continued

Disease/Condition	Part of Plant Used in Therapy	Recommended Form	Recommended German Dosage	Recommended US Dosage	Warnings	Notes	See Page
Chamomile, *Chamomilla recutita* (continued)							
Inflammations of the mouth and throat in children	Flowers	Gargle	Pour 250 mL boiling water onto 2 tsp herb	Same			248
Eczema	Flowers	Compress	Apply to affected areas 3 times/day for 1–2 hours, replace as soon as it becomes warm and dry	Same		Use a strong infusion	266
Chaste tree, *Vitex agnus castus*							
Menopausal complaints. Premenstrual syndrome (PMS)	Fruit	Extract	30–40 mg/day	Use a 1 : 5 tincture (1–2 mL, morning and evening) or a standardized extract in capsules or tablets (for instance 400 mg standardized to 5000 ppm agnuside/6000 ppm aucubin), take 1 capsule daily between meals	Do not use during pregnancy or nursing; in breast cancer		44

PMS		Oral	1 mL tincture first thing in the morning	Same as above	Do not use during pregnancy or nursing; in breast cancer	49

Chinese rhubarb, *Rheum palmatum*

Constipation	Rhubarb root	Tablets	2, 4, or 6 tablets each evening, as necessary	Same	Do not use during pregnancy or nursing; abdominal pain of unclear origin; acute inflammatory bowel disease; or in children younger than 12 years	196
Moderate constipaton	Rhubarb root	Tea	1 tsp powdered root in 1 cup boiling water. Sweeten to taste with honey, licorice or sweetener. 2 cups each evening	The traditional Chinese medical dose is 3–12 g a day in a decoction, often with other herbs	Do not use during pregnancy or nursing; abdominal pain of unclear origin; acute inflammatory bowel disease; or in children younger than 12 years	198

Table 5 Continued

Cinquefoil (Tormentil), *Potentilla erecta*

Disease/Condition	Part of Plant Used in Therapy	Recommended Form	Recommended German Dosage	Recommended US Dosage	Warnings	Notes	See Page
Inflammation and mild suppuration of the gums	Rhizome	Tincture	Apply undiluted to gums, 2–3 times/day	Same			161
Chronic gingivitis and periodontal disease	Rhizome	Tincture	Dilute 1 tsp in 1 glass of water and rinse or apply undiluted to gums, 2–3 times/day	Same			161
Inflammations of the mouth and throat	Rhizome	Tincture	(1 : 10) Gargle with 10–20 drops in a glass of water, several times/day or apply undiluted to affected areas	Same			121
Diarrhea	Rhizome	Tea	3–4 g in 150 mL hot water One cup, between meals, 2–3 times/day Daily dose: 4–6 g herb	Same			121
Subacute and chronic proctitis	Rhizome	Irrigation	1 tsp tincture in 1 cup of chamomile tea	Same			188

Clove, *Syzygium aromaticum*

Inflammations of the mouth and throat	Flower buds	Mouthwash/gargle	Solution 1–5% oil, several times/day	Add several drops of clove oil to each 1 mL of peppermint or myrrh tincture; add to 4 ounces of water and gargle	49
Topical pain reliever in dental medicine	Flower buds	Oil	Undiluted	Apply 1–3 drops of clove oil to affected tooth as needed	50
Acute stomatitis (painful)	Essential oil	Mouthwash or gargle	1 tbsp in a cup of water, 3–10 times/day	Add several drops of clove oil to each 1 mL of peppermint or myrrh tincture; add to 4 ounces of water and gargle	162

Coffee, *Coffea arabica*

Migraine headaches. Decreased performance	Seed	Coffee	500 mg caffeine/day		One cup (150 mL) of brewed coffee contains about 60–150 mg of caffeine; a cup of tea contains about 50 mg; 2 tablets of Excedrin contain about 130 mg	51

Table 5 Continued

Disease/Condition	Part of Plant Used in Therapy	Recommended Form	Recommended German Dosage	Recommended US Dosage	Warnings	Notes	See Page
Coffee, *Coffea arabica* (continued)							
Diarrhea. Inflammations of the mouth and throat. Gingivitis and periodontal diseases. Diseases of the lips, mouth and tongue	Coffee charcoal (roasted outer parts of seed)	Powder	Daily dose: 9 g ground herb. One dose = 3 g powder	Same			51
Comfrey, *Symphytum officinale*							
Leg ulcerations	Root	Ointment	Apply locally to edges of ulcer	Same	Do not use during pregnancy and nursing. Use only on intact skin	Allantoin, the cell-proliferant, wound-healing compound from comfrey is not soluble in oil; neither is the mucilage; It is recommended to use a comfrey cream (like the one from Bioforce), rather than an oil-based ointment that contains neither of these compounds	281

Blunt trauma		Root	Compress	Apply locally to affected area for 1–2 hours, 3 times/day. Do not cover with airtight material	Same	Do not use during pregnancy and nursing, use only on intact skin	Crush fresh comfrey root or leaves, or soak dried roots until soft; blend with enough water to make a liquidy paste; apply as indicated and wrap with a cloth soaked in the tea as indicated	279
Condurango, *Marsdenia condurango*							
Anorexia. Dyspeptic complaints		Bark	Drink	One cup of tea or one liqueur glassful condurango wine 30 min. before meals. Daily dose 2–4 g herb	Make a tea with 2–4 g or add 2–4 mL of the 1 : 5 tincture to 2–4 ounces of water and drink several times daily before meals		52
Coriander, *Coriandrum sativum*							
Anorexia; dyspeptic complaints	Fruit	Tea	1 g fresh herb in 150 mL water. One cup, between meals, 3 times/day. Daily dose: 3 g herb	Same	Make an infusion.		175

Table 5 Continued

Dandelion, *Taraxacum officinale*

Disease/Condition	Part of Plant Used in Therapy	Recommended Form	Recommended German Dosage	Recommended US Dosage	Warnings	Notes	See Page
Chronic biliary dyskinesia with dyspepsia and anorexia	Root and aerial parts	Tea	1–2 tsp chopped herb in 1 cup cold water, boil. 1 cup each morning and evening for 4–6 weeks	Simmer 2–8 g for 30 minutes, steep for 15 minutes, strain; Drink 1–3 cups a day after meals. Chinese medical dose is 9–30 g of the roots and leaves together as a daily dose prepared by decoction.			54
Chronic biliary dyskinesia, dyspepsia. Anorexia	Root and aerial parts	Tincture	20 drops in water after the noon and evening meals	5–10 mL (1 : 5 tincture) in a little water, several times a day before meals	Do not use in biliary obstructive disease		185
		Juice	Adults 1 tbsp after meals, 2–3 times/day. Children 1 tsp after meals, 2–3 times/day	1–2 tsp before meals	Do not use in biliary obstructive disease		185

Indication	Part	Form	Dosage		Contraindication	Page
		Tablets	1–2 tablets with water or dissolve in water and drink	Follow manufacturer's directions; potency and formulation of dandelion leaf and root product in capsules and tablets vary	Do not use in biliary obstructive disease	Standardized extracts are available, for instance taraxacin	185
		Tea	3–4 g (1 tbsp) chopped herb in 150 mL water. One cup morning and at night	Decoct 6–9 g as a daily dose	Do not use in biliary obstructive disease	185
Irritable bladder	Root and aerial parts	Tea	1 cup, 3–5 times/day	See above	Do not use in biliary obstructive disease	204

Devil's claw, *Harpagophytum procumbens*

Indication	Part	Form	Dosage		Contraindication	Page
Anorexia. Dyspeptic complaints. Supportive treatment of degenerative diseases of connective tissue	Root	Tea	4.5 g (1 tsp) in 300 mL boiled water. Divide into 3 portions to be taken throughout the day. Daily dose: 4.5 g	Same	Do not use during pregnancy and nursing and in gastric or duodenal ulcers	95
Anorexia. Dyspeptic complaints. Supportive treatment of degenerative tissue diseases	Root	Tincture	Dilute 1 tbsp with 250 mL water. Use as gargle or compress	2–5 mL (1 : 5 tincture) in a little water, 2–3 times/day	Do not use during pregnancy and nursing and in gastric or duodenal ulcers	95

5

Table 5 Continued

Disease/Condition	Part of Plant Used in Therapy	Recommended Form	Recommended German Dosage	Recommended US Dosage	Warnings	Notes	See Page
Devil's claw, *Harpagophytum procumbens* (continued)							
General rheumatic complaints	Root	Tea	2 cups boiling water onto 1 tbsp finely chopped root. Divide into three portions, to be taken before meals	1.5–3.0 g as a decoction, 2–3 times/ day (up to 9.0 g/day of the dried secondary tubers)	Do not use during pregnancy and nursing and in gastric or duodenal ulcers		55
Dog rose, *Rosa canina*							
Prevention and treatment of upper respiratory tract infections	Fruit (rose hip peel)	Tea	2–5 g herb in 1 cup of boiled water. One cup, several times/day	Same			152
Echinacea (Pale coneflower), *Echinacea pallida*							
To strengthen immune defenses of infection-prone children	Root	Tincture	20–50 drops of tincture several times/day	Same			246
Chronic, recurrent respiratory tract and urinary tract infections	Root	Liquid	30–40 drops, 3–4 times/day	1–3 mL in a little water 2–3 times/ day away from meals			227

Indication	Part	Form	Dosage	Dosage	Notes	Page
		Lozenges, tablets, capsules	1–2 single doses, 3 times/day or as directed			227
During the first symptoms of common cold	Root	Tincture	2–4 mL added to water, taken orally, 4–5 times daily	2–4 mL of the 1:5 tincture in a little water or tea, 4–5 times/day as needed up to 2 weeks	Do not use during pregnancy or in conditions of reduced immune system function due to hematological or virus-induced disorders or due to application of immunosuppressants	153
Supportive treatment of colds or flu-like infections	Root	Tincture	1:5 parts for max. 2 weeks	2–4 mL of the 1:5 tincture in a little water or tea 4–5 times/day as needed up to 2 weeks		153

Echinacea (Purple echinacea, Purple coneflower), *Echinacea purpurea*

Indication	Part	Form	Dosage	Dosage	Notes	Page
Chronic, recurrent respiratory tract and urinary tract infections	Leaves	Liquid	30–40 drops, 3–4 times/day	1–3 mL, 3–4 times a day in a little water for up to 2 weeks	Hypersensitivity to echinacea and related plants; immunosuppression due to	227

5

5

Table 5 Continued

Echinacea (Purple echinacea, Purple coneflower), *Echinacea purpurea* (continued)

Disease/Condition	Part of Plant Used in Therapy	Recommended Form	Recommended German Dosage	Recommended US Dosage	Warnings	Notes	See Page
					application of immunosuppressive drugs; hematological disorders or chronic virus infections		
		Lozenges, tablets, capsules	1–2 single doses, 3 times/day or as directed	Same	Hypersensitivity to echinacea and related plants; immunosuppression due to application of immunosuppressive drugs; hematological disorders or chronic virus infections		227
To strengthen immune defense of infection-prone children	Leaves	Tincture	20–50 drops of tincture several times/day	See above	Hypersensitivity to echinacea and related plants; immunosuppression due to application of immunosuppressive drugs; hematological disorders or chronic virus infections		246

Chronic bronchitis	Leaves	Tincture	2–4 mL added to water, taken orally, 4–5 times/day	Same		157
Colds and fever. Urinary tract infections. Coughs and bronchitis. Decreased resistance to infections. Runny nose. Wounds and burns (external use)	Leaves	Expressed juice	6–9 mL for max. 2 weeks	Same	Hypersensitivity to echinacea and related plants; immunosuppression due to application of immunosuppressive drugs; hematological disorders or chronic virus infections	57
Chronic infections of the upper respiratory tract	Leaves	Liquids	30–40 drops, 3–4 times/day	Many kinds of hydroalcoholic tinctures are available; generally, for acute infections, double the manufacturer's dose for up to a week or 10 days		153
		Solids	1–2 lozenges, tablets or capsules, 3 times/day	Follow the manufacturer's instructions for standardized extracts; up to double dose as needed for up to 10 days		153
Chronic venous ulcers	Leaves	Ointment	Apply locally to edges of ulcer	Follow manufacturer's label instructions	Hypersensitivity to echinacea and related plants	281

Table 5 Continued

Disease/Condition	Part of Plant Used in Therapy	Recommended Form	Recommended German Dosage	Recommended US Dosage	Warnings	Notes	See Page
English ivy, *Hedera helix*							
Coughs and bronchitis	Leaves		Commercial preparations only	Syrups prepared from the fresh, new growth are available			59
English lavender, *Lavandula angustifolia*							
Restless anxiety, pain-related restlessness, difficulty in falling asleep, stress, anxiety. Hypertension. Hyperthyroidism. Postinfarction debility. Terminal illness	Essential oil	Body wash	5 drops lavender oil in ½ cup milk or 1 L lavender infusion (3 tbsp lavender flower in 1 L boiling water for 5 min). 3–4 L warm water	Same			307
Anorexia. Dyspeptic complaints. Circulatory disorders. Nervous complaints and insomnia	Flowers	Tea	1–2 tsp (1–2 g) flowers in 150 mL water. Daily dose: 3–5 g herb (3 cups/day)	Same			59

		Bath additive	100 g flower in 2 L hot water; add to bath water	Same	59
		Infusion for external use	Handful of flowers in 1 L water; boil; add another 1 L water.	Same	59
		Oil	1–4 drops on, e. g., sugar cube	Or add 1–4 drops to hot water or herb tea to avoid sugar	59
Sleep disorders	Flowers	Tea	1 cup water onto 1 tsp herb. 2–3 cups during the day and 1 cup before retiring	Same	59
Nervous anxiety, tension and restlessness	Flowers	Vaporizer	1–2 times daily	Use the essential oil in a commercial vaporizer; inhale the steam for a few minutes, twice daily	212
Nervousness, anxiety, difficulty in falling asleep or sleeping through the night, cough, bronchitis	Essential oil	Compress	1 tbsp 1 % lavender oil or 1 tbsp sunflower or olive oil + 5 drops 100 % lavender oil. Warm compress on hot water bottle. Compress for 30 minutes. Can be left on longer	Same; apply the lavender compress to the affected area and then lay on the hot water bottle	306

5

Table 5 Continued

Disease/Condition	Part of Plant Used in Therapy	Recommended Form	Recommended German Dosage	Recommended US Dosage	Warnings	Notes	See Page
English plantain, *Plantago lanceolata*							
Colds and fever; coughs and bronchitis; runny nose	Aerial parts/leaves	Tea	2–4 g chopped herb in water. 2 tsp = ca. 3 g herb. One cup, several times/day. Daily dose: 3–6 g herb	Simmer 2–4 g of the dried and coarsely cut herb in 1 pint of water. Drink 1 cup 3–5 times a day			60
Catarrhal disorders of the respiratory tract and inflammations of the mouth and throat	Aerial parts/leaves	Juice extract	Mix juice with equal parts honey, boil. 3–6 g/day	Same			60
Inflammations of the mouth and throat	Aerial parts/leaves	Mouthwash/gargle	Rinse mouth several times/day with tea infusion	See above			60
Eucalyptus, *Eucalyptus globulus*							
Cystitis; retention of urine	Essential oil	Compress	1 tbsp 10 % eucalyptus oil or 1 tbsp sunflower or olive oil + 5 drops 100 % eucalyptus oil. Heat compress on hot	Same			303

			water bottle. Duration of treatment 30 minutes, or until wrap becomes too cool. Twice daily			
CAD-related pain	Leaves	Liniment	Apply alcohol-based liniment several times daily			134
Coughs, bronchitis	Leaves	Tea	Infuse 2 – 6 g of the dried leaves in 1 pint of boiled water and drink ½ cup every 2 – 3 hours	1.5 – 2 g in 150 mL water. 4 – 6 g/day		61
Coughs, bronchitis. Rheumatic complaints	Essential oil	Drops	Take 1 – 3 drops of the essential oil in a little water or tea, several times daily	3 – 6 drops in 150 mL water several times/day. Daily dose: 0.3 – 0.6 g (0 – 2 g = 10 drops)	Do not overdose, do not use local applications in children up to 2 years	62
		Inhalation	Same	2 – 3 drops in boiling water	Do not overdose, do not use local applications in children up to 2 years / Commercial steam enhalers are available from pharmacies	62
		Liniment	Same	20 % liniment rubbed onto skin	Do not overdose, do not use local applications in children up to 2 years	62

Table 5 Continued

Disease/Condition	Part of Plant Used in Therapy	Recommended Form	Recommended German Dosage	Recommended US Dosage	Warnings	Notes	See Page
Eucalyptus, *Eucalyptus globulus* (continued)							
Bronchial asthma	Essential oil	Capsules	2 capsules, 3 times/day	Commercial products are available—250 mg containing essential oil in a soybean oil carrier.	Do not overdose		160
European elder, *Sambucus nigra*							
Fever and colds; mild cases of flu. Coughs and bronchitis (supportive)	Flower	Tea	2 tsp (3–4 g) flower in 150 mL water. 1–2 cups, several times/day. Daily dose: 10–15 g herb	Same		Make an infusion	63
European goldenrod, *Solidago virgaurea*							
Irrigation therapy, kidney flush, prevention of urinary calculi and renal gravel	Flowering aerial parts	Tea	1–2 tsp (3–5 g) in 150 mL water. One cup, between meals, 2–4 times/day. Daily dose: 6–12 g/day	Same	Do not use in renal or cardiac edema		64
Dysuria	Flowering aerial parts	Tea	1 cup, 3–5 times/day	Same	Do not use in renal or cardiac edema		202

European mistletoe, *Viscum album*

Cancer-related symptoms	Young twigs including leaves, flowers, and fruit	Commercial preparation as available in Europe	Parenterally, either s.c. or i.v. Dose 0.5 – 1 ng of ML-1* /kg* body weight, 1 – 2 times/ week, for 3 months. Break for 4 – 8 weeks, then repeat cycle	Same	229
Hypertension (adjuvant treatment)	Young twigs including leaves, flowers, and fruit	Tea	Pour 1 cup cold water onto 2.5 g (1 tsp) of chopped herb. 1 – 2 cups/day. Daily dose: 10 g	Same; let the chopped herb and stems infuse in the water overnight	94
				The berries are toxic	
Rheumatism	Young twigs including leaves, flowers, and fruit	Fluid extract	1 : 1. 1 – 3 mL three times/day		94
		Tincture	1 : 5. 0.5 mL three times/day	Take 1 – 2 mL of a 1 : 5 tincture, 2 – 3 times/day	94

* ML-1: Mistletoe lektin-1

5

Table 5 Continued

Fennel, *Foeniculum vulgare* Miller

Disease/Condition	Part of Plant Used in Therapy	Recommended Form	Recommended German Dosage	Recommended US Dosage	Warnings	Notes	See Page
Dyspeptic complaints. Coughs and bronchitis. Catarrh of the upper respiratory tract in children	Fruit (seeds)	Syrup	10–20 g/day	Take 1 tsp as needed after meals up to 3 times	Do not use during pregnancy or in infants and children	Make an elixir by adding 1 ounce of the 1 : 5 hydroalcoholic tincture (at least 75 % ethanol) to 4 ounces of sweet base	65
		Tea	2–5 g in 150 mL water. One cup between meals, 2–4 times/day. Daily dose: 5–7 g	Same			65
	Essential oil	Oil	2–5 drops, diluted in water after meals. 0.1–0.6 mL/day	Same	Do not use during pregnancy or in infants and children		65
	Essential oil, fruit	Tincture	0.8–2 mL (30 drops) 3 times/day	Same	Do not use during pregnancy or in infants and children		65

Digestive problems; flatulence; cramps; hiccups; nausea and vomiting	Essential oil	Wrap	1 tbsp 10% fennel oil or 1 tbsp olive oil + 5 drops 100% fennel oil. Heat on hot water bottle	Add 5–10 drops of fennel essential oil to 1 pint of hot water, stir vigorously; soak cloth in	301
			Compress for 30 minutes. Can be left on longer	solution and apply warm over abdominal area	
Roemheld's complex with poor evacuation of the bowels	Fruit (seeds)	Tea	1–2 tsp in 1 cup of boiling water. 1 cup mornings and evenings.	Therapeutic dose in traditional Chinese medicine is 6–9 g/ day as an infusion: 1 cup twice daily after meals	178
Infant dyspepsia	Fruit (seeds)	Tea	1 cup of boiled water on 1 tsp crushed seeds. 1–2 cups, 5 times/day	Make the infusion as indicated and give 2–3 droppersful (2–3 mL) to 2 tsp by mouth several times a day	192
	Essential oil	Oil	2–4 drops in small amount of water, 5 times/day. 150–200 g/kg body weight/day	Add 1–2 drops of sweet fennel oil to 2 ounces of water and give 1 or 2 droppersful of the solution by mouth after feeds	Do not use during pregnancy or in infants and children	Fennel appears to be safe for infants in moderate doses	192
Flatulence, dyspepsia, or diarrhea in infants	Fruit (seeds)	Tea	2 tsp crushed herb in 150 mL boiling water	Drink 1 cup several times a day after meals		252

5

5 Table 5 Continued

Disease/Condition	Part of Plant Used in Therapy	Recommended Form	Recommended German Dosage	Recommended US Dosage	Warnings	Notes	See Page
Fenugreek, *Trigonella foenum-graecum*							
Furuncles (boils)	Seed	Poultice	50 g with 1 L warm water. Apply to affected areas	Same			271
Flax, *Linum usatissimum*							
Constipation	Seeds (linseed)	Seeds	1 tbsp whole or crushed flaxseed taken in 150 mL water 2–3 times/day	Same	Do not use in acute enteritis, or in obstructive intestinal diseases	Use a coffee grinder to powder seeds freshly for each dose; store seeds whole	66
Chronic constipation	Seeds (linseed)	Medication	2–4 tbsp mixed with stewed fruit, hot cereal, etc. 1–3 times/day	Same	Do not use in acute enteritis or in obstructive intestinal disease	Coarsly grind the seeds before use	199
Chronic gastritis, chronic enteritis	Seeds (linseed)	Gruel	2–3 tbsp ground or chopped seed	Soak 2–3 tsp in a cup of warm water and drink morning and evening	Do not use in acute enteritis, or in obstructive intestinal diseases		66

Chronic esophagitis, chronic gastritis	Seeds (linseed)	Gruel	2 tbsp in ½ L water and boil; strain. 3–4 sips, several times/day	Same	Do not use in acute enteritis, and in obstructive intestinal diseases	172
Acute proctitis	Seeds (linseed)	Irrigation	1 tsp herb in 150 mL water	Same	Grind the seeds in a coffee grinder, infuse in warm water for 30 minutes, strain and use as a rectal irrigation	187
Inflammatory skin diseases	Seeds (linseed)	Poultice	Mix 125 g flaxseed with 1 cup water. Apply hot, wet poultice to affected area twice daily	Same		66
Furuncles (boils)	Seeds (linseed)	Compress	Small linen bag one-third filled with linseed, sewn together, then boiled briefly. Squeeze gently and apply to affected areas while as hot as possible	Same		271
Sinusitis, i.e., inflammation of nasal and/or frontal sinuses. Dermatitis	Seeds (linseed)	Poultice	300 g linseed (whole or cracked) in 600 mL water. Bring to boil. Makes 6–8 poultices. 20–30 minutes, 1–3 times daily	Same	Coarsly grind the seeds for quicker extraction	292

Table 5 Continued

Disease/Condition	Part of Plant Used in Therapy	Recommended Form	Recommended German Dosage	Recommended US Dosage	Warnings	Notes	See Page
Frangula (Alder buckthorn), *Rhamnus frangula*							
Chronic constipation	Bark	Extract	20–40 drops each evening	Take 2–5 mL of the tincture morning and evening as needed for occasional constipation; for more than 10 days, reduce to 1–2 mL	Do not use during pregnancy and nursing; in children younger than 12 years; acute enteritis. No long-term application		198
Constipation	Bark	Tea	2 g in 150 mL water. One cup mornings and evenings	Same	Do not use during pregnancy and nursing; in children younger than 12 years; acute enteritis. No long-term application		67
	Bark	Suspension	0.6 g content	Same	Do not use during pregnancy and nursing; in children younger than 12 years; acute enteritis. No long-term application		67

Fumitory, *Fumaria officinalis*

Gastrointestinal spasms with gall bladder dyskinesia	Flowering aerial parts	Tea	2 tsp herb in 1 cup boiled water. 1 cup with meals, 3 times/day	Make an infusion by adding 4–8 g to a quart of water; strain. Drink 1 cup 3 times/day	183
Liver and gallbladder complaints. Cholelithiasis. Cholecystitis. Diseases of the liver. Other diseases of the gallbaldder/biliary tract	Flowering aerial parts	Tea	2–3 g in 150 mL water. 1 cup/day 30 minutes before meals	Same as above	68
		Juice	2–3 tsp/day, cold infusion (maceration) or hot infusion. (2.4–3.5 g/day)	Same	68
		Tincture	1 : 5, 75% menstruum with dried herb. 2–4 mL 3 times/day	Same	68
		Triturated plant material	1 tsp, 3 times/day. Daily dose 6 g	Same	68

5

Table 5 Continued

Disease/Condition	Part of Plant Used in Therapy	Recommended Form	Recommended German Dosage	Recommended US Dosage	Warnings	Notes	See Page
Garlic, *Allium sativum*							
Prevention of arteriosclerosis. Mild hypertension. Minor infections.	Bulb	Oral	4 g fresh garlic, i.e., 1–2 fresh bulbs per day or corresponding dose of commercial preparation (garlic powder)	Crush 1–2 cloves of fresh garlic and let stand in the air for 15 minutes; mix into food and eat daily. 1–2 capsules of a commercial preparation standardized to "allicin potential" daily	Do not use during nursing. May cause reduced thrombocyte function in high doses	Aged garlic is not effective for antibiotic or antiparasitic effects; may be useful for cardiovascular benefits, but not as good as fresh garlic	70
Ginger, *Zingiber officinale* Rosc.							
Anorexia. Travel sickness. Dyspeptic complaints	Rhizome	Tea	0.5–1 g powder in boiled water, or sliced fresh rhizome, strained (1 tsp = ca. 3 g) One dose 0.3–1.5 g. Daily dose: 2–5 g	3–9 g of the dried herb as a daily dose, taken twice daily is the traditional Chinese medical dose. Use 2–4 g for mild-moderate symptoms	Do not use for vomiting during pregnancy	Fresh ginger tea is not contraindicated during pregnancy for relieving morning sickness according to the most reliable traditional Chinese medical sources. Do not take dried ginger or extracts during pregnancy	71

Anorexia and insufficient peristalsis	Rhizome	Tea	Pour 1 cup of hot water on to 1 tsp powdered herb. 1 cup 15–30 minutes before meals	Same, but preferably use dried and coarsely cut dried rhizome	Do not use for vomiting during pregnancy	See above	167
		Tincture	10–20 drops in ½–1 glass water. 15–30 minutes before meals	0.5–3.0 mL of the tincture in a little water, depending on the strength of the preparation; otherwise as indicated	Do not use for vomiting during pregnancy	See above	167
Chronic joint disease; rheumatism; gout; back pain; muscle tension; shoulder pain; acute shoulder-arm syndrome. Psoriasis with joint involvement. To promote excretion. Chronic bronchitis	Rhizome	Wrap	3 tbsp fresh grated rhizome or 2 tbsp powdered dry root. Steep in 500 mL hot water. Dip cotton cloth in ginger water until completely soaked. Apply to treated area after treatment. Once daily	Steep ginger in boiled water for 30 minutes, or simmer lightly for 15 minutes and steep for 20 minutes for stronger tea. Apply compress wet; after the compress cools it should get hot again from the action of the ginger for full effectiveness			309

5

Table 5 Continued

Disease/Condition	Part of Plant Used in Therapy	Recommended Form	Recommended German Dosage	Recommended US Dosage	Warnings	Notes	See Page
Ginkgo, *Ginkgo biloba*							
Symptomatic treatment of cerebro-organic impairment of mental performance	Leaves	Ginkgo biloba extract	120–240 mg divided into 2–3 portions daily	Same			72
Vertigo. Tinnitus. Circulatory disorders	Leaves	Ginkgo biloba extract	120–160 mg/day, divided into 2–3 portions daily	Same			72
Grape, *Vitis vinifera*							
Chronic venous insufficiency	Red leaves	Ointment	Apply gently to affected areas, several times/day	Same			146
Grass flowers* , *Graminis flos*							
Rheumatic pain	Flowering parts	Compress	Heat to 42 °C and apply to affected area for 40 minutes	Same			308

---

* Grass flowers are probably commercially not available in North America. Substitute Wild Oats (*Avena fatua* or *Avena sativa*).

Indication	Part	Form	Preparation	Children	Notes	Page
		Bath additive	Add 500 g to 4–5 L of water and boil. Strain and add to bathwater	Same		286
Rheumatoid diseases; muscle tension; arthrosis. Menstrual cramping. Chronic liver disease. Vegetative dystonia	Flowering parts	Pillow	Half-fill cloth bag with flowers. Sew ends. Pour water into pot and heat to boiling. Steam-heat pillow for 30 minutes. Apply pillow for 20–40 minutes, until too cool. 1–2 times daily	Same		286
Muscle pain and tension, sore muscles, pulled muscles and contusions, massages after sports, connective tissue massages	Hay flower	Tincture	Apply up to 4 times/day	Same		286

Guarana, *Paulina cupana*

Indication	Part	Form	Preparation	Children	Notes	Page
Headache	Seeds	Drops	5–10 drops every 30 minutes, up to 20 drops if necessary. For chronic pain, 5–10 drops, 3 times/day	Same	Do not overdose, especially if coffeine-sensitive	219

5

Table 5 Continued

Disease/Condition	Part of Plant Used in Therapy	Recommended Form	Recommended German Dosage	Recommended US Dosage	Warnings	Notes	See Page
Hawthorn, *Crataegus laevigata*							
Functional heart disorders	Leaves and flowers	Tincture	15 drops, 3 times/day	1–2 mL, 3 times/day in a little water		In addition to standard treatment	137
Supportive treatment of heart failure (NYHA class I–II). Strengthening tonic for prevention of heart irregularities and congestive heart failure	Leaves and flowers	Extract	One dose 2–3 times/day. Daily dose: 900 mg extract	Standardized extract is commonly recommended. The dose of a product containing 1.8% vitexin-4 rhamnoside is 100–250 mg, 3 times/day			74
CAD	Leaves and flowers	Extract	One oral dose 2–3 times/day. Daily dose ca. 900 mg	Standardized extract is commonly recommended. The dose of a product containing 1.8% vitexin-4 rhamnoside is 100–250 mg, 3 times/day		In addition to standard treatment	135
Prevention and treatment of early-stage CAD; mild hypertension	Leaves and flowers	Tea	2 tsp herb in 150 boiling water. 2 times/day	4–6 g dried leaves and flowers simmered in 1 pint water for 30 minutes. Drink ½–1 cup, twice daily		Rather weak preparation	135

Prevention and treatment of early-stage CAD	Leaves and flowers	Extract	1–2 capsules or tablets	Standardized extract is commonly recommended. The dose of a product containing 1.8 % vitexin-4 rhamnoside is 100–250 mg, 3 times/day	135
		Tincture	10–20 drops	1–2 mL, 3 times/ day in a little water	

Heartsease (Wild pansy), *Viola tricolor*

Skin inflammations	Flowering aerial parts	Compress	1 tsp chopped herb in 1 cup hot water. Apply to affected areas of skin	Same	75
Dermatitis	Flowering aerial parts	Compress	1 tsp chopped herb in 1 cup hot water. Apply 2–3 times/ day	Same	273
Itching (pruritus), especially in elderly people	Flowering aerial parts	Compress	1 tsp chopped herb in 1 cup hot water; strain	Same	273
Allergy, eczema-related itching, itching associated with liver or kidney diseases	Flowering aerial parts	Body wash	Steep 3 tbsp wild pansy in 1 L boiling water for 5 minutes. Add 3–4 L cold water to yield	Same	320

Disease/Condition	Part of Plant Used in Therapy	Recommended Form	Recommended German Dosage	Recommended US Dosage	Warnings	Notes	See Page
Heartsease (Wild pansy), *Viola tricolor* (continued)							
			a water temperature of 30–35 °C. Wash 1–3 times daily, depending on the severity of symptoms				
High mallow, *Malva sylvestris*							
Coughs and bronchitis. Inflammations of the mouth and throat	Flowers	Tea	1.5–2 g chopped herb in 1 cup boiled water 1 cup 2–3 times/day. Daily dose: 5 g herb	Same		Fresh flowers are preferred if available	89
Coughs and bronchitis. Inflammations of the mouth and throat	Leaves	Tea	3–5 g (2 tsp) in 150 mL water. One cup, 1–2 times/day. Daily dose: 5 g herb	Same			90
Acute stomatitis (with less severe pain). Pharyngitis	Leaves	Tea as mouthwash or gargle	3–6 times/day	2–3 tsp herb as an infusion in 150 mL water, filter and use as a gargle			162

Chronic stomatitis; chronic pharyngitis; smoker's catarrh	Leaves	Demulcent mouthwash		Same as above		163
Acute proctitis	Flowers	Irrigation	1 tsp herb in 150 mL water	2–3 tsp as an infusion, filter and use as an irrigation		187
Hops, _Humulus lupulus_						
Insomnia, nervous tension	Cones	Tea	1–2 g single dose before retiring	Infuse 2–4 g of the dried female cones in a pint of water for 20 minutes, strain. Drink 1 cup before bed	Combine with other herbal sleep-inducers	76
Nervous tension	Cones	Tincture	1–2 mL one dose	2–4 mL in a little water as needed		76
Nervous tension	Cones	Tea	2–3 cups (1 tbsp) during the daytime and before retiring	Infuse 2–4 g of the dried female cones in a pint of water for 20 minutes; strain. Drink 1 cup 2–3 times/day		76
Sleep disorders	Cones	Tea	Pour 1 cup water onto 1 tsp herbs. 2–3 cups during the day and 1 cup before retiring	Infuse 2–4 g of the dried female cones in a pint of water for 20 minutes; strain. Drink 1 cup 2–3 times/day; 1 cup before bed	Hops acts as a diuretic which can cause wakefulness during the night for some individuals. Combine with other sleep-inducing herbs	210

5

Table 5 Continued

Disease/Condition	Part of Plant Used in Therapy	Recommended Form	Recommended German Dosage	Recommended US Dosage	Warnings	Notes	See Page
Horehound, _Marrubium vulgare_							
Coughs and bronchitis. Inflammations of the mouth and throat	Aerial parts	Cough lozenges. Syrup	2–4 mL 3 times/day	Follow the directions on commercial lozenges and syrups containing horehound	Do not use during pregnancy	The herb is extremely bitter and most manufacturers keep total concentration low, limiting effectiveness	76
Anorexia, dyspeptic complaints	Aerial parts	Syrup	2–6 tbsp/day	Follow the directions on commercial syrups containing horehound	Do not use during pregnancy	The herb is extremely bitter and most manufacturers keep total concentration low, limiting effectiveness	76
Horse chestnut, _Aesculus hippocastanus_							
Anal fissures	Seeds	Ointment	Topical application as needed	Follow label directions on commercial products	Do not use in children younger than 12 years		188
Complaints associated with chronic venous insufficiency. Posttraumatic or postoperative soft-tissue swelling	Seeds	Ointment	Apply gently to skin. Daily dose: 100 mg of aescin	Follow label directions on commercial products.	Do not use in children younger than 12 years		77

Chronic venous insufficiency	Seeds	Extract	One oral 50 mg dose, twice/day	Standardized extracts usually contain about 50 mg of aescin (16–20%) for each capsule or tablet; take 1–3/day with food	146

Horseradish, _Armoracia rusticana_

Sinusitis, i. e., inflammation of the nasal and/or frontal sinuses, cough and bronchitis	Root	Poultice	2 tbsp grated root at room temperature, wrapped in compress. Wipe sparingly with olive oil afterwards. Initially 2–5 minutes, 1–2 times daily	Same	293
Cystitis	Root	Poultice	4 tbsp grated root. Spread 1–2 cm thick layer of grated horseradish onto compress. Fold over edges and secure with tape. Leave on no longer than 4–5 mins, check for skin irritation. Wipe skin with olive oil	Same	304

Table 5 Continued

Disease/Condition	Part of Plant Used in Therapy	Recommended Form	Recommended German Dosage	Recommended US Dosage	Warnings	Notes	See Page
Horsetail, *Equisetum arvense*							
Inflammatory skin diseases	Sterile green stems	Bath additive	100 g herb to 10 L of bathwater. Boil herb for 5–10 minutes in small amount of water, then steep for 15 minutes. Strain and add to bathwater	Same			
Urinary tract infections; renal or urinary calculi	Sterile green stems	Tea	2–3 g herb in 150–200 mL water One cup, beween meals, several times/day Daily dose: 6 g herb	Traditional dose in Chinese medical prescriptions is 3–9 g of the dried herb as a decoction, twice daily	Do not use in cardiac or renal edema		
Dysuria, irritable bladder	Sterile green stems	Tea	1 cup (2–3 g herb), 3–5 times/day	Make a decoction with 3–9 g of the dried herb and drink a cup several times a day			78
Wounds and burns	Sterile green stems	Compress	10 g in 1 L water	Make a decoction, soak a cloth with the strong tea and apply to minor wounds and burns			78

Iceland moss, *Cetraria islandica*

	Iceland moss	Tea	1.5–2.5 g (1–2 tsp) chopped in boiled water. Daily dose: 4–6 g herb. One dose = 1.5 g herb	Same		79
Anorexia. Dyspeptic complaints. Coughs and bronchitis. Inflammations of the mouth and throat						

Indian plantain, *Plantago ovata*

	Seed, husks	Medication	2 tsp, 3 times/day for 1–3 days. Afterwards, 3 times/day as needed	Same	Do not use without enough water; in people with swallowing problems; in obstructive disease of the intestines	192
Recurrent diarrhea						
Preternatural anus	Seed, husks	Medication	Swallow 1–2 tsp whole, with at least 1 glass water	Same	Do not use without enough water; in people with swallowing problems; in obstructive disease of the intestines	193
Crohn's disease	Seed, husks	Medication	Granulated husks: Take 1 tsp or 1 packet, mixed with a glass of water, 2–6 times/day	Same	Do not use without enough water; in people with swallowing problems; in obstructive disease of the intestines	193

5

Table 5 Continued

Disease/Condition	Part of Plant Used in Therapy	Recommended Form	Recommended German Dosage	Recommended US Dosage	Warnings	Notes	See Page
Indian plantain, *Plantago ovata* (continued)							
Chronic constipation. Hyperlipidemia	Seed, husks		Commercial products as directed	Same	Do not use without enough water; in people with swallowing problems; in obstructive disease of the intestines		106
Irritable bowel syndrome, diverticulosis	Husks	Medication	2 tsp granulated product with at least 1–2 glasses water, 1 hour before retiring. Additional dose of 1 tsp before breakfast, if necessary	Same	Do not use in severe diabetes mellitus, inflammatory bowel disease, or obstruction in the intestinal tract		195
Java tea, *Orthosiphon aristatus*							
Urinary tract infections. Renal or urinary calculi	Leaves	Tea	2 g herb in 150 mL water One cup, several times/day Daily dose: 6–12 g herb	Same	Do not use in cardiac or renal edema		80
Dysuria, irritable bladder	Leaves	Tea	1 cup, 3–5 times/day	Same	Do not use in cardiac or renal edema		204

Juniper, *Juniperus communis*

Anorexia. Dyspeptic complaints. For aquaresis in unspecific inflammations of the lower urinary tract	Fruit (berries)	Infusion	1 tsp berries in 1 cup of boiled water. One cup, 3 times/ day. 2 – 10 g (maximum dose) herb, corresponding to 20 – 100 mg of the essential oil	Same	Do not overdose. Do not use during pregnancy and in inflammatory renal diseases	81
	Fruit (berries)	Tincture	20 – 30 drops, 2 – 3 times/day. 2 – 10 g (maximum dose) herb, corresponding to 20 – 100 mg of the essential oil	Same	Do not overdose Do not use during pregnancy and in inflammatory renal diseases	81
Blunt trauma	Fruit (berries)	Compress	Apply locally to affected area for 1 – 2 hours, 3 times/day. Do not cover with airtight material	Same	Do not use in dermatitis and wounds	278
		Liniment	Apply 3 times/day. Especially effective when warmed prior to use	Same	Do not use in dermatitis and wounds	278

■ 5 ■

Table 5 Continued

Disease/Condition	Part of Plant Used in Therapy	Recommended Form	Recommended German Dosage	Recommended US Dosage	Warnings	Notes	See Page
Kava, *Piper methysticum*							
Nervous tension, states of tension and anxiety	Rhizome	Extracts	60–120 mg commercially available herb preparations	Tinctures (1–3 mL 2–5 times daily) Tea (6–12 g in decoction, 1 cup several times a day) Standardized extracts (1–2 gel caps extract standardized to 60–80% kava lactones) in capsules or tablets are widely available	Concerns about hepatotoxicity surfaced in 2002 in Europe; some reports to FDA in North America, but not substantiated. Reliable analysis of the case reports by medical experts makes it likely that kava is not hepatotoxic per se, but rare allergic or idiosyncratic reactions are possible, along with confounding interactions with other hepatotoxic substances (i. e. aspirin, alcohol), or that high-potency kava products can possibly create problems when a		82

Nervous anxiety, tension and restlessness	Rhizome		Oral daily dose: 60–120 mg kava pyrones	As above	patient has pre-existing liver disease. Products should be labeled accordingly
					212
Nervous restlessness in older children; anxiety disorders with depression	Rhizome		Use as recommended by manufacturer	As above	See above. Do not use during pregnancy or nursing. Do not use for treatment of depression
					257

Lemon, *Citrus limon*

Budding throat inflammation with difficulty in swallowing, chronic throat inflammation	Fruit	Wrap	1 lemon, 500 mL hot water. Apply wrap to neck until it becomes too cool	Slice or blend lemon in the water, place the hot pulp into a cloth and apply to the affected area until cool	See above
					313

5

Table 5 Continued

Disease/Condition	Part of Plant Used in Therapy	Recommended Form	Recommended German Dosage	Recommended US Dosage	Warnings	Notes	See Page
Lemon balm, *Melissa officinalis*							
General nervousness and sleeplessness	Leaves	Tea	1.5–4.5 g in 1 cup hot water. One cup, several times/day. Daily dose: 1.5–4.5 g herb	2–5 g of the dried flowering tops are infused for 20 minutes in boiled water in a covered pot. Drink 4–5 cups a day as needed.		Mild in nature, use *ad libitum* within reason.	84
Sleep disorders	Leaves	Tea	Pour 1 cup water onto 1 tsp herbs. 2–3 cups during the day and 1 cup before retiring	Same as above			210
Nervousness and sleep disorders	Leaves	Bath additive	10 g leaves in 2 L hot water for 5 minutes. Strain and add to bathwater	Same			285
Nervousness, tension and restlessness	Leaves	Spirit	2 tsp in 150 mL water daily	Same		The spirit of melissa contains 75 % ethanol; contraindicated for alcoholics and patients with liver disorders	212

Anxiety-related heart consciousness or stomach complaints	Leaves	Tea	1–2 tsp in 150 mL boiling water. Drink warm before retiring, sweeten with honey if desired	2–5 g of the dried flowering tops are infused for 20 minutes in boiled water in a covered pot. Drink 4–5 cups a day as needed	137
Herpes simplex labialis	Leaves	Creme	10–20 mg creme per cm² of affected skin, 2–4 times/day	Apply moderately to the affected areas several times a day	164

Lesser centaury, *Centaurium minus*

Anorexia. Dyspeptic complaints	Flowering aerial parts	Tea	2–3 g in 150 mL boiled water, ½ hour before meals. Up to 6 g/day	Same	Do not use in gastric or duodenal ulcers	85
	Flowering aerial parts	Tincture	1 : 5 tincture: 2–5 g/day	20 drops to 2 mL in a little water (1 : 5 tincture), before meals	Do not use in gastric or duodenal ulcers	85
Chronic stomatitis; chronic pharyngitis; smoker's catarrh; persistent "lump" in the throat or need to clear one's throat	Flowering aerial parts	Bitter mouthwash	1–2 tsp tea mixture to 1 L of water	Mix 1–2 mL in 2 ounces of water. Gargle every 2–3 hours		164

5

Table 5 Continued

Disease/Condition	Part of Plant Used in Therapy	Recommended Form	Recommended German Dosage	Recommended US Dosage	Warnings	Notes	See Page
Lesser galangal, Alpinia officinarum							
Roemheld's complex. Anorexia	Rhizome	Tea	Pour 1 cup boiled water onto 1 tsp chopped or powdered herb. 1 cup, 15–30 minutes before each meal	Same			178
	Rhizome	Tincture	(1 : 10): 10 drops in lukewarm water 3 times/day 15 minutes before meals	Add 2–4 mL 1 : 10 tincture to 4 ounces of warm water and drink before meals			178
Licorice, Glycyrrhiza glabra L.							
Gastritis. Coughs and bronchitis	Root	Tea	2–4 g (1 tsp = 3 g) in boiling water One cup, after meals, 2–3 times/day Daily dose: 5–15 g herb	Same. The traditional Chinese medical dose used in prescriptions is 2–12 g, almost always in combination with other herbs in a prescription	Do not use during pregnancy; in cholestatic liver disease; in hypokalemia; in severe renal or hepatic insufficiency. Do not use for more than 8 weeks		86

Catarrh of the upper respiratory tract	Root	Succus liquiritae	0.5 – 1 g herb Daily dose: 5 – 15 g	Same	Do not use during pregnancy; in cholestatic liver disease; in hypokalemia; in severe renal or hepatic insufficiency. Do not use for more than 8 weeks	86
Peptic ulcers	Root	Succus liquiritae	1.5 – 3 g herb Daily dose: 5 – 15 g	Same	Do not use during pregnancy; in cholestatic liver disease; in hypokalemia; in severe renal or hepatic insufficiency. Do not use for more than 8 weeks	86
Ulcers with nocturnal pain and localized epigastric hunger pain	Root	Extract	1 tsp diluted in water up to 4 times/day	Same	Do not use during pregnancy; in cholestatic liver disease; in hypokalemia; in severe renal or hepatic insufficiency. Do not use for more than 8 weeks	171
Non-ulcer-related dyspepsia	Root	Tea	½ tsp in 1 cup boiled water 1 cup, 3 – 4 times/day	Same	Do not use during pregnancy; in cholestatic liver disease; in hypokalemia; in severe renal or hepatic insufficiency. Do not use for more than 8 weeks	172

5

Table 5 Continued

Disease/Condition	Part of Plant Used in Therapy	Recommended Form	Recommended German Dosage	Recommended US Dosage	Warnings	Notes	See Page
Licorice, *Glycyrrhiza glabra* L. (continued)							
		Extract	1 tsp in 1 cup water 3–4 times/day	Same	Do not use during pregnancy; in cholestatic liver disease; in hypokalemia; in severe renal or hepatic insufficiency. Do not use for more than 8 weeks		172
Lily-of-the-valley, *Convallaria majalis*							
CAD	Flowering aerial parts	Tincture (DAB 8)	One oral dose, 2–3 times/day, individualized dose setting required.	KD**: 5–30 drops of the tincture (1:10); BPC*: 1 in 8 hydroalcoholic extract, dose, 0.3–1.2 mL, approximately 10–40 drops	Contains cardiac glycosides; toxic; use with caution		135

* BPC = British Pharmaceutical Codex, Published by the Council of the Pharmaceutical Society of Great Britain, 1911
** KD = King's American Dispensatory, Harvery Wickes Felter and John Uri Lloyd, Eclectic Medical Publications, 1898

Functional heart disorders	Flowering aerial parts	Tincture (DAB 8)	30 drops, 3 times/day	See above	Contains cardiac glycosides; toxic; use with caution		137
Heart failure (NYHA I and II). Cardiac arrhythmias. Nervous heart disorders	Flowering aerial parts	Tincture (DAB 8)	1:10 One dose = 2.0 mL Daily dose: 6.0 mL	See above	Do not overdose		87
		Fluid extract (DAB 8)	1:1 One dose = 2.0 mL Daily dose 6.0 mL	See above	Do not overdose		87
		Dry extract (DAB 8)	4:1 One dose = 0.05. Daily dose: 0.15	See above	Do not overdose		87

Linden (Lime), *Tilia* spp.

Cold and associated cough	Flowers	Tea	2 g herb in 1 cup boiled water (1 tsp = 1.5 g herb). Best taken in the afternoon. Daily dose: 2–4 g herb	2–4 g as an infusion or 1:5 tincture, 1–2 mL, several times daily		Drink as hot as possible	88
Diaphoretic (sweating inducer)	Flowers	Tea	2 tsp per cup	See above		Drink as hot as possible	152

5

5

Table 5 Continued

Disease/Condition	Part of Plant Used in Therapy	Recommended Form	Recommended German Dosage	Recommended US Dosage	Warnings	Notes	See Page
Lovage, *Levisticum officinale*							
Urinary tract infections. Renal or urinary calculi	Root	Tea	2 g herb in 1 cup boiled water. One cup, between meals, several times/day. Daily dose: 4–8 g herb	Strong infusion made with 2–3 g of the dried, coarsely ground or cut herb	Do not use during pregnancy; in renal or cardiac edema; in renal insufficiency or inflammatory diseases of the urinary tract		88
Urolithiasis	Root	Tea	1 cup, 3–5 times/ day	See above	Do not use during pregnancy; in renal or cardiac edema; in renal insufficiency or inflammatory diseases of the urinary tract		205
Marigold (calendula), *Calendula officinalis*							
Poor wound healing; dirty wounds; leg ulceration; radiation ulcers; decubitus ulcers grade II/III; complex wound healing disorders (e.g., in diabetes); poor heal-	Flowers	Dressing	70% calendular tincture, Ringer solution; draw into syringe, apply to compress and soak for 3 mins. Change dressings every 12	Same			315

			or 24 hours, according to manufacturer's instructions	
Deep decubitus ulcers stage III/IV; wounds with frayed edges and deep pockets; wounds due to tumors; weeping deep wounds; proctological wounds; deep radiation ulcers; bite and stab wounds	Flowers	Dressing	8.5 mL Ringer solution and 1.5 mL 70 % calendular tincture. Change every 24 hours or whenever exudate from wound seeps through the dressing	Same	315
Leg ulcerations	Flowers	Ointment	Apply locally to edges of ulcer	Same	280
Inflammations of the mouth and throat	Flowers	Gargle	2 tsp herb in 150 mL boiling water	Same	90
		Mouthwash / gargle	2–3 g (1–2 tsp) in 150 mL hot water. Gargle several times/day	Same	90
Burns and wounds	Flowers	Compress	Apply fresh several times/day	Same	90

Row notes: Calendula creams and salves are also widely available (280); Steep for 15 minutes, strain (90); Steep 5–10 fresh or dried flowers in 1 pint of boiled water for 20 minutes; strain and cool (90)

5

Table 5 Continued

Disease/Condition	Part of Plant Used in Therapy	Recommended Form	Recommended German Dosage	Recommended US Dosage	Warnings	Notes	See Page
Marshmallow, Althaea officinalis							
Dry cough; irritations of the mouth and throat	Leaves	Tea	1–2 g in hot water One cup several times/day. Daily dose: 5 g	Make a strong tea with 3–5 g in 1 pint hot water Drink 1 cup several times a day			91
	Root	Tea	6 g in 150 mL water One cup several times/day	Infuse 2–6 g of the coarsely cut or powdered root in 1 pint of warm water for an hour and drink throughout the day. An infusion in boiled water for 15 minutes is also used			91
Inflammations of the mouth and throat	Root	Mouthwash	6 g in 150 mL water	Same as above			91
Chronic stomatitis, chronic pharyngitis, smoker's catarrh	Root	Demulcent mouthwash	Same as above	Same as above			163

Paroxysmal cough in cases of catarrhal disorders of the upperrespiratorytract in children	Root	Tea	1 tsp herb with 150 mL cold water. Warm before use	Same as above	250

Meadowsweet, *Filipendula ulmaria*

Colds and fever. Coughs and bronchitis	Flowers	Tea	1 tsp (1.4 g herb) in boiled water. One cup, several times/day	4–6 g of the dried herb is infused in boiled water for 20 minutes; drink several cups a day as needed; or a 1 : 5 tincture, 2–4 mL in a little water several times daily	92

Milk Thistle (Marian), *Silybum marianum*

Dyspeptic complaints. Liver and gall bladder complaints	Fruit	Tea	3 g crushed fruit in cold water, then boil. Daily dose: 200–400 mg sily marin, in a divided dose, around meal times	The decoction contains few of the hepatoprotective flavanolignans as they are poorly soluble in water. Either the tincture (2–4 mL in a little water several times/day) or the standardized extract (1–3 tablets or capsules twice	93

5

Table 5 Continued

Milk Thistle (Marian), *Silybum marianum* (continued)

Disease/Condition	Part of Plant Used in Therapy	Recommended Form	Recommended German Dosage	Recommended US Dosage	Warnings	Notes	See Page
				daily) are recommended			
Liver damage associated dyspeptic complaints	Fruit	Tea	1 tsp combined with 1 tsp peppermint leaf in 1 cup boiled water Drink on an empty stomach	See above			181
		Tincture	Add 2–4 mL to 1 cup peppermint tea. One cup, 3–4 times/day	2–4 mL in a little water as needed, several times daily			181
Chronic infectious hepatitis, toxic liver damage, cirrhosis of the liver	Fruit		Selected commercial products	1–3 capsules or tablets of a standardized extract (80% flavanolignans, calculated as silybinin), twice daily (140–560 mg/day)			181

Motherwort, *Leonurus cardiaca*

Functional heart disorders; use only as an additive to other cardiac remedies	Aerial parts	Tea	2 tsp in 1 cup boiling water. One cup 2–3 times/day	Same	Do not use during pregnancy	137

Mullein, *Verbascum densiflorum*

Dry, unproductive cough, bronchitis	Flowers	Tea	1.5–2 g (3–4 tsp) of the flowers in 150 mL boiled water. Daily dose: 3–4 g herb			95

Myrrh, *Commiphora molmol*

Local inflammation of mouth and throat	Myrrh	Tincture	Mixture 1 : 5 Apply to affected areas 2–3 times/day	Dilute the tincture of myrrh in water and use as a gargle	Do not use during pregnancy	162

Nasturium, *Tropaeolum majus*

Urinary tract infections. Coughs, acute or chronic bronchitis. Cystitis	Aerial parts including leaves, flowers, and seeds	Tea infusion	30 g herb/L of water. One cup, 2–3 times/day	Same	Do not overdose. Do not use in children younger than 2 years or in renal disease	96
		Juice	Daily dose: 30 g	Same		

5

Table 5 Continued

Oak, *Quercus robur*

Disease/Condition	Part of Plant Used in Therapy	Recommended Form	Recommended German Dosage	Recommended US Dosage	Warnings	Notes	See Page
Unspecific acute diarrhea	Bark	Tea	1 g in water (1 tsp = 3 g) Daily dose: 3 g dried bark	Same			99
Acute diarrhea of any origin	Bark	Tea	½ tsp herb in 1 cup cold water; boil. 1 cup, 3 times/day	Same		Quercus alba or white oak bark is more readily available in North America; substitute	191
Topical treatment of inflammations of the mouth and throat	Bark	Gargle	2 tbsp in 3 cups water. Gargle several times/day	Same			99
Acute hemorrhoidal inflammation	Bark	Compress	Boil 1 small handful in 1 L water. Apply compresses for 1 hour 2 – 3 times/day. Infusion can also be used as sitz-bath	Same			188
Acute diarrhea of any origin	Bark	Tea	½ tsp chopped bark in 1 cup water, boil. 1 cup, 30 minutes before each meal	Same			191

Indication	Part	Form	Preparation		Notes	Page
Eczema	Bark	Compress	Boil 2 tbsp (10 g) herb in 500 mL water. Allow to cool	Same		266
Furuncles (boils)	Bark	Compress	2 tbsp chopped herb in 3 cups water, boil. Steep for 5 minutes. Apply hot to affected region several times/day	Same		271
Leg ulcerations	Bark	Compress	Boil 2 tbsp in 500 mL water for 15 minutes, then strain. Use undiluted in compresses	Same		281
Inflammatory skin diseases	Bark	Bath additive	5 g herb to 1 L of water, boil and steep for 15–20 minutes. Strain and add to bath water	Same	Do not use in large wounds, heart insufficiency (NYHA III and IV), or severe hypertension	288
Inflammatory skin complaints of various causes. Topical treatment of mild inflammation of the genital and anal region	Bark	Bath additive	5 g to 1 L water 1 bath/week initially, then 2–3/week thereafter	Same	Do not use in large wounds	99

5

Table 5 Continued

Disease/Condition	Part of Plant Used in Therapy	Recommended Form	Recommended German Dosage	Recommended US Dosage	Warnings	Notes	See Page
Oat, *Avena sativa*							
Inflammatory skin diseases	Oatstraw	Bath additive	Pour 4 L boiling water onto 100 g herb and cool. Strain and add to bath water	Same	Do not use in large wounds, heart insufficiency (NYHA III and IV), or severe hypertension		289
Olive, *Olea europaea*							
Chronic gastritis in very underweight or weak patients	Olive oil	Oil	1 tbsp each morning, slowly sipped	Same			172
Onion, *Allium cepa*							
Blunt trauma, iatrogenic wounds	Bulb	Poultice	Stir finely chopped onion, water and a little salt to a pulp and apply to affected area	Same			279
	Bulb (juice)	Compress	Apply locally to affected area for 1–2 hours, 3 times/day. Do not cover with airtight material	Same			279

Oregon grape (Mountain grape), *Mahonia aquifolium*

| Eczema, boils and acne. Psoriasis | Root | Fluid extract | Max. 1–2 mL, 3 times/day | Same | |

Papaya, *Carica papaya*

| Dyspeptic disorders | Fruit | Tablets/tinctures | Commercial products recommended | Follow manufacturer's directions; digestive enzyme products vary widely in their composition and potency | 101 |

Parsley, *Petroselinum crispum*

| Urinary tract infections. Renal or urinary calculi | Aerial parts | Tea | 1 cup 2–3 times/day. Daily dose: 6 g herb | Same | Do not use during pregnancy, in known allergy against parsley, or inflammatory renal diseases. Do not use in cardiac or renal edema | |

| Urolithiasis | Aerial parts | Tea | 1 cup, 3–5 times/day | Same | Do not use during pregnancy, in known allergy against parsley, or inflammatory renal diseases. Do not use in cardiac or renal edema | 205 |

Table 5 Continued

Disease/Condition	Part of Plant Used in Therapy	Recommended Form	Recommended German Dosage	Recommended US Dosage	Warnings	Notes	See Page
Parsley, _Petroselinum crispum_ (continued)							
Irritable bladder	Root	Tea	1 cup, 3–5 times/day	Simmer 2–4 g of the dried and coarsely cut root in 1 pint of water. Drink 1 cup 3–5 times a day	Do not use during pregnancy, in known allergy against parsley, or inflammatory renal diseases. Do not use in cardiac or renal edema		204
Passion Flower, _Passiflora incarnata_							
States of nervous unrest	Aerial parts	Tea	2 g (1 tsp) in 150 mL hot water One cup, 2–3 times/day and 30 minutes before retiring. Daily dose 4–8 g			Passion flower tea is very mild	102
Nervous restlessness in children	Aerial parts		Use as recommended by manufacturer	Take 1–2 mL of a 1:5 tincture in a little water, several times daily			258

Sleep disorders	Aerial parts	Tea	Pour 1 cup water onto 1 tsp herbs. 2–3 cups during the day and 1 cup before retiring	Same		210
Peppermint, _Mentha piperita_						
Tension headache	Essential oil	Ointment	Rub into the skin as often as needed	Same; or use 2–3 drops of the essential oil; or cut the essential oil 50–50 with sweet almond oil and rub in		218
		Oil	Massage a few drops into the skin	Same	Asthma. Do not use in children below the age of 2 years	218
Headache	Essential oil	Oil	Apply topically, 2–3 times/day	Apply 2–3 drops of the essential oil or dilute to suit needs in sweet almond oil		218
Acute rhinitis	Essential oil	Oil	2–4 drops in boiling water. Inhale several times/day, or 1 drop directly below the nostrils (school-aged children and adults only)	Same	Asthma	148

5

Peppermint, *Mentha piperita* (continued)

Disease/Condition	Part of Plant Used in Therapy	Recommended Form	Recommended German Dosage	Recommended US Dosage	Warnings	Notes	See Page
Body temperature over 39 °C	Essential oil	Body wash	3 tbsp peppermint leaf, 1 L boiling water. Steep for 5 minutes. Strain and add to 3–4 L wash water. Repeat as necessary, when temperature rises above 39 °C	Same	Asthma. Do not use in children below the age of 2 years		314
Dyspeptic complaints. Liver and gallbladder complaints	Peppermint leaf	Tea	3–6 g (1 tbsp) in 150 mL boiled water. One cup, between meals, 3–4 times/day	Same	Cholecystitis, severe hepatic problems, obstruction of biliary tract		102
Beginning stages of liver damage associated with dyspepsia, sensations of pressure, fullness in the right upper quadrant, and decreasing physical exercise capacity	Leaves	Tea	1 tsp combined with 1 tsp milk thistle fruit in 1 cup boiled water. Drink on an empty stomach	Add 1 capsule of a standardized milk thistle product (80 % flavanolignans calculated as silybinin) to a cup of peppermint tea	Cholecystitis; severe hepatic problems; obstruction of biliary tract.	The active flavanolignans are not soluble in water, rather in ethanol, so a tea of milk thistle seeds is not an effective preparation. High ethanolic (95 %) extracts of the seeds are commonly sold in North America,	181

Indication	Part used	Form	Dosage		Contraindications	
					and these contain typically about 2–5% flavanolignans.	
Spastic functional epigastric syndrome	Leaves	Tea	Pour 1 cup of hot water onto 1–2 tsp herb. 1 cup after or between meals	Same	Cholecystitis; severe hepatic problems; obstruction of biliary tract	178
	Leaves/oil	Tincture	10 drops in 1 glass water (two doses)	Same; or add 1–2 drops of the essential oil to a cup of hot water and drink after meals	Asthma. Do not use in children below the age of 2 years	178
Spastic epigastric pain due to functional problems (only in older children)	Leaves	Tea	Pour 150 mL boiling water onto 1 tsp herb. Drink hot	Same	Cholecystitis; severe hepatic problems; obstruction of biliary tract	251
Dyspeptic complaints. Colds and fever, runny nose. Coughs and bronchitis. Decreased resistance to infections. Liver and gallbladder complaints. Inflammations of the mouth and throat	Essential oil	Oil	6–12 drops Daily dose for irritable colon: 0.6 mL Individual dose in enteric-coated preparations: 0.2 mL	Same	Cholecystitis; severe hepatic problems; obstruction of biliary tract	103
		Inhalation	3–4 drops in hot water	Same	Asthma. Do not use in children below the age of 2 years	103

5

Table 5 Continued

Disease/Condition	Part of Plant Used in Therapy	Recommended Form	Recommended German Dosage	Recommended US Dosage	Warnings	Notes	See Page
Peppermint, *Mentha piperita* (continued)							
		Liniment	Apply several drops to affected area 2–4 times/day. Pediatric use: 5–15 drops to chest and back	Same	Asthma. Do not use in children below the age of 2 years		103
Gastric anacidity, achylia, and anorexia (in the elderly)	Peppermint	Tea	1 tsp in 1 cup water 1 cup, before meals, 2 times/day	Same			167
***Picea* sp.**							
Catarrhal disorders of the upper respiratory tract in children	Spruce needle oil	Oil	1 g in hot water; inhale 3–5 times/day	Same	Do not use in asthma bronchiale or whooping cough		250
Acute bronchitis	Spruce needle oil	Ointment; inhalation	Apply to skin or use for inhalations several times/day	Same	Do not use in asthma bronchiale or whooping cough		157

Pineapple, *Ananas comosus*

Dyspepsia	Bromelain	Tablets/tinctures	One 500 mg tablet before meals is a common dose		178

Pine tree, *Pinus* spp.

Muscle pain and tension, sore muscles; pulled muscles and contusions; massages after sports; connective-tissue massages	Needles → pine needle oil	Creme	Apply up to 4 times/ day	Same	Do not use in asthma, whooping cough	234
Rheumatism Arthropathies. Neuralgia, neuritis, radiculopathy	Needles → pine needle oil	Bath additive	Add 100 g ethanolic extract to bath water	Same	Asthma; whooping cough; large wounds; acute dermatitis; cardiac insufficiency (NYHA III and IV)	105, 286
		Ointment	Rub onto affected areas	Same	Asthma; whooping cough	234
	Needles → pine needle oil	Bath additive	0.025 g/L of water	Same	Asthma; whooping cough; large wounds; acute dermatitis; cardiac insufficiency (NYHA III and IV)	286
	Needles → pine needle oil	Oil	A few drops on affected area	Same	Asthma; whooping cough	234

5

Table 5 Continued

Pine tree, *Pinus* spp. (continued)

Disease/Condition	Part of Plant Used in Therapy	Recommended Form	Recommended German Dosage	Recommended US Dosage	Warnings	Notes	See Page
	Needles → pine needle oil	Ointment	10–50 % ointment several times/day	Same	Asthma; whooping cough		234
Acute bronchitis, cough, fever and common cold	Needles → pine needle oil	Ointment, inhalation	Apply to skin or use for inhalations several times/day	Same	Do not use in asthma, whooping cough; may induce bronchspasms. Only apply to healthy skin		157
Coughs, acute bronchitis. Decreased resistance to infections. Inflammations of the mouth/throat. Acute upper/lower respiratory tract infections. Acute rhinopharyngitis, tonsillitis. (Acute) Obstructive laryngitis, pharyngitis, tracheitis	Needles → pine needle oil	Inhalation	9–10 drops in 2 cups hot water several times/day	Same	Asthma; whooping cough		104

Primula, *Primula veris*

Acute and chronic coughs, bronchitis	Flowers	Tea	1.3 g (1 tsp) in boiled water. One cup, several times/day, especially mornings and before retiring. Daily dose: 3 g herb	Do not use in known allergy against primrose	106
	Root	Tea	0.2–0.5 g herb (3.5 g = 1 tsp). One cup every 2–3 hours. Daily dose: 1 g herb	Simmer 2–5 g of the coarsely ground or chopped root in 1 pint of water. Drink ½ cup several times a day as needed	106

Psyllium, *Plantago arenaria*

Irritable colon, chronic constipation. Diarrhea. Intestinal diseases in which stool softening is desired to facilitate defecation	Seeds	Seeds	5 g crushed seeds in 150 mL water. 12–40 g/day	Do not use in severe diabetes mellitus inflammatory bowel disease, or obstruction in the intestinal tract	107

5

Table 5 Continued

Pumpkin, *Cucurbita pepo*

Disease/Condition	Part of Plant Used in Therapy	Recommended Form	Recommended German Dosage	Recommended US Dosage	Warnings	Notes	See Page
Prostate complaints associated with adenoma; benign prostatic hyperplasia, irritable bladder	Seed	Powder	1–2 heaped tsp mornings and at night. Chew, swallow with fluid, or mix with food. Daily dose: 10 g ground seeds	Same		Powder the seed just before use	108
Irritable bladder	Seeds	Medication	As recommended by manufacturer	Same			204
Benign prostatic hyperplasia	Seeds	Medication	As recommended by manufacturer, generally 1–3 times/day	Take 1–2 capsules of standardized seeds extract (80 mg, 85% essential fatty acids), 2–3 times/day			208

Purple butterbur, *Petasites hybridus*

Disease/Condition	Part of Plant Used in Therapy	Recommended Form	Recommended German Dosage	Recommended US Dosage	Warnings	Notes	See Page
Migraine	Root	Capsules	1–3 times/day as needed. To prevent new attacks: 2 capsules twice/day for a period of 4 months. Use com-	Capsules and tablets containing a standardized extract (minimum of 7.5 mg of petasin	Avoid during pregnancy. Avoid internal use for more than a week of any extracts that are	Pyrrolizidine-free tinctures and standardized extracts are available and are to be preferred	219

		mercial products as directed	and isopetasin); adult dosage ranges from 50 – 100 mg twice daily with meals	not "pyrrolizidine alkaloid-free"	
Headaches	Root	Extract	Use only industrially manufactured extracts. Dosage according to manufacturer's instructions	See above	108
Renal or urinary calculi	Root	Extract	Use only industrially manufactured extracts. Dosage according to manufacturer's instructions	See above	108
Radish, *Raphanus sativus*					
Cough, bronchitis	Root	Juice	1 tbsp, 2 – 3 times/ day (commercial juice)	Same	155
Chronic biliary dyskinesia with frequent dyspepsia and constipation.	Root	Juice	Mix with flaxseed meal or gruel. Drink 100 – 150 mL, divided into small portions, for 4 – 5 days, then break for 2 – 3 days	Same Do not use in cholecystolithiasis.	184

5

Table 5 Continued

Disease/Condition	Part of Plant Used in Therapy	Recommended Form	Recommended German Dosage	Recommended US Dosage	Warnings	Notes	See Page
Raspberry, *Rubus idaeus*							
Dyspepsia	Leaves	Powder	1 coffee spoonful, 3–5 times/day	3–6 g of leaf powder in warm water, 3–5 times/day			176
Red cinchona, *Cinchona pubescens*							
Anorexia	Bark	Tincture	20 drops in lukewarm water, 30 minutes before each meal	The dose of a 1:5 tincture is about 2–4 mL (maximum therapeutic dose, BPC*)	Do not use during pregnancy. Do not overdose: may cause thrombocytopenia	Add about 10% glycerin during maceration. As a bitter tonic, take 20 drops to 2 mL in a little water before meals	166
Red squill, *Urginea maritima*							
Heart failure (NYHA I and II). Cardiac arrhythmias. Nervous heart disorders	Bulb	Powder	0.1–0.5 g (DAB 10)	Dried bulb 60–200 mg or by infusion three times daily (Newall) 1:10 tincture, 10 drops to 1 mL	Do not overdose. One dose = 60–200 mg Daily dose: 180–200 mg		111

* BPC = British Pharmaceutical Codex, Published by the Council of the Pharmaceutical Society of Great Britain, 1911

Indication	Part	Preparation	Dose		Instructions	
		Extract	Not available	2–6 drops of the 1:1 fluid extract (Osol A, Farrar G. 1955)	Do not overdose. One dose = 60–200 mg Daily dose: 180–200 mg	111
		Fluid extract	0.03–2.0 mL	Same as above	Do not overdose. One dose = 60–200 mg Daily dose: 180–200 mg	111
		Tincture	0.3–2.0 mL	Same as above	Do not overdose. One dose = 60–200 mg Daily dose: 180–200 mg	111
Heart failure NYHA II	Bulb	Any of the above	One oral dose, 2–3 times/day. Individualized dose setting required	Same as above	Do not overdose. One dose = 60–200 mg Daily dose: 180–200 mg	133

Table 5 Continued

Disease/Condition	Part of Plant Used in Therapy	Recommended Form	Recommended German Dosage	Recommended US Dosage	Warnings	Notes	See Page
Rhatany, *Krameria lappacea*							
Abrasions. Bleeding through spontaneous skin fissures during cortisone treatment. Ureteral bleeding due to in-dwelling catheters. Fever blisters/herpes zoster. Efflorescences. Oozing. Hemorrhages in hemophiliacs	Root	Tincture	Clean wound with undiluted tincture. Apply several times a day as needed	Same			318
Nosebleeds	Root	Tincture	Soak tampon or small sterile cotton ball with tincture and insert into nostril	Same			318
Gum inflammations; inflammations of the mouth and throat	Root	Tea	1.5–2 g (1 tsp) powder in 1 cup boiled water. Rinse mouth or gargle 2–3 times/day	Add 2–4 mL of the tincture to a little water and use as a rinse 1–2 times/day			112

Rosemary, _Rosmarinus officinalis_

Hypotension; venous insufficiency; chronic debility and convalescence, for patients with perceptual disorders (basal stimulation)	Leafy shoots with flowers	Body wash	Same	Mix 5 drops rosemary essential oil with ½ cup of milk and add to warm water. 1–2 times/day, as needed		291
		Body wash	Same	Steep 3 tbsp rosemary leaf in 1 L of water for 15 minutes, allow to cool to 28–32 °C, then pour into washbowl. 1–2 times/day, as needed		291
Dyspeptic complaints. Supportive treatment of rheumatic diseases. Circulatory complaints	Leafy shoots with flowers	Tea	Same	2 g (1 tsp) chopped herb in boiled water. One cup, several times/day. Daily dose: 4–6 g herb	Do not use during pregnancy	112
		Oil	Same	Semisolid and liquid analgesic preparations containing 6–10 % essential oil. Apply externally 2–3 times/day	Do not use during pregnancy	113

5

Table 5 Continued

Disease/Condition	Part of Plant Used in Therapy	Recommended Form	Recommended German Dosage	Recommended US Dosage	Warnings	Notes	See Page
Rosemary, _Rosmarinus officinalis_ (continued)							
		Bath additive	Steep 50 g herb to 1 L water. Add to bath water or use for sitz bath	Same			113
Hypotension	Leafy shoots with flowers	Tincture	(1 : 5) 5 drops in warm water. 15 minutes before meals, 3 times/day	Add 20 – 40 drops to ½ cup of warm water and drink before each meal	Do not use during pregnancy		140
Circulatory disorders	Leafy shoots with flowers	Bath additive	Steep 50 g leaves in 1 L of hot water for 30 minutes; strain and add to bath water. Bath in the morning	Same			284
Rheumatic pain	Leafy shoots with flowers	Bath additive	Steep 50 g in 1 L of hot water for 30 minutes; strain and add to bath water. Bath 2 – 3 times/ week	Same			286

Round-leaved sundew, *Drosera rotundifolia*

Paroxysmal cough and dry cough in cases of catarrheal disorders of the upper respiratory tract in children	Aerial parts with root fragments	Tincture 1 : 10	5 drops, 3 times/ day	Take 0.5 – 1.0 mL of a 1 : 5 tincture in a little water several times a day	250
Cough and bronchitis	Aerial parts with root fragments	Tea	1 – 2 g herb in boiled water One cup, 3 – 4 times/day Mean daily dose: 3 g herb	Same	118, 156
	Aerial parts with root fragments	Tincture	1 – 3 mL, 2 – 3 times/ day	Same	118, 156

Sage, *Salvia officinalis*

Anorexia	Leaves	Tea	1 – 2 g herb in 150 mL hot water. One cup, several times/day. Drink warm	Infuse 2 – 4 g in boiled water for 20 minutes. Drink ½ – 1 cup before meals	114
Inflammations of the mouth and throat	Leaves	Mouthwash/gargle	2.5 g herb in 100 mL hot water Use several times/ day	Infuse 2 – 4 g in boiled water for 20 minutes. Gargle several times a day	114

5

Table 5 Continued

Disease/Condition	Part of Plant Used in Therapy	Recommended Form	Recommended German Dosage	Recommended US Dosage	Warnings	Notes	See Page
Sage, *Salvia officinalis* (continued)							
Inflammations of the mouth and throat in children	Leaves	Gargle	Pour 250 mL boiling water onto 1 tsp herb	Same			248
Chronic stomatitis; chronic pharyngitis; smoker's catarrh	Leaves	Demulcent mouthwash	2.5 g herb in 100 mL hot water. Use several times/day	Same as above			163
Acute febrile infections in children	Leaves	Tea	Pour 250 mL boiling water onto 1 heaped tsp herb	Same			246
Excessive perspiration (hyperhidrosis)	Leaves	Tea	1–2 g herb in 150 mL hot water. One cup, several times/day. Allow to cool before drinking	Infuse 2–4 g in boiled water for 20 minutes. Drink ½–1 cup before meals			114
		Tincture	1 tsp in small amount of water. Take before meals	Add 2–4 mL of a 1:5 tincture to a little water and take before meals			275
		Extract	(1:1): 1 tsp in a little water	Same as above			275

St. John's wort, *Hypericum perforatum*

Herpes simplex labialis, wounds and burns	Essential oil	Creme	10–20 mg creme per cm² of affected skin, 2–4 times/day	Same; the infused red oil is also widely used topically	164, 277
Depressive mood, anxiety	Flowering aerial parts	Tea	2 tsp in 150 mL boiled water. One cup mornings and evenings	Same	very mild effect 215
				Do not use during pregnancy and nursing; in children below the age of 12 years; in severe depression; in hypersensitivity to sunlight. Do not apply concomitantly with ciclosporin, indinavir, or anticoagulants of the warfarin type	
Nervous restlessness, anxiety disorders with depression Psychovegetative syndrome	Flowering aerial parts	Extract	Use as recommended by manufacturer Standardized extract (0.3 hypericin and/or 3 % hyperforin) Take 1–2 capsules or tablets morning and evening	Do not use during pregnancy and nursing; in children below the age of 12 years; in severe depression; in hypersensitivity to sunlight. Do not apply concomitantly with ciclosporin, indinavir, or anticoagulants of the warfarin type	215

Table 5 Continued

Disease/Condition	Part of Plant Used in Therapy	Recommended Form	Recommended German Dosage	Recommended US Dosage	Warnings	Notes	See Page
St. John's wort, *Hypericum perforatum* (continued)							
Contusions, wounds, burns	Flowering aerial parts	Tincture	Extract 20 g in 100 g 70% ethanol, filtered 2–4 g/day externally	Apply dark red tincture or oil to affected areas 2–3 times/day			115
Acute proctitis	Flowering aerial parts	Enema	Inject twice daily with an irrigator. (No concrete dosage information given)	Inject 1 ounce of the red infused oil of Hypericum flowering tops once or twice daily			187
Saw palmetto, *Serenoa repens*							
Urinary tract infections. Benign prostatic hyperplasia grades I and II	Fruit (berries)	Extract	Daily dose: 1–2 g or 320 mg lipophilic extract	Many standardized extracts available, for instance to 90% free fatty acids. Take 1–2 softgel caps with 160 mg extract twice daily		Extracts made with supercritical carbon are superior to hexane-extracted fruit products	116
Benign prostatic hyperplasia		Medication	As recommended by manufacturer, usually 1–3 times/day	Same as above			208

Senna, *Senna angustifolia*

Roemheld's complex with poor evacuation of the bowels	Leaves/fruit (pods)	Tea	1 – 2 tsp in 1 cup of boiling water 1 cup mornings and evenings	Same	Do not use during pregnancy or nursing; abdominal pain of unclear origin; ileus; acute inflammatory bowel disease; or in children younger than 12 years	178
Severe bowel irritation and severe constipation	Leaves/fruit (pods)	Tea	1 tsp chopped leaves in 1 cup of cold water Evening use only	Same	Do not use during pregnancy or nursing; abdominal pain of unclear origin; ileus; acute inflammatory bowel disease; or in children younger than 12 years	198

Siberian ginseng (Eleuthero), *Eleutherococcus senticosus*

Decreased resistance to infections. Decreased performance. Prevention or supportive treatment of jet lag	Root	Fluid extract (1 : 1)	3 – 5 drops in water several times/day Daily dose: 2 – 3 g herb	1 – 3 mL in water, several times daily	Standardized extracts are available in liquid form or in capsules or tablets (for instance, to 0.8 total eleutherosides). Take 1 capsule or tablet twice daily	58

Table 5 Continued

Disease/Condition	Part of Plant Used in Therapy	Recommended Form	Recommended German Dosage	Recommended US Dosage	Warnings	Notes	See Page
Siberian ginseng (Eleuthero), *Eleutherococcus senticosus* (continued)							
Exhaustion, convalescence, subjective fatigue, and debility. Decreased mental performance and/or decreased concentration capacity	Root	Extract	3–5 drops in glass of water, 3–5 times/day	See above			228
Silverweed (Goosewort), *Potentilla anserina*							
Unspecific diarrhea. Inflammations of the mouth and throat. PMS	Flowering aerial parts	Tea	2 g in 1 cup water (1 tsp = ca. 0.7 g) One cup between meals, 3 times/day Daily dose 4–6 g	Same			117
Inflammations of the mouth and throat	Flowering aerial parts	Mouthwash	4 g in ½ L water, several times/day	Same			161
Inflammations of the mouth and throat in children	Flowering aerial parts	Gargle	4 g chopped herb in 500 mL hot water	Same			247

Spring adonis, *Adonis vernalis*

				Active constituents are poorly soluble in water (USD25)	133, 136
Heart failure (NYHA I–II), cardiac arrhythmia, nervous heart disorders	Aerial parts	Extract	One oral dose, 2–3 times/day Individualized dose setting required. Daily dose: 0.5–3 g/day	60–300 mg dried herb, 2 times/day "It is usually prescribed: ten drops in four ounces of water, a teaspoonful every two hours." (Felter 1922)	Do not overdose

Stinging nettle, *Urtica dioica*

Rheumatic complaints. Urinary tract infections. Renal or urinary calculi	Leaves	Tea	1.5 g (2 tsp) in boiled water. One cup, several times a day 1 tsp = ca. 0.8 g) Daily dose: 4–6 g	Infuse 2–4 g in boiled water, strain, and drink	Do not use in renal or cardiac edema	97
Rheumatic pain	Leaves	Tincture/spirit	1:10	2–5 mL (1:5 tincture) in a little water, 2–3 times/day	External use only	97
Dysuria, irritable bladder, rheumatic pain	Leaves	Tea	1 cup, 3–5 times/day	Infuse 2–4 g in boiled water, strain and drink		202, 204, 233
Prostate problems. Irritable bladder	Root	Tea	1.5 g (1 heaped tsp) in 200 mL cold water. Daily dose: 4–6 g/day	Infuse 2–4 g in 1 pint of boiled water for 20 minutes, strain, and drink 2–3 cups/day		98

5

Table 5 Continued

Disease/Condition	Part of Plant Used in Therapy	Recommended Form	Recommended German Dosage	Recommended US Dosage	Warnings	Notes	See Page
Stinging nettle, _Urtica dioica_ (continued)							
Rheumatic complaints	Leaves	Capsule, tablet	120 mg extract twice/day. Daily dose: 4–6 herb	Standardized extracts of the leaves are available and vary in guaranteed compounds. Follow manufacturer's instructions, but double the dose for acute conditions			233
Benign prostatic hyperplasia	Root	Medication	As recommended by manufacturer. Generally 1–3 times/day	Standardized extracts of the roots and rhizomes are available and vary in guaranteed compounds. Follow manufacturer's instructions			98, 207
Thuja, _Thuja occidentalis_							
Colds and fever. Decreased resistance to infections	Leaves	Extract	1–2 mL, 3 times/day	Tea infusion made by steeping 1 tsp dried leaves/cup of boiled water for 20 minutes is best	Do not use during pregnancy		119

Psoriasis, warts	Leaves	Tincture	Max. 0.5 g. Paint onto affected site	Apply several drops to the wart(s) several times daily	119

Thyme, _Thymus vulgaris_

Coughs and bronchitis	Leaves and flowers	Tea	1.5–2 g (1–1½ tsp) in 1 cup boiled water One cup, several times/day Daily dose: 10 g herb with 0.3 % phenol content	Infuse 1–4 g of the dried herb in 1 pint of water Drink ½–1 cup several times a day	120
Acute bronchitis	Leaves and flowers	Ointment; inhalation	Apply to skin or use for inhalations several times/day	Same	155
Supportive treatment of acute and chronic respiratory tract diseases. Dermatosis-related pruritus	Leaves and flowers	Compress	Prepare using 5 % infusion	Same	120
		Bath additive	500 g herb in 4 L boiled water. Add to bath water	Same	120

The first row (above Psoriasis) continues text:
form (up to 3–4 times daily).
Avoid hydroalcoholic tincture for internal use

Do not use during pregnancy

Do not use in large skin lesions

Table 5 Continued

Disease/Condition	Part of Plant Used in Therapy	Recommended Form	Recommended German Dosage	Recommended US Dosage	Warnings	Notes	See Page
Thyme, *Thymus vulgaris* (continued)							
Colds, bronchitis, asthma, whooping cough. To dissolve viscous mucus, promote secretolysis after extubation. Chronic obstructive respiratory tract disease	Leaves and flowers	Compress	Mix 1 tbsp sunflower oil with 5 drops thyme oil. Compress for 30 minutes. Use warm	Same		Thyme oil can be irritating to the skin; check for individual sensitivity	294
Coughs, Asthma	Leaves and flowers	Chest wrap	½ L boiling water to 1 tbsp thyme leaf. Steep for 5 minutes. Apply wrap for 20–30 minutes	Same			296
Paroxysmal cough in cases of catarrhal disorders of the upper respiratory tract in children	Leaves and flowers	Syrup	1 tsp 5 times/day	Same			249
Inflammatory skin diseases	Leaves and flowers	Bath additive	Add 1 g to 1 L of bath water	Add 2–4 g to 1 quart of boiled water; infuse for 30 minutes; add to bath	Do not use in large skin lesions		288

Turmeric, *Curcuma longa*

Gastrointestinal spasms with gall bladder dyskinesia	Root	Tea	1 cup boiled water onto 1–2 tsp chopped root 1 cup before meals	Same In traditional Chinese herbal prescriptions, 4.5–9 g	Do not use in obstruction of biliary system	183
		Tincture	10–15 drops in small amount of water 3 times/day	1–2 mL in a little water, several times a day before meals	Do not use in obstruction of biliary system	183
Anorexia. Dyspeptic complaints	Root	Tea	0.5–1 g (1 tsp) in 1 cup boiled water Drink between meals. 2 g herb/day	Same In traditional Chinese herbal prescriptions, 4.5–9 g	Do not use in obstruction of biliary system	122

Uva-ursi (Bearberry), *Arctostaphylos uva-ursi*

Urinary tract infections. Cystitis	Leaves	Tea	2 g dried leaves, finely chopped in 150 mL boiled water. Daily dose: 10 g herb	1.5–4 g of dried leaves, daily dose as an infusion. Drink ½ cup 2–3 times daily	Do not use during pregnancy and nursing, or in children below the age of 12 years	123

Uzara, *Xysmalobium undulatum*

Acute, unspecific diarrhea	Root	Tablets	Industrially produced. Use according to manufacturer's instructions	Same	Do not use together with cardiac glycosides	124

5

Table 5 Continued

Disease/Condition	Part of Plant Used in Therapy	Recommended Form	Recommended German Dosage	Recommended US Dosage	Warnings	Notes	See Page
Uzara, *Xysmalobium undulatum* (continued)							
			Daily dose: 45–90 mg glycosides				
	Root	Tincture	Industrially produced. Use according to manufacturer's instructions. Daily dose: 45–90 mg glycosides	Same	Do not use together with cardiac glycosides		124
Unspecific acute diarrhea in children	Root	Solution or tablets	Use as recommended by manufacturer	Same	Do not use together with cardiac glycosides		124
Valerian, *Valeriana officinalis*							
Difficulty in falling asleep due to nervous tension. Restlessness, anxiety, nervous agitation. Lack of concentration, decreased mental performance	Root	Tincture	1 : 5 tincture. 15–20 drops several times/day	1–3 mL of the tincture made from fresh rhizomes and roots, several times a day in a little water or chamomile tea; 30 minutes before bedtime	Do not use together with alcohol		125

Indication	Part	Form	Dosage		Warning	Page
	Root	Extract	2–3 g once to several times a day	Standardized extracts of the roots and rhizomes are available and vary in guaranteed compounds. Follow manufacturer's instructions, but double the dose for acute conditions; for instance, 0.8–1% Valeric acid or valerenic acid, 200 mg	Do not use together with alcohol	125
	Root	Tea	3–5g in ca. 150 mL hot water 2–3 cups/day + 1 cup before retiring Daily dose: 15 g	Same	Do not use together with alcohol	125
Sleep disorders	Root	Tea	1 cup water onto 1 tsp herbs 2–3 cups during the day and 1 cup before retiring	Same	Do not use together with alcohol	210
Nervous restlessness in older children	Root	Commercial preparations	Use as recommended by manufacturer	Standardized extract or tincture made from fresh rhizomes and roots. Follow manufacturer's instructions; double dose for acute conditions	Do not use together with alcohol	257

Table 5 Continued

Disease/Condition	Part of Plant Used in Therapy	Recommended Form	Recommended German Dosage	Recommended US Dosage	Warnings	Notes	See Page
Valerian, *Valeriana officinalis*(continued)							
Functional heart disorders	Root	Tincture	20 drops, 3 times/day	Tincture made from fresh roots and rhizomes, 1–3 mL in a little water or chamomile tea several times daily	Do not use together with alcohol		137
Functional heart disorders with anxiety	Root	Tincture	15 drops, 3 times/day	See above	Do not use together with alcohol		137
Virginia bugleweed, *Lycopus virginicus*							
PMS. Sleep disorders. Restlessness	Aerial parts	Oral	As recommended by manufacturer	1–2 mL of a 1 : 5 tincture in a little water several times daily	Do not use concurrently with thyroid hormones	Tinctures of varying strengths are on the market; adjust dose accordingly	237
White cabbage, *Brassica oleracea*							
Blister- and pustule-forming skin diseases, acne, impetigo, erysipelas, phlegmons, gangrene,	Leaves	Compress	Pack open wounds with puréed cabbage leaves or thinly sliced (1–2 mm) cabbage leaves	Same			321

abscess, felons, urticaria, acute atopic dermatitis			Do not extend over the wound. Cover with gauze. Change dressing frequently	
Infected wounds, insect bites, bite wounds, burns, mastitis, lymph congeston, thrombophlebitis, leg ulceration, gout, primary chronic polyarthritis, suppurative arthritis	Leaves	Compress	Apply puréed leaves to wound. Do not extend over the edges of the wound. Leave on for 1–12 hours	Same	321
Herpes zoster	Leaves	Juice	Apply juice of puréed leaves to lesions. Do not extend over the edges of the wound	Same	321

White deadnettle, *Lamium album*

Inflammations of the mouth and throat, also in children	Flowers	Gargle	2 tsp herb in 150 mL boiling water	Same	127

■ **5** ■

Table 5 Continued

Disease/Condition	Part of Plant Used in Therapy	Recommended Form	Recommended German Dosage	Recommended US Dosage	Warnings	Notes	See Page
White deadnettle, *Lamium album* (continued)							
Coughs and bronchitis. Inflammations of the mouth and throat	Flowers	Tea	1 g herb in 150 mL hot water Sip slowly Daily dose: 3 g	Same			127
Skin inflammations	Flowers	Sitz bath	Add 5 g herb in 1 L hot water. Add water as needed	Same			127
Skin inflammations. Coughs and bronchitis	Flowers	Compress	50 g chopped herb in 500 mL hot water	Same			127
White mustard, *Sinapis alba*							
Acute pneumonia, pleuritis, bronchitis, asthma. Prevention of pneumonia, breathing problems	Seed	Wrap	4 tbsp mustard powder as poultice soaked in warm water for 2–3 minutes 1st wrap: 2–3 minutes 2nd wrap: 3–4 minutes. Maximum 12 minutes. Apply once/day	Same	Caution: severe burns can result from prolonged exposure; cut ground mustard seed 50–50 with wheat flour or kudzu root powder to reduce strength Do not use in children below the age of 6 years.		297

				Do not apply to skin lesions	
Budding colds, sinusitis, tonsillitis, headaches	Seed	Footbath	2 tbsp mustard powder and small foot tub (water up to ankle). Keep water at a constant 37 °C. Treat for 10–20 minutes depending on skin tolerance and severity of disease. Rinse feet with lukewarm water. Dry well. Apply oil afterwards	Same	See above	312
Coughs and bronchitis, Rheumatic complaints. Head colds	Seed	Poultices	4 tbsp powdered herb with water. Apply to skin for 10–15 minutes for adults; 5–10 minutes for children. Daily dose: 60–240 g	Same	See above	128
	Seed	Bath additive	150 g mustard flour in bag; add to bath water	Same	Do not use in children below the age of 6 years. Do not apply to skin lesions	128
	Seed	Footbaths	20–30 g mustard flour per L of water	Same		128

Table 5 Continued

Disease/Condition	Part of Plant Used in Therapy	Recommended Form	Recommended German Dosage	Recommended US Dosage	Warnings	Notes	See Page
Witch hazel, *Hamamelis virginiana*							
Acute hemorrhoidal inflammation	Bark/leaves	Ointment	Apply after sitz-bath	Apply commercial cream, ointment, or liquid preparation; water-based cream might be more effective			188
Chronic hemorrhoids	Bark/leaves	Ointment	Apply thinly several times/day, as needed	See above			188
		Suppositories	1–2/day	Same			188
Hemorrhoids. Skininflammations. Varicose veins. Wounds and burns	Bark/leaves	Rinses and compresses	5–10 g in 250 mL water	Soak a compress in the strong tea and apply for 20–30 minutes at a time			128
		Gargle	2–3 g in 150 mL water, several times/day	Gargle a few ounces of the decoction, several times daily; or add 1–2 mL to 2 ounces of water			128
Hemorrhoids	Bark/leaves	Suppositories	0.1–1 g suppository 3 times/day	Same			128

Wormwood, _Artemisia absinthium_

Anorexia. Dyspeptic complaints. Biliary dyskinesia	Flowering aerial parts	Tea	One cup, 30 minutes before meals, 3 times/day. Daily dose: 2–3 g herb	Same	Do not use chronically	Make the tea as an infusion	129
		Tincture	10–30 drops in 150 mL water. 3 times/day	Same	Do not use chronically	Infusion is safer than tincture because of the low thujone content (not very water-soluble)	129
Biliary dyskinesia	Flowering aerial parts	Tea	1 tsp chopped herb (or tea bag) in 1 cup water 1 cup, 3 times/day	Same	Do not use chronically		183 ff
		Tincture	10–30 drops in small amount of water 3 times/day	Same	Do not use chronically		183 ff
Gastroenteritis with torpidity	Flowering aerial parts	Tincture	30 drops in water, 3 times/day	Same	Do not use chronically		191
Gastric anacidity, achylia, and anorexia (in the elderly)	Flowering aerial parts	Tea	1 tsp in 1 cup water 1 cup, before meals, 2 times/day	Same	Do not use chronically		167

Disease/Condition	Part of Plant Used in Therapy	Recommended Form	Recommended German Dosage	Recommended US Dosage	Warnings	Notes	See Page
Wormwood, _Artemisia absinthium_ (continued)							
Debility, fatigue, adaptive and functional disorders. Postflu asthenia. Postsurgical and postinfective conditions	Flowering aerial parts	Tea	1 tsp chopped herb in 1 cup boiling water (or tea bags)	Same	Do not use chronically		221
Yarrow, _Achillea millefolium_							
Inflammatory skin diseases	Flowering aerial parts	Bath additive	Add 100 g herb to 20 L of bath water	Same			228
Liver diseases; metabolic disorders; to stimulate liver activity; to promote digestion after heavy meals; constipation; depression; atopic dermatitis	Flowering aerial parts	Wrap	1 tbsp herb, ½ L boiling water. Steep for 5 minutes, strain and keep warm. Wrap 20–30 minutes until wrap has cooled	Pour boiling water over 2–5 tbsp of the dried flowering tops; steep for 15 minutes. Soak cloth in the tea and apply to affected spot until cool. Repeat several times for 20 minutes or so, once or twice daily			302

Indication	Part	Form	Dosage		Notes		Page
Anorexia; dyspeptic complaints; liver and gallbladder complaints	Flowering aerial parts	Tea	2–5 g in water One cup, between meals, 3–4 times/day	Place the dried flowering tops in boiled water in a closed pan			131
Spasmodic pain in the minor pelvis	Flowering aerial parts	Bath additive	100 g herb in 1–2 L water. Then add to bath water	Same			131
Yellow gentian, _Gentiana lutea_							
Secondary nocturnal enuresis in children	Root	Tincture	10–20 drops in water at noontime and in the evening	20 drops to 2 mL in a little water (1:5 tincture), before meals			255
Anorexia; dyspeptic complaints	Root	Tea	½ tsp (1–2 g) in 150 mL water. 1 cup several times/day	Same	Do not use with gastric or duodenal ulcers	Take bitter herbs for digestive enhancement generally before meals	166
	Root	Tincture	1:5 with 45 % ethanol: 1–4 mL, 3 times/day before meals. 2–4 g/day	Same	Do not use with gastric or duodenal ulcers		166
Chronic stomatitis, chronic pharyngitis, smoker's catarrh	Root	Bitter mouthwash	1–2 tsp tea mixture to 1 L of water	Same	Do not use with gastric or duodenal ulcers		163
Gastroenteritis with torpidity	Root	Tincture	1–3 mL in a little water 2–3 times/day before meals	30 drops in water, 3 times/day	Do not use with gastric or duodenal ulcers		191

5

Table 5 Continued

Yellow sweetclover (Melilot), *Melilotus officinalis*

Disease/Condition	Part of Plant Used in Therapy	Recommended Form	Recommended German Dosage	Recommended US Dosage	Warnings	Notes	See Page
Chronic venous insufficiency. Hemorrhoids	Flower	Extract	Up to 30 mg per day (oral)	Take 1–2 mL of a 1 : 5 tincture of the recently dried flowering tops, several times daily	Do not overdose	Tincture is most readily available in North America	146

Herbal Medicine Associations

Company	Address	City	State / Province	Postal Code	Country	Email	URL	Phone	Toll Free	Fax
American Association of Ayurvedic Medicine	PO Box 1382	South Lancaster	MA	01561	USA			(978) 368-7446		
American Botanical Council (ABC)	PO Box 144345	Austin	TX	78714 4345	USA	abc@herbalgram.org	http://www.herbalgram.org/	(512) 926-4900		(512) 926-2345
American Herb Association (AHA)	PO Box 1673	Nevada City	CA	95959	USA		www.ips.net/ahaherb	(530) 265-9552		(916) 265-9552
American Herbal Products Association (AHPA)	8484 Georgia Ave, Suite 370	Silver Spring	MD	20910	USA	ahpa@ahpa.org	http://www.ahpa.org/	301-588-1171		301-588-1174
American Herbalists Guild (AHG)	1931 Gaddis Road	Canton	GA	30115	USA	ahgoffice@earthlink.net	http://www.americanherbalistsguild.com/	(770) 751-6021		(770) 751-7472
American Institute of Ayurvedic Sciences	2115 112th Ave., NE	Bellevue	WA	98004	USA			(206) 453-8022		
American Spice Trade Association	PO Box 1267, 580 Sylvan Ave.	Englewood Cliffs	NJ	07632	USA			(201) 568-2163		(201) 568-7318

Herbal Medicine Associations

Company	Address	City	State / Province	Postal Code	Country	Email	URL	Phone	Toll Free	Fax
Australian Unani Medicine Society, Inc.	PO Box 346	Elizabeth	S. Australia	5112-	Australia	unani@traditionalmedicine.net.au	www.traditionalmedicine.net.au/unani.htm			
Ayurvedic Institute	11311 Menaul NE, Suite A	Albuquerque	NM	87112-	USA			(505) 291-9698		
Ayurvedic Institute	PO Box 23445	Albuquerque	NM	87192-1445	USA					
British Herbal Medical Association	Sun House, Church Street	Stroud	Gloucester	GL5 1JL	UK		www.ex.ac.uk/phytonet/bhma.html	+44-1-453-751389		
Canadian Herb Society	5251 Oak Street	Vancouver	BC	V6M 4H1	Canada	info@herbsociety.ca	www.herbsociety.ca			
Canadian Herbalists' Association of British Columbia							www.chaof.bc.ca			
Chinese Medical Association of Suppliers (CMAS)	8th Floor 87-90 Albert Embankment	London		SE1 7UD	UK		www.cmas.org.uk			

Herbal Medicine Associations

Company	Address	City	State / Province	Postal Code	Country	Email	URL	Phone	Toll Free	Fax
Flower Essence Society (FES)	PO Box 459	Nevada City	CA	95959	USA	mail@flowersociety.org	www.flowersociety.org	(530) 265-9163	(800) 736-9222	(530) 265-0584
Herb Growing and Marketing Network	PO Box 245	Silver Springs	PA	17575 0245	USA			(717) 393-3295		(717) 393-9261
Herb Research Foundation (HRF)	1007 Pearl Street, Suite 200	Boulder	CO	80302	USA	info@herbs.org	www.herbs.org/	(303) 449-2265	(800) 748-2617	(303) 449-7849
Herb Society of America, Inc.	9019 Kirtland Chardon Road	Mentor	OH	44060	USA			(216) 256-0514		(216) 256-0541
Herbs Northwest	1546 W. Jewett Blvd.	White Salmon	WA	98672	USA					
International Aromatherapy and Herb Association (IAHA)	3541 W. Acapulco Lane	Phoenix	AZ	85053	USA	jeffreys@aztec.asu.edu	aztec.asu.edu/iaha/index.html	(602) 938-4439		
International Federation of Aromatherapists (IFA)	182 Chiswick High Road	London		W4 1PP	UK	i.f.a@ic24.net	www.int-fed-aromatherapy.co.uk			
International Herb Association	PO Box 317	Mundelein	IL	60060	USA			(847) 949-4372		

5

Herbal Medicine Associations

Company	Address	City	State / Province	Postal Code	Country	Email	URL	Phone	Toll Free	Fax
National Association for Holistic Aromatherapy (NAHA)	4509 Interlake Ave N., #233	Seattle	WA	98103 6773	USA	info@naha.org	www.naha.org/	(206) 547-2164	888-ASK-NAHA	(206) 547-2680
National Institute of Medicinal Herbalists (NIMH)	56 Longbrook Street	Exeter	Devon	EX4 6AH	UK	nimh@ukexeter.freeserve.co.uk	www.nimh.org.uk	(44/0) 1392 426022		(44/0) 1392 498963
Native Plant Society of Oregon	1605 SE 36th Ave.	Portland	OR	97214	USA		www.NPSOregon.org	(503) 232-7405		
Northeast Herbal Association	PO Box 479	Milton	NY	12547	USA			(914) 795-5431		
Ortho-McNeil Pharmaceutical, Inc.	9218 Oxted	San Antonio	TX	78250	USA			(210) 647-7398		(210) 682-4866
Pacific Institute of Aromatherapy (PIA)	PO Box 6723	San Rafael	CA	94903	USA			(415) 479-9120		(415) 479-0614
Pharmacotherapy Journal	American College of Clinical Pharmacy, 3101 Broadway, Suite 380	Kansas City	MO	64111	USA	accp@accp.com	www.accp.com	(617) 636-5390		(617) 636-5318

Addresses

Herbal Medicine Associations

Company	Address	City	State / Province	Postal Code	Country	Email	URL	Phone	Toll Free	Fax
Rocky Mountain Herbalist Coalition	412 Boulder Street	Boulder	CO	80302	USA					

5

Please note that numbers beginning 1-800 are toll-free when dialling from the USA (only).

Company	Address	URL	Unstandardized Powdered Extracts (capsules or tablets)	Unstandardized Tinctures Liquid Extracts	Standardized Tinctures	Standardized Powdered Extracts (capsules or tablets)	Bulk Powdered Extracts	Loose Herbs (Teas)	Essential Oils	Custom	Notes
Manufacturers											
Botanicals International Nutraceuticals	2550 El Presidio Street Long Beach CA 90810-1193 USA Phone +1-310-669-2100 Fax: 1-310-637-3644 Email: contact@botanicals.com	www.botanicals.com	×				×	×	×	Will formulate and produce special powders and tea combinations to customer specifications	Specialize in straight cut teas and powders
eWellness	7750 Zionsville Rd. Suite 850 IN 46268-5116 USA Phone: +1-800-472-0604 Fax: +1-317-704-3303 Email: info@wellness.com	www.ewellness.com									Dressing products (see section 24.2) Suppliers of Cutinova dressings

Company	Address	URL	Unstandardized Powdered Extracts (capsules or tablets)	Unstandardized Tinctures Liquid Extracts	Standardized Tinctures	Standardized Powdered Extracts (capsules or tablets)	Bulk Powdered Extracts	Loose Herbs (Teas)	Essential Oils	Custom	Notes
Health Concerns	8001 Capwell Drive Oakland CA 94621 USA Phone: +1-800-233-9355 Fax: +1-510-639-9140 Email: info@healthconcerns.com service@healthconcerns.com	www.healthconcerns.com				×					Herbal products based on traditional Chinese formulas. Separate catalog for professional clients
Herbal Extract Co.	PO Box 1425 Narre Warren Victoria Australia 3805 Phone: +61-3-9796-7966 Fax: +61-3-9704-0601 Email:	www.oborne.com.au		×							Distributed by www.oborne.com.au Manufacture standardized saw palmetto extract. Professional clients only

Company	Address	URL	Unstandardized Powdered Extracts (capsules or tablets)	Unstandardized Tinctures Liquid Extracts	Standardized Tinctures	Standardized Powdered Extracts (capsules or tablets)	Bulk Powdered Extracts	Loose Herbs (Teas)	Essential Oils	Custom	Notes
Herbalist & Alchemist, Inc.	51 S. Wandling Ave. Washington NJ 07882 USA Phone: +1-800-611-8235 +1-908-689-9020 Fax: +1-908-689-9071 Email: herbalist@nac.net	www.herbalist-alchemist.com	x	x		x		x			Specialize in single herbal extracts and compounds. Also carry tea blends and Chinese bulk herbs
Herb Pharm	PO Box 116 Williams OR 97544 USA Phone: +1-800-348-4372 Fax: +1-800-545-7392 Email: info@herb-pharm.com	www.herb-pharm.com	x	x		x			x		Specialize in single herbal liquid extracts and compounds

5

Addresses

Company	Address	URL	Unstandardized Powdered Extracts (capsules or tablets)	Unstandardized Tinctures Liquid Extracts	Standardized Tinctures	Standardized Powdered Extracts (capsules or tablets)	Bulk Powdered Extracts	Loose Herbs (Teas)	Essential Oils	Custom	Notes
KW Botanicals	165 Tunstead Avenue San Anselmo CA 94960-2616 USA Phone: +1-415-459-4066 　　　　+1-888-459-4066 Fax:　　+1-415-459-2243 　　　　+1-877-459-2243 Email: kw@kwbotanicals.com	www.kwbotanicals.com		×					×	Custom formulation service for practitioners	Professional clients only
MMS Pro Professional Products, Inc.	10 Mountain Springs Parkway Springville UT 84663 USA Phone: +1-800-240-9912 Fax:　+1-800-718-7238 Email: info@mmspro.com	www.mmspro.com	×	×		×					Distributed by Emerson Ecologics, Inc. Professional clients only

Company	Address	URL	Unstandardized Powdered Extracts (capsules or tablets)	Unstandardized Tinctures Liquid Extracts	Standardized Tinctures	Standardized Powdered Extracts (capsules or tablets)	Bulk Powdered Extracts	Loose Herbs (Teas)	Essential Oils	Custom	Notes
Medi Herb Pty., Ltd.	P.O. Box 713 Warwick Queensland 4370 Australia or 124 McEvoy Street Warwick Queensland 4370 Australia Phone: +61-7-4661-0700 Fax: +61-7-4661-0788 Email:Cust.service@ mediherb.com.au	www.mediherb.com		×	×	×					Distributed by Standard Process in USA, and by Professional Herb Services in New Zealand. Professional clients only

Company	Address	URL	Essential Oils	Loose Herbs (Teas)	Bulk Powdered Extracts	Standardized Powdered Extracts (capsules or tablets)	Standardized Tinctures	Unstandardized Tinctures Liquid Extracts	Unstandardized Powdered Extracts (capsules or tablets)	Custom	Notes
Metagenics, Inc.	100 Avenida La Pata San Clemente CA 92673 USA Phone: +1-800-692-9400 +1-949-366-0818 Fax: +1-949-366-0853 +1-949-366-2859	www.metagenics.com				×					Via distributors only
Napiers Direct	35 Hamilton Place Edinburgh EH3 5BA UK Phone: +44-131-343-6683 Fax: +44-131-343-1152 Email: napiers.direct@talk21.com	www.napiers.net	×	×				×	×		TCM and Ayurvedic herbal preparations and vitamin formulations. Professional clients only

Company	Address	URL	Unstandardized Powdered Extracts (capsules or tablets)	Unstandardized Tinctures Liquid Extracts	Standardized Tinctures	Standardized Powdered Extracts (capsules or tablets)	Bulk Powdered Extracts	Loose Herbs (Teas)	Essential Oils	Custom	Notes
Nature's Way	10 Mountain Springs Parkway Springville Utah 84663 USA Phone: +1-801-489-1500 Fax: +1-801-489-1700	www.naturesway.com		×	×	×					Online only
NewChapter, Inc.	NewChapter, Inc. Corporate Headquarters 22 High Street Brattleboro VT 05301 USA Phone: +1-800-543-7279 Fax: +1-800-470-0247 Email: info@new-chapter.com	www.new-chapter.com		×	×						Vitamin and herb complexes

Company	Address	URL	Essential Oils	Loose Herbs (Teas)	Bulk Powdered Extracts	Standardized Powdered Extracts (capsules or tablets)	Standardized Tinctures	Unstandardized Tinctures Liquid Extracts	Unstandardized Powdered Extracts (capsules or tablets)	Custom	Notes
North American Medicinal Mushroom Extracts	Box 1780 Gibsons British Columbia Canada V0N 1V0 Phone: +1-604-886-7799 Fax: +1-604-886-9626 Email: info@nammex.com	www.nammex.com			×	×			×	Mycelium for producing medicinal compounds, especially polysaccharides	Online only
NuHerbs Co.	3820 Penniman Ave Oakland CA 94619 USA Phone: +1-800-899-4307 Fax: +1-800-550-1928 Email: herbal@nuherbs.com	www.nuherbs.com			×	×				Will powder, char, or honey the herbs to customer's specification	Specialize in Chinese herb complexes and professional GMP formulas. Professional clients only

Company	Address	URL	Unstandardized Powdered Extracts (capsules or tablets)	Unstandardized Tinctures Liquid Extracts	Standardized Tinctures	Standardized Powdered Extracts (capsules or tablets)	Bulk Powdered Extracts	Loose Herbs (Teas)	Essential Oils	Custom	Notes
Pharmaceutical Plant Company Pty., Ltd.	Unit 2 24 London Drive Bayswater Victoria 3153 Australia Phone: +61-3-9762-3777 Fax: +61-3-9762-9992 Email: ppc1@bigpond.net.au							×			
Potters Herbal Medicines	Leyland Mill Lane Wigan WN1 2SB UK Phone: +44-1942-405100 Fax: +44-1942-820255 Email: info@pottersherbals.co.uk	www.pottersherbals.co.uk	×	×							Professional clients only

Company	Address	URL	Unstandardized Powdered Extracts (capsules or tablets)	Unstandardized Tinctures Liquid Extracts	Standardized Tinctures	Standardized Powdered Extracts (capsules or tablets)	Bulk Powdered Extracts	Loose Herbs (Teas)	Essential Oils	Custom	Notes
Rainbow Light Nutritional Systems, Inc.	125 McPherson Street Santa Cruz CA 95060 USA Phone: +1-800-635-1233 +1-831-429-8989 Fax: +1-831-429-0189 Email: info@rlns.com	www.rainbowlight.com	×	×	×	×					Standardized herbal tinctures and capsules, and vitamin and herbal complexes

5

Company	Address	URL	Unstandardized Powdered Extracts (capsules or tablets)	Unstandardized Tinctures Liquid Extracts	Standardized Tinctures	Standardized Powdered Extracts (capsules or tablets)	Bulk Powdered Extracts	Loose Herbs (Teas)	Essential Oils	Custom	Notes
Distributors											
Allegro Medical	1733 E. McKillps Suite 110 Tempe AZ 85281 USA Phone: +1-800-861-3211 Fax: +1-480-990-3211 Email: chood@allegro-medical.com	www.allegromedical.com									Dressing products (see section 24.2) Distribute Bard's Algi-DERM
Becker Natural	6876 Main St. Red Creek RedCreek NY 13143 USA Phone: 315-754-6221 Email: jbecker@becker-natural.com	www.beckerpharm.com		×	×			×			Distribute Scientific Botanicals

Company	Address	URL	Unstandardized Powdered Extracts (capsules or tablets)	Unstandardized Tinctures Liquid Extracts	Standardized Tinctures	Standardized Powdered Extracts (capsules or tablets)	Bulk Powdered Extracts	Loose Herbs (Teas)	Essential Oils	Custom	Notes
Emerson Ecologics, Inc.	7 Commerce Drive Bedford NH 03110 USA Phone: +1-800-654-4432 +1-603-656-9778 Fax: +1-800-718-7238 +1-603-656-9797 Email: cs@emersonecologics.com	www.emersonecologics.com	×	×	×	×	×		×		Distribute MMS Pro
Herbal Doctor Remedies	497 Cumbre Street Monterey Park CA 91754 USA Phone: +1-800-600-0808 Fax: +1-323-263-3182 Email: herb-doc@herb-doc.com	www.herb-doc.com	×	×				×			Distribute Plum Flower brand. Professional clients only

5

Company	Address	URL	Unstandardized Powdered Extracts (capsules or tablets)	Unstandardized Tinctures Liquid Extracts	Standardized Tinctures	Standardized Powdered Extracts (capsules or tablets)	Bulk Powdered Extracts	Loose Herbs (Teas)	Essential Oils	Custom	Notes
Integrative Therapeutics	9775 S.W. Commerce Cir. C5 Wilsonville OR 97070 USA Phone: +1-800-931-1709 Fax: +1-800-380-8189 +1-503-582-0467 Email: edservices@ integrativeinc.com	www.integrativeinc.com	×		×	×					Distribute Tyler Encapsula-tions, NF For-mulas, Phyto-Pharmica and Vitaline Formu-lations. Professional clients only
Life-Span Holdings Pty Ltd	Life-Span NSW/ACT/WA 2/15 Carrington Road Castle Hill NSW 2154 Australia Phone: +1-300-654-336 +61-2-9634-3122 Fax: +61-2-9634-2301 Email: lifespan@lifespan. com aunsworders@ lifespan.com.au	www.lifespan.com.au	×	×	×	×	×	×	×		Professional clients only

Company	Address	URL	Unstandardized Powdered Extracts (capsules or tablets)	Unstandardized Tinctures Liquid Extracts	Standardized Tinctures	Standardized Powdered Extracts (capsules or tablets)	Bulk Powdered Extracts	Loose Herbs (Teas)	Essential Oils	Custom	Notes
Mayway Corp.	1338 Mandela Parkway Oakland CA 94607 USA Phone: +1-800-2MAYWAY (+1-800-262-9929) +1-510-208-3113 Fax: +1-800-909-2828 +1-510-208-3069 Email: sales@mayway.com	www.mayway.com	×			×	×	×			Distribute Chinese herbs and herbal products, including Plum Flower brand and Min Shan brand. Professional clients only

5

Company	Address	URL	Unstandardized Powdered Extracts (capsules or tablets)	Unstandardized Tinctures Liquid Extracts	Standardized Tinctures	Standardized Powdered Extracts (capsules or tablets)	Bulk Powdered Extracts	Loose Herbs (Teas)	Essential Oils	Custom	Notes
Mayway UK Corp.	43 Waterside Trading Centre Trumpers Way Hanwell London W7 2QD UK Phone: +44-0208-893-6873 Fax: +44-0208-893-6874 Email: admin@mayway.demon.co.uk	www.mayway.demon.co.uk	×			×	×	×			Distribute Chinese herbs and herbal products, including Plum Flower brand and Min Shan brand. Professional clients only

Company	Address	URL	Unstandardized Powdered Extracts (capsules or tablets)	Unstandardized Tinctures Liquid Extracts	Standardized Tinctures	Standardized Powdered Extracts (capsules or tablets)	Bulk Powdered Extracts	Loose Herbs (Teas)	Essential Oils	Custom	Notes
Oborne Health Supplies	P.O. Box 165 13 Harker Street Burwood Victoria Australia 3125 Phone: +61-3-8831-3818 Fax: +61-3-8831-3898 Email: info@oborne.com.au	www.oborne.com.au		×			×		×		

5

Company	Address	URL	Unstandardized Powdered Extracts (capsules or tablets)	Unstandardized Tinctures Liquid Extracts	Standardized Tinctures	Standardized Powdered Extracts (capsules or tablets)	Bulk Powdered Extracts	Loose Herbs (Teas)	Essential Oils	Custom	Notes
Professional Herb Services, Ltd.	Unit 5 44 Clarence Street Addington Christchurch New Zealand Phone: +64-3-338-8166 Fax: +64-3-336-8146 Email: paulm@ proherb.co.nz sales@ proherb.co.nz			×	×	×	×		×		Distribute MediHerb products in New Zealand. Professional clients only
Singing Brook Farm	99 Harvey Road Worthington MA 01908 Phone: +1-888-540-1600 Email: info@wiseways.com	www.wiseways.com									Witch hazel suppositories

5

Company	Address	URL	Unstandardized Powdered Extracts (capsules or tablets)	Unstandardized Tinctures Liquid Extracts	Standardized Tinctures	Standardized Powdered Extracts (capsules or tablets)	Bulk Powdered Extracts	Loose Herbs (Teas)	Essential Oils	Custom	Notes
Standard Process, Inc.	1200 W. Royal Lee Drive P.O. Box 904 Palmyra WI 53156-0904 USA Phone: +1-800-848-5061 +1-262-495-2122 Fax: +1-262-495-2512 Email: info@standard-process.com	www.standardprocess.com	×	×		×					Distribute MediHerb products in the USA. Specialize in vitamin and herbal formulations. Professional clients only.
Viable Herbal Solutions	PO Box 969 Morrisville PA 19067-0969 Phone: +1-800-505-9475 +1-215-337-8182 Fax: +1-800-505-9476 -1-215-337-8186 Email: vhssales@viable-herbal.com										Bulk bittersweet twigs

Company	Address	URL	Unstandardized Powdered Extracts (capsules or tablets)	Unstandardized Tinctures Liquid Extracts	Standardized Tinctures	Standardized Powdered Extracts (capsules or tablets)	Bulk Powdered Extracts	Loose Herbs (Teas)	Essential Oils	Custom	Notes
Westons	P.O. Box 1646 Hassocks BN6 9GS UK Phone: +44-1273-846504 Fax: +44-1273-846901 Email: sales@westons.com	www.westons.com									Supply Sorbalgon dressings

Bisset NG, Wichtl M: Herbal Drugs and Phytopharmaceuticals: A Handbook for Practice on a Scientific Basis. Medpharm Scientific Publishers, 1994.

E/S/C/O/P Monographs: The Scientific Foundations for Herbal Medicinal Brodnets – Second edition. Thieme Verlag, Stuttgart, New York, 2003.

Blumenthal M (Ed) The ABC Clinical Guide to Herbs. Austin TX: American Botanical Counsil, 2003

Felter HW: The Eclectic Materia Medica: Pharmacology and Therapeutics. John K Scudder 1922.

Frohne D, Pfänder JH: Giftpflanzen, ein Handbuch für Apotheker, Toxikologen und Biologen. 4. Aufl., Wissenschaftliche Verlagsgesellschaft Stuttgart 1997.

Gruenwald J, Brendler T, Jaenicke C (Eds.): Physician's Desk Reference for Herbal Medicines, 2nd Ed. Medical Economics Co. Montvale, 2000.

Hänsel R, Keller K, Rimpler H, Schneider G (Eds):Hagers Handbuch der pharmazeutischen Praxis. 5. Aufl. Bde 4–6 (Drogen), Springer Verlag Berlin, Heidelberg, New York 1992–1994.

McGuffin M, Hobbs C, Upton R, Goldberg A: Botanical Safety Handbook. Boca Raton, FL, 1997.

Osol A, Farrar G: The Dispensatory of the United States of America. 25th Ed. JB Lippincott, Philadelphia 1955.

Roth L, Daunderer M, Kormann K: Giftpflanzen, Pflanzengifte. 4. Aufl., Ecomed Fachverlag Landsberg/Lech 1993.

Schulz V, Hänsel R, Tyler V: Rational Phytotherapy: A Physician's Guide to Herbal Medicine. 4th Ed. Springer Verlag, Berlin, 2001.

Steinegger E, Hänsel R: Pharmakognosie. 5. Aufl., Springer Verlag Heidelberg 1992.

Teuscher E: Biogene Arzneimittel. 5. Aufl., Wissenschaftl. Verlagsgesellschaft Stuttgart 1997.

http://www.ars-grin.gov/duke/index.html	Dr. Jim Duke's site
http://www.botanical.com	A Modern Herbal Homepage
http://www.christopherhobbs.com	Author's website
http://www.dakotacom.net/~bear/herb.html	A very complete botanical and herbal site with numerous links
http://www.escop.com	European Scientific Cooperative on Phytotherapy (ESCOP)
http://www.eudra.org/emea.html	European Medicines Evaluation Agency (EMEA)
http://www.fimed.org	The Foundation for Integrated Medicine (FIM)
http://www.herbalgram.org/	The American Botanical Council
http://www.irch.org	The International Register of Consultant Herbalists
http://www.itis.usda.gov/itis_query.html	To check taxonomy and current name for plants
http://www.medherb.com	A good source of herbal information and links
http://metalab.unc.edu/herbmed	Henriette's Herbal Homepage
http://www.mioti.org	MIOTI Medical Information on the Internet
http://www.open.gov.uk/mca/mix249.htm	Medicines Control Agency UK (MCA)
http://rccm.org.uk	Research Council for Complementary Medicine
http://rchm.co.uk	Register of Chinese Herbal Medicine
http://www.umd.umich.edu/cgi-bin/herb/	Dr. Dan Moerman's ethnobotanical site
http://www.users.globalnet.co.uk/~ehpa/index.htm	European Herbal Practitioners Association
http://www.who.int	World Health Organization (WHO)
http://www.dg3.eudra.org/eudralex/vol-1/home.htm	Directorate General III

Note: page numbers in *italics* refer to figures and tables